Certification Review for Nurse Anesthesia

Shari M. Burns, CRNA, Ed.D.
Program Director/Professor
Nurse Anesthesia Program
Midwestern University,
Glendale, Arizona

With Contributors
Jacob D. Hantla, CRNA, MS
Arizona Heart Anesthesia
Phoenix, Arizona

F. Scott Imus, CRNA, MS
Assistant Professor
Nurse Anesthesia Program
Midwestern University
Glendale, Arizona

Shaun Mendel, CRNA, MS
Assistant Director/Assistant Professor
Nurse Anesthesia Program
Midwestern University
Glendale, Arizona

Michael MacKinnon, CRNA, MSN
MacKinnon Anesthesia PLLC
Phoenix, Arizona

Christol Williams, CRNA, DNAP
Assistant Professor
Nurse Anesthesia Program
Midwestern University
Glendale, Arizona

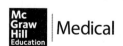 Medical

New York Chicago San Francisco Athens London Madrid Mexico City
Milan New Delhi Singapore Sydney Toronto

Certification Review for Nurse Anesthesia

1 2 3 4 5 6 7 8 9 0   QVS/QVS   18 17 16 15 14

ISBN 978-0-07-182766-9
MHID 0-07-182766-8

Notice

Medicine is an ever-changing science. As new research and clinical experience broaden our knowledge, changes in treatment and drug therapy are required. The authors and the publisher of this work have checked with sources believed to be reliable in their efforts to provide information that is complete and generally in accord with the standards accepted at the time of publication. However, in view of the possibility of human error or changes in medical sciences, neither the authors nor the publisher nor any other party who has been involved in the preparation or publication of this work warrants that the information contained herein is in every respect accurate or complete, and they disclaim all responsibility for any errors or omissions or for the results obtained from use of the information contained in this work. Readers are encouraged to confirm the information contained herein with other sources. For example and in particular, readers are advised to check the product information sheet included in the package of each drug they plan to administer to be certain that the information contained in this work is accurate and that changes have not been made in the recommended dose or in the contraindications for administration. This recommendation is of particular importance in connection with new or infrequently used drugs.

This book was set in Adobe Garamond Pro by Aptara, Inc.
The editors were Brian Belval and Regina Y. Brown.
The production supervisor was Catherine H. Saggese.
Production management was provided by Amit Kashyap.
Quad Graphics was printer and binder.

This book is printed on acid-free paper.

Library of Congress Cataloging-in-Publication Data
Burns, Shari, author.
 Certification review for nurse anesthesia / Shari Burns. – First edition.
   p. ; cm.
Includes index.
ISBN 978-0-07-182766-9 (pbk. : alk. paper) – ISBN 0-07-182766-8 (pbk. : alk. paper)
I. Title.
[DNLM: 1. Anesthesia–nursing–Examination Questions. 2. Nurse Anesthetists–Examination Questions. WY 18.2]
RD82.3
617.9'6076–dc23
                                                                                        2014004105

McGraw-Hill books are available at special quantity discounts to use as premiums and sales promotions, or for use in corporate training programs. To contact a representative please visit the Contact Us pages at www.mhprofessional.com.

Contents

Preface

Building a solid foundation of knowledge is pivotal for practice as a Certified Registered Nurse Anesthetist (CRNA). Continuous changes in science, pharmacology, and technology necessitate the need to consistently strive to build upon material learned through classroom, simulation, and clinical rotations. Even with years of practice, seasoned CRNAs strive to consistently update knowledge to improve anesthetic care. The purpose of this book is twofold: (1) to provide a strong resource for graduating student nurse anesthetists that assists in preparation for the National Certification Examination (NCE) and (2) to offer current, comprehensive review material for seasoned CRNAs.

The review book is based upon the content areas tested by the National Board of Certification and Recertification of Nurse Anesthetists (NBCRNA). The NBCRNA's quest to promote patient safety is laudable. The review questions foster knowledge acquisition providing a foundation for safe anesthetic practice. Basic Science; Equipment, Instrumentation, and Technology; and Basic and Advanced Principles serve as the focus for each chapter. The intent of the content-based questions provides you with the ability to identify strengths and gaps in your knowledge base. Rationale for the correct responses is provided along with current anesthesia references including the newest edition of *Morgan and Mikhail's Clinical Anesthesiology* (5th ed.). New York, NY: Lange Medical Books McGraw-Hill. Question formats include multiple choice, multiple response, and calculation. The questions are intentionally not grouped according to specific topics in order to provide a review that mirrors a real test environment. Enjoy the review!

Acknowledgments

Many thanks to nurse anesthesia colleagues, faculty, and students who reviewed items contained in this review book. Contributions by clinical and academic faculty fostered a comprehensive review for students and practicing nurse anesthetists.

Special thanks to Jacqueline Smith, Ph.D., Dean, College of Health Sciences, Glendale, and the Midwestern University Nurse Anesthesia Program faculty for unwavering support and encouragement and to Alanna Connelly, Program Coordinator, for countless hours of formatting and editing. This work is dedicated to the nurse anesthesia profession and today's students who aspire to continue the tradition of providing safe anesthetic care. Finally, I thank my dear family.

CHAPTER 1

Basic Sciences
Questions

1. What results when alpha-1 receptors are activated?

   (A) Presynaptic nerve terminals are stimulated.
   (B) Adenylate cyclase activity is inhibited.
   (C) Negative feedback loop inhibits norepinephrine release.
   (D) Intracellular calcium ion concentration increases.

2. Which initial intervention is correct if pulmonary embolism is suspected?

   (A) Discontinue intravenous fluids
   (B) Increase FiO_2
   (C) Extubate the patient
   (D) Discontinue inotropic support

3. Which anticholinergic increases heart rate the most?

   (A) Scopolamine
   (B) Glycopyrrolate
   (C) Atropine
   (D) Pyridostigmine

4. What is the normal V/Q ratio?

   (A) 1
   (B) 0.8
   (C) 2
   (D) 0.5

5. What is the underlying pathology of cor pulmonale?

   (A) Pulmonary hypertension
   (B) Decreased pulmonary vascular resistance
   (C) Systemic hypertension
   (D) Orthostatic hypotension

6. What is the blood to gas partition coefficient of halothane?

   (A) 0.47
   (B) 0.65
   (C) 1.4
   (D) 2.4

7. Which inhalational agent is a halogenated alkane?

   (A) Halothane
   (B) Nitrous oxide
   (C) Desflurane
   (D) Sevoflurane

8. How would you classify a patient with repeated blood pressure measurements ranging from 160/100 to 179/109?

   (A) High normal
   (B) Stage 1 hypertension
   (C) Stage 2 hypertension
   (D) Stage 3 hypertension

9. Which condition is NOT associated with precipitating unstable angina?

   (A) Polycythemia
   (B) Anemia
   (C) Thyrotoxicosis
   (D) Emotional stress

10. Which neuromuscular blocking drug is contraindicated during the care of a patient with Guillain-Barré syndrome?

    (A) Succinylcholine
    (B) Rocuronium
    (C) Atracurium
    (D) Pancuronium

11. Which two lung pathologies are forms of chronic obstructive pulmonary disease (COPD)?

    Select (2) two

    (A) Asthma
    (B) Chronic bronchitis
    (C) Aspiration pneumonitis
    (D) Emphysema

12. Which is a normal functional residual capacity?

    (A) 500 mL
    (B) 1,200 mL
    (C) 2,300 mL
    (D) 1,100 mL

13. What are the **three** most common used pharmacological agents for treating ischemic heart disease?

    (A) Nitrates, alpha blockers, and ACE-inhibitors
    (B) Nitrates, beta-blockers, and calcium channel blockers
    (C) Beta-blockers, calcium channel blockers, and ACE-inhibitors
    (D) Calcium channel blockers, nitrates, and ARBs

14. Which narcotic does not cause histamine release?

    (A) Fentanyl
    (B) Morphine
    (C) Hydromorphone
    (D) Meperidine

15. Which of the following occurs following administration of morphine?

    (A) Increased hypoxic drive
    (B) Decreased apneic threshold
    (C) Decreased hypoxic drive
    (D) Decreased $PaCO_2$

16. The patient is shivering in the post–anesthesia care unit. Which intravenous medication will you use?

    (A) Meperidine (10 to 25 mg)
    (B) Fentanyl (25 μg)
    (C) Morphine (5 mg)
    (D) Hyromorphone (5 mg)

17. A patient with mitral stenosis is asymptomatic with occasional mild symptoms with exertion. Which mitral valve area is associated with these symptoms?

    (A) 0.2-0.5 cm^2
    (B) 0.5-1.0 cm^2
    (C) 1.5-2.0 cm^2
    (D) 2.0-2.5 cm^2

18. Which term describes full drug activation of a receptor?

    (A) Antagonist
    (B) Partial agonist
    (C) Agonist
    (D) Noncompetitive antagonist

19. A 60-year-old female with mitral stenosis has the following post-induction vital signs: HR 125, BP 70/45 followed by sudden supraventricular tachycardia (SVT). What will you do first?

    (A) Cardioversion
    (B) Ephedrine
    (C) Phenylephrine
    (D) Vasopressin

20. Which adrenergic agonist affects the heart rate the greatest?

    (A) Norepinephrine
    (B) Dobutamine
    (C) Ephedrine
    (D) Isoproterenol

21. What is the onset of analgesia following administration of epidural morphine 5 mg?

    (A) 30-60 minutes
    (B) 15-30 minutes
    (C) 5-15 minutes
    (D) >60 minutes

22. Which of the following local anesthetics and dosages are used for cesarean section with spinal anesthesia?

    (A) Lidocaine (100 mg)
    (B) Tetracaine (14 mg)
    (C) Bupivacaine (12 mg)
    (D) Mepivacaine (16 mg)

23. Which anticholinergic is classified as a quaternary amine?

    (A) Scopolamine

    (B) Atropine

    (C) Neostigmine

    (D) Glycopyrrolate

24. Which anticholinergic cannot cross the blood-brain barrier?

    (A) Glycopyrrolate

    (B) Atropine

    (C) Scopolamine

    (D) Scopolamine and atropine

25. Which variable increases minimum alveolar concentration (MAC)?

    (A) Hypernatremia

    (B) Hyperthermia

    (C) Acute intoxication

    (D) Ketamine

26. Which factors will exacerbate mitral regurgitation?

    (A) Tachycardia and acute increases in afterload.

    (B) Tachycardia and acute decreases in afterload.

    (C) Bradycardia and acute increases in afterload.

    (D) Bradycardia and acute decreases in afterload.

27. Which volumes are included in vital capacity?

    (A) Tidal volume and residual volume

    (B) Residual volume and expiratory reserve volume

    (C) Expiratory reserve volume and inspiratory capacity volume

    (D) Inspiratory capacity volume and residual volume

28. Your patient's hemodynamic profile is as follows: HR = 100 beats/minute, cardiac output (CO) = 5.0 L/min, end-diastolic volume (EDV) = 100 mL. **Calculate the ejection fraction and write the answer in the box below:**

    [   ] %

29. What classic triad of symptoms is associated with aortic stenosis with a valve area <1 cm^2?

    (A) Hypotension, dyspnea on exertion, and pulmonary congestion

    (B) Hoarseness, chest pain, and pulmonary emboli

    (C) Chest pains, arrhythmias, and embolic events

    (D) Dyspnea on exertion, angina, and exertional syncope

30. How does the elimination half-time of remifentanil differ from alfentanil?

    (A) Elimination half-time is longer for remifentanil.

    (B) Elimination half-time is shorter for alfentanil.

    (C) Elimination half-time is similar for alfentanil and remifentanyl.

    (D) Elimination half-time is shorter for remifentanil.

31. One goal during a general anesthetic is to decrease the neuroendocrine stress response to surgical stimulation. Which medication will be helpful?

    (A) Vecuronium

    (B) Midazolam

    (C) Lidocaine

    (D) Fentanyl

32. You administered meperidine IV. Immediately following administration the patient developed profound hypotension, hyperpyrexia, and respiratory arrest. What drug interaction do you suspect?

    (A) Interaction with monoamine oxidase inhibitors (MAOs)

    (B) Interaction with erythromycin

    (C) Interaction with sodium pentothal

    (D) Interaction with etomidate

33. What is the normal aortic valve area?

    (A) 0.5-1.0 cm^2

    (B) 1.0-1.5 cm^2

    (C) 1.5-2.5 cm^2

    (D) 2.5-3.5 cm^2

34. For which severity of aortic stenosis is spinal anesthesia contraindicated?

    (A) 0.5-1.0 cm^2
    (B) 1.0-1.5 cm^2
    (C) 1.5-2.5 cm^2
    (D) 2.5-3.5 cm^2

35. Which agent results in an increased heart rate during inhalational anesthesia?

    (A) Desflurane 0.75 MAC
    (B) Sevoflurane >1.5 MAC
    (C) Desflurane 0.5 MAC
    (D) Sevoflurane <1 MAC

36. The anesthetic plan includes an inhalational induction. Which inhalational agent is the **least** desirable for a patient with chronic bronchitis and a 50-pack-year history of smoking?

    (A) Desflurane
    (B) Sevoflurane
    (C) Halothane
    (D) Nitrous oxide

37. Which local anesthetic is metabolized by O-toluidine?

    (A) Nesacaine
    (B) Cocaine
    (C) Prilocaine
    (D) Mepivacaine

38. Which local anesthetic is linked to methemoglobinemia?

    (A) Prilocaine
    (B) EMLA
    (C) Lidocaine
    (D) Cocaine

39. Which risk factor contributes to myocardial ischemia in a patient with aortic regurgitation?

    (A) Heart rate 40-50 beats/minute.
    (B) Heart rate 50-70 beats /minute.
    (C) Heart rate 80-100 beats/minute.
    (D) Heart rate 110-120 beats/minute.

40. Prior to general anesthesia the patient reports taking daily imipramine. What is your most serious concern for this patient?

    (A) Dry mouth
    (B) Sedation
    (C) Orthostatic hypotension
    (D) Sympathomimetic activity

41. Where is the primary location of hepatic microsomal enzymes?

    (A) Hepatic smooth endoplasmic reticulum
    (B) Kidneys
    (C) Gastrointestinal system
    (D) Small intestine

42. In which valvular disease is the pulmonary capillary wedge pressure (PCWP) an overestimation of the left ventricular end-diastolic pressure (LVEDP)?

    (A) Mitral stenosis
    (B) Mitral regurgitation
    (C) Aortic stenosis
    (D) Aortic regurgitation

43. Which of the following medications block alpha- and beta receptors?

    (A) Phentolamine
    (B) Isoproterenol
    (C) Propranolol
    (D) Labetalol

44. The patient arrives in the operating room following a motor vehicle accident. 40% of the body is burned. When is it permissible to use succinylcholine?

    Select (2) two
    (A) Within 8 hours of injury.
    (B) Within 48 hours of injury.
    (C) After 48 hours of injury.
    (D) No succinylcholine is used for patients with burns.

45. What variables are needed to calculate systemic vascular resistance (SVR)?

    (A) Body surface area, cardiac output, and central venous pressure

    (B) Mean arterial pressure, heart rate, and pulmonary capillary wedge pressure

    (C) Mean arterial pressure, cardiac output, and pulmonary capillary wedge pressure

    (D) Mean arterial pressure, cardiac output, and central venous pressure

46. The patient is scheduled for a tympanoplasty. Which inhalational agent will you avoid?

    (A) Sevoflurane

    (B) Nitrous oxide

    (C) Desflurane

    (D) Isoflurane

47. Which agent increases the cerebral metabolic rate for oxygen ($CMRO_2$)?

    (A) Halothane

    (B) Isoflurane

    (C) Sevoflurane

    (D) Nitrous oxide

48. Which hemodynamic event will decrease coronary perfusion pressure the most?

    (A) Decreased systolic blood pressure

    (B) Decrease in left ventricular end-diastolic pressure (LVEDP)

    (C) Increase in pulmonary capillary wedge pressure (PCWP)

    (D) Increase in diastolic blood pressure

49. Which antibiotic is classified as a beta-lactam?

    (A) Penicillin

    (B) Gentamicin

    (C) Erythromycin

    (D) Ciprofloxacin

50. To avoid hypotension and possible cardiac arrest what is the best method for administering IV vancomycin?

    (A) >60 minutes

    (B) <30 minutes

    (C) >20 minutes

    (D) <10 minutes

51. What is the most common cause of myocardial remodeling?

    (A) Congenital heart disease

    (B) Myocardial ischemic injury

    (C) Chronic lung disease

    (D) Cardiomyopathy

52. A 55-year-old male with congestive heart failure, status post–cardiac transplantation is now undergoing elective surgery for hernia repair. Thirty-minutes into the case, his heart rate drops to 28. What medication will you give for bradycardia?

    (A) Atropine

    (B) Ephedrine

    (C) Isoproterenol

    (D) Dexmedetomidine

53. The patient with renal disease is scheduled for an exploratory laparotomy. What muscle relaxant is the best choice for this patient?

    (A) Vecuronium

    (B) Pancuronium

    (C) Rocuronium

    (D) Cisatracurium

54. The patient's glomerular filtration rate is 20 mL/min. What condition most likely exists?

    (A) Acute glomerulonephritis

    (B) Uremia

    (C) Renal calculi

    (D) Acute kidney failure

55. What arterial line waveform might you observe in a patient with severe aortic regurgitation?

    (A) Pulsus paradoxus

    (B) Pulsus alternans

    (C) Pulsus bisferiens

    (D) Anacrotic pulse

56. Which characteristic describes a typical patient with diastolic heart failure?

    (A) Left ventricular ejection fraction less than 40%
    (B) Dilated left ventricular cavity size
    (C) Persistent atrial fibrillation
    (D) Fourth heart sound

57. How does the mechanism of action of methylxanthines affect patients with asthma?

    (A) Blocks degranulation of mast cells
    (B) Bronchodilates via B_2 receptors
    (C) Bronchodilates via B_1 receptors
    (D) Inhibits phosphodiesterase

58. A 42-year-old female with multiple sclerosis is scheduled for major surgery with general anesthesia. She has been taking corticosteroid therapy. Which approximate equivalent dose achieves the anti-inflammatory potency of prednisone 50 mg?

    (A) 8 mg dexamethasone
    (B) 100 mg methylprednisolone
    (C) 25 mg prednisolone
    (D) 300 mg cortisone

59. A patient with rheumatoid arthritis has been receiving long-term corticosteroid therapy and infliximab. Which statement best describes the major anesthetic implication for this drug regimen?

    (A) Avoiding anesthetic drugs that are excreted via kidneys
    (B) Administering PO dose of infliximab via NGT intraoperatively
    (C) Paying meticulous attention to sterile techniques
    (D) Monitoring intraoperative labs for hypoglycemia

60. A patient with a prosthetic heart valve presents for a scheduled total abdominal hysterectomy with a heparin infusion. How far in advance of surgery will you recommend this heparin be discontinued?

    (A) 2-4 hours
    (B) 4-6 hours
    (C) 24 hours
    (D) 48 hours

61. What is the predicted FEV_1/FVC ratio for a patient whose history includes a 55-pack-year history of smoking with wheezing on auscultation?

    (A) FEV_1/FVC ratio of >0.7
    (B) FEV_1/FVC ratio equal to 0.8
    (C) FEV_1/FVC ratio of >0.9
    (D) FEV_1/FVC ratio of <0.7

62. Where do local anesthetics exert their primary mechanism of action?

    (A) Sodium channel alpha subunit
    (B) Calcium channel
    (C) Vanilloid 1 channel
    (D) Potassium channel

63. Which neuromuscular blocker is considered an acetylcholine (ACh) receptor agonist?

    (A) Vecuronium
    (B) Rocuronium
    (C) Cisatracurium
    (D) Succinylcholine

64. What do you expect when administering neuromuscular blockers to patients with myasthenia gravis?

    (A) Up-regulation
    (B) Profound response to succinylcholine
    (C) Down-regulation
    (D) Decreased sensitivity to vecuronium

65. Which fibers are most sensitive to local anesthetics?

    (A) A-alpha fibers
    (B) Small unmyelinated C fibers
    (C) A-gamma
    (D) C fibers

66. Which ratio of the forced expiratory volume in the first second of exhalation (FEV_1) to the total forced vital capacity (FVC) would signify the greatest degree of obstruction?

    (A) FEV_1/FVC ratio of 80%
    (B) FEV_1/FVC ratio of 40%
    (C) FEV_1/FVC ratio of 20%
    (D) FEV_1/FVC ratio of 60%

67. What compensatory mechanism is commonly seen with aortic regurgitation?

(A) Eccentric hypertrophy
(B) Dilated annulus of aortic valve
(C) Concentric hypertrophy
(D) Elevated brain natriuretic peptide

68. Which pharmacological agent is contraindicated in the patient with Wolff-Parkinson-White (WPW) syndrome exhibiting atrial fibrillation?

(A) Atropine
(B) Diltiazem
(C) Verapamil
(D) Metoprolol

69. Your patient has mitral valve prolapse. What is the most common arrhythmia associated with this disease?

(A) Paroxysmal supraventricular tachycardia
(B) Atrial fibrillation
(C) Premature ventricular contraction
(D) Junctional tachycardia

70. From where do the cardiac sympathetic fibers originate?

(A) T1-T4
(B) T2-T4
(C) T3-T6
(D) T4-T8

71. Which statement about coronary blood flow is incorrect?

(A) At rest, approximately 4-5% of the cardiac output passes through the coronary vessels.
(B) The left ventricle is perfused almost entirely during diastole.
(C) The right ventricle is perfused during systole and diastole.
(D) Increases in the aortic pressure can reduce coronary perfusion pressure.

72. What is indicated by a V/Q ratio that is equal to infinity?

(A) Dead space
(B) Shunting
(C) Normal V/Q ratio
(D) Inadequate ventilation

73. As compared to other anticholinergics, what are scopolamine's sedative effects?

(A) Less than atropine
(B) Greater than glycopyrrolate
(C) Same as atropine
(D) Same as atropine and glycopyrrolate

74. Who studied the relationship between volume and temperature when pressure remains constant?

(A) Boyle
(B) Charles
(C) Gay-Lussac
(D) Dalton

75. Which factor most negatively affects myocardial oxygen consumption?

(A) Cardiac volume work
(B) Electrical activity
(C) Heart rate
(D) Wall stress

76. What is the functional residual capacity for an adult patient in the supine position following induction of general anesthesia?

(A) 500 mL
(B) 800 mL
(C) 1300 mL
(D) 2300 mL

77. What is the normal coronary blood flow at rest?

(A) 175-200 mL/min
(B) 200-225 mL/min
(C) 225-250 mL/min
(D) 250-275 mL/min

78. If a 64-kg woman receives a standard initial dose of dantrolene during malignant hyperthermia crisis, how many grams of mannitol have been administered?

(A) 12
(B) 16
(C) 20
(D) 24

79. Which statement about protamine is incorrect?

(A) A hypotensive reaction can be treated with incremental doses of phenylephrine.

(B) Administering protamine over 10-15 minutes will decrease risk of hypotension reaction.

(C) The normal dose is 10 mg of protamine for every 100 units of heparin.

(D) Supplementary doses of 50-100 mg can be administered to reverse residual anticoagulation.

80. What two pathologies can increase alveolar dead space?

Select (2) two

(A) Mucus plug

(B) Pulmonary embolism

(C) Decreased cardiac output

(D) Hypoventilation

81. How is residual volume defined?

(A) Maximum volume of air expired from resting end-expiratory level

(B) Maximum volume of air inspired from the resting end inspiratory level

(C) Normal breath

(D) Volume remaining after maximal exhalation

82. Which patient does not pose an increased risk for an allergic reaction to protamine sulfate?

(A) A patient who has a history of two previous cardiac catheterizations.

(B) A patient who is currently undergoing aortic valve replacement.

(C) A diabetic patient on maintenance NPH insulin therapy.

(D) A patient who is maintained on a weekly hemodialysis regimen.

83. Compared to neostigmine, what is the onset of action of pyridostigmine?

(A) Longer than neostigmine

(B) Same as neostigmine

(C) Slower than neostigmine

(D) Clinically inconsequential

84. Which condition potentiates neuromuscular blockade?

(A) Hypomagnesemia

(B) Hypercalcemia

(C) Hyperkalemia

(D) Hypothermia

85. What is the result of acetylcholine acting on the muscarinic receptor (M2) in the sinoatrial node?

Select (3) three

(A) Positive dromotropic effects

(B) Negative dromotropic effects

(C) Positive chronotropic effects

(D) Negative chronotropic effects

(E) Positive inotropic effects

(F) Negative inotropic effects

86. Which paradoxical cardiac wall motion, when diagnosed with transesophageal echocardiography (TEE) is indicative of myocardial infarction?

(A) Dyskinesia

(B) Hypokinesia

(C) Akinesia

(D) Hyperkinesia

87. You plan a standard induction for an 80-kg patient scheduled for cholecystectomy. What induction dose of cisatracurium will you use?

(A) 16 mg

(B) 8 mg

(C) 1.6 mg

(D) 0.8 mg

88. Following topical administration of a local anesthetic you note erythema, skin blanching, and edema. Which local anesthetic did you apply?

(A) Chloroprocaine

(B) Tetracaine

(C) Ropivacaine

(D) EMLA

89. Which rate of systemic absorption of local anesthetics is true?

   (A) Intravenous > tracheal > intercostal > para-cervical > epidural > brachial plexus > sciatic > subcutaneous
   (B) Tracheal > intercostal > intravenous > para-cervical > epidural > brachial plexus > sciatic > subcutaneous
   (C) Intravenous < tracheal < intercostal < para-cervical < epidural < brachial plexus < sciatic < subcutaneous
   (D) Tracheal < intercostal < intravenous < para-cervical < epidural < brachial plexus < sciatic < subcutaneous

90. What do you expect when adding epinephrine to local anesthetic?

   (A) Vasodilation at the site of injection
   (B) Increased absorption
   (C) Decreased duration of action
   (D) Vasoconstriction at the site of injection

91. During surgery for a bowel obstruction, you note persistent tachycardia and hypertension. What neuromuscular blocker was most likely used?

   (A) Rocuronium
   (B) Cisatracurium
   (C) Atracurium
   (D) Pancuronium

92. Which factor is a relative contraindication to pulmonary artery (PA) catheterization?

   (A) Left bundle branch block
   (B) Right bundle branch block
   (C) A patient in septic shock
   (D) A patient undergoing thoracic aortic aneurysm repair

93. Which statement about the central venous waveform *a* wave is correct?

   (A) It is produced by the passive filling of the right atrium.
   (B) It is produced by right atrial contraction.
   (C) It is produced by the closure of the tricuspid valve.
   (D) It is produced by the venous return against a closed tricuspid valve.

94. Which statement is false regarding nitric oxide (NO)?

   (A) NO regulates pulmonary vascular resistance.
   (B) NO inhibits platelet activation.
   (C) NO regulates systemic vascular resistance.
   (D) NO is an exogenous neurotransmitter.

95. The patient is taking gabapentin. In which patient would you decrease the dose?

   (A) Hepatic compromised patients
   (B) Cardiac compromised patients
   (C) Renal compromised patients
   (D) Respiratory compromised patients

96. Which statement about monitoring the CVP waveform in a patient with atrial fibrillation is correct?

   (A) There are large *v* waves.
   (B) The *v* waves are absent.
   (C) There are giant, "cannon" *a* waves.
   (D) The *a* waves are absent.

97. Which pathologic state will not cause giant, "cannon" *a* waves on the CVP waveform?

   (A) Tricuspid stenosis
   (B) Tricuspid regurgitation
   (C) Mitral stenosis
   (D) Ventricular hypertrophy

98. The patient received streptokinase. When is surgery permitted?

   (A) 3 days following administration
   (B) 5 days following administration
   (C) 7 days following administration
   (D) 10 days following administration

99. Where does acetazolamide exert its action?

   (A) Proximal convoluted tubule
   (B) Ascending loop of Henle
   (C) Distal convoluted tubule
   (D) Collecting ducts

100. Which hemodynamic profile is consistent with pulmonary embolism?

	CVP	PCWP
(A)	High	High
(B)	High	Normal
(C)	High	Low
(D)	Normal	High

101. Which antibiotic would you avoid in patients with myasthenia gravis?

(A) Chloramphenicol

(B) Amphotericin B

(C) Ciprofloxacin

(D) Gentamicin

102. Which chemotherapeutic agent is strongly associated with pulmonary fibrosis?

(A) 5-FU

(B) Cyclophosphamide

(C) Doxorubicin

(D) Bleomycin

103. Which hemodynamic profile reflects chronic left ventricular failure?

	CVP	PCWP
(A)	High	High
(B)	High	Normal
(C)	High	Low
(D)	Normal	High

104. In which West zone must the tip of the pulmonary artery catheter lie in order for the pulmonary artery wedge pressure (PAWP) measurement to be accurate?

(A) 1

(B) II

(C) III

(D) IV

105. How do codeine and morphine differ?

(A) Codeine undergoes O-demethylation.

(B) Codeine is less antitussive than morphine.

(C) Codeine undergoes 2 glucuronide conjugation.

(D) Codeine's equipotent dose is 1.5 mg.

106. What is the characteristic pulmonary artery catheter (PAC) pressure waveform that tells you the catheter has entered the pulmonary artery?

(A) A sharp, upstroke/down stroke waveform with the highest point reaching the 10 mmHg point.

(B) A brisk upstroke followed by a steep down stroke returning to mean central venous pressure levels.

(C) A brisk upstroke followed by a notched, sloping down stroke with acute rise in diastolic pressure.

(D) An undulating waveform that occurs near the 10 mmHg point.

107. Which statement about correlation of the CVP waveform and the EKG waveform is incorrect?

(A) The *a* wave follows the P wave on the ECG.

(B) The *c* wave immediately follows the start of the QRS complex on ECG.

(C) The *v* wave appears shortly after the start of the T wave on the ECG.

(D) The *y* descent occurs during the QRS complex on the ECG.

108. During induction of anesthesia you note the inability to ventilate the patient. The chest wall appears rigid. Which medication did you administer?

(A) Sufentanil

(B) Versed

(C) Etomidate

(D) Methohexital

109. Which of the following is inhibited by opioids?

(A) Coupling to G proteins

(B) Binding to agonists

(C) Voltage gated sodium channels

(D) Activation of adenylyl cyclase

110. How do COX-1 and COX-2 enzymes differ?

(A) COX 1 responds to inflammation.

(B) COX-1 inhibition increases thrombosis.

(C) COX-2 inhibition increases heart attack risk.

(D) COX-1 sites attract large molecules.

111. If amiodarone is not available, what antiarrhythmic will you use to treat unsuccessful defibrillation?

    (A) Lidocaine
    (B) Diltiazem
    (C) Dobutamine
    (D) Magnesium

112. What is the mechanism of action of aspirin?

    (A) Irreversible inhibition of COX-2
    (B) Low binding to plasma proteins
    (C) Plasma esterase hydrolysis
    (D) Irreversible inhibition of COX-1

113. Which central line site has the shortest distance to the junction of the vena cava and the right atrium?

    (A) Left internal jugular
    (B) Right internal jugular
    (C) Subclavian vein
    (D) Right median basilic vein

114. What is the hallmark sign of a catheter-induced pulmonary artery rupture?

    (A) Hypotension
    (B) Hypoxemia
    (C) Hemoptysis
    (D) Arrhythmias

115. Which law of physics explains why an increase in left ventricular wall thickness will reduce ventricular wall tension?

    (A) La Place's Law
    (B) Ohm's Law
    (C) Poiseuille's Law
    (D) Fick's Law

116. Which cardiovascular reflex does not result in an efferent vagal response?

    (A) Baroreceptor reflex
    (B) Bainbridge reflex
    (C) Valsalva maneuver
    (D) Oculocardiac reflex

117. Which herbal remedy does not delay awakening from anesthesia?

    (A) Valerian
    (B) Kava kava
    (C) St. John's wort
    (D) Garlic

118. While floating a pulmonary artery catheter via the right internal jugular, the patient monitor shows a run of ventricular tachycardia. Which insertion depth is most likely to induce this arrhythmia?

    (A) 15 cm
    (B) 22 cm
    (C) 28 cm
    (D) 45 cm

119. At what dose is the onset of action of rocuronium similar to that of succinylcholine for rapid sequence intubation?

    (A) 0.9-1.2 mg/kg
    (B) 1.5-2.0 mg/kg
    (C) 2.0-2.5 mg/kg
    (D) >2.5 mg/kg

120. What is the primary neurotransmitter of the parasympathetic nervous system?

    (A) Norepinephrine
    (B) Acetylcholine
    (C) Acetylcoenzyme A
    (D) Muscarine

121. Which is correct about the CVP waveform in a patient with tricuspid regurgitation?

    (A) Decreasing CVP pressure implies worsening right ventricular dysfunction.
    (B) The x descent is usually absent.
    (C) Giant, "cannon" a-waves are apparent.
    (D) The v-waves become diminished.

122. Which sympathomimetic amine structurally related to amphetamine may cause cardiac arrhythmias, myocardial infarction, and stroke?

    (A) Echinacea
    (B) Ma huang
    (C) Ginkgo biloba
    (D) Ginseng

123. How does hydromorphone differ from morphine?

    (A) Hydromorphone is more potent.
    (B) Hydromorphone has a shorter duration of action.
    (C) Hydormorphone is less potent.
    (D) Hydromorphone is less lipid soluble.

124. What should be used to reconstitute a standard vial of dantrolene?

    (A) 60 mL normal saline
    (B) 100 mL normal saline
    (C) 60 mL sterile water
    (D) 100 mL sterile water

125. Preoperatively, you learn that the patient is taking warfarin. Which herbal remedy poses the potential for bleeding?

    (A) Ginkgo biloba
    (B) Evening primrose
    (C) Kola nut
    (D) Goldenseal

126. Which antibiotic should not be administered during pregnancy?

    (A) Penicillin
    (B) Aminoglycosides
    (C) Tetracycline
    (D) Erythromycin

127. How is emphysema characterized?

    (A) Narrowing of small airways by inflammation and mucus.
    (B) Destruction of parenchyma that leads to loss of surface area, elastic recoil, and structural support to maintain the airway.
    (C) Antigen binding to immunoglobulin E on the surface of mast cells causes degranulation.
    (D) Reversible enlargement of the airways distal to terminal bronchioles with damage of the alveolar septa.

128. Preoperatively, the patient shares that they were treated with vincristine for Hodgkin's disease. What side effect would you expect?

    (A) Paresthesias
    (B) Coagulopathy
    (C) Magnesium wasting
    (D) Arthralgias

129. A 70-kg adult patient with mitral valve prolapse is scheduled for an exploratory laparotomy. If the patient has history of anaphylaxis to penicillin, what antibiotic prophylaxis will you administer?

    (A) Cefazolin 1 g IV
    (B) Clindamycin 600 mg IV
    (C) Ampicillin 2 g IV
    (D) Amoxicillin 2 g IV

130. A 70-year-old female is undergoing a large bowel resection when the following hemodynamic profile is obtained: BP 100/80, cardiac output 6 L/min. and central venous pressure 3 mmHg. What is the systemic vascular resistance?

    (A) 504 dynes/sec/cm^5
    (B) 1,120 dynes/sec/cm^5
    (C) 1,160 dynes/sec/cm^5
    (D) 2,200 dynes/sec/cm^5

131. What has been firmly established as the primary environmental risk factor associated with emphysema and bronchitis?

    (A) Homozygous α_1-antitrypsin
    (B) Cigarette smoking
    (C) Antigen binding to immunoglobulin E
    (D) Drug toxicity with bleomycin and nitrofurantoin

132. What is the most significant precipitating factor leading to obstructive sleep apnea (OSA)?

    (A) History of stroke
    (B) History of type II diabetes
    (C) Obesity
    (D) Hypertension

133. By what mechanism do local anesthetics depress cardiac contractility?

    (A) By increasing Ca^{2+} influx and release into the myocardial cell.
    (B) By decreasing Ca^{2+} influx and release into the myocardial cell.
    (C) By enhancing the intracellular levels of cAMP of the myocardial cell.
    (D) By enhancing the intracellular levels of cGMP of the myocardial cell.

134. Which local anesthetic agent depresses cardiac contractility the least?

    (A) Bupivacaine
    (B) Tetracaine
    (C) Ropivacaine
    (D) Lidocaine

135. A patient is scheduled for a general anesthetic. You plan to induce with propofol. What is the best dose for a 70-kg male?

    (A) 350 mg
    (B) 100 mg
    (C) 250 mg
    (D) 200 mg

136. What clinical sign is not consistent with Cushing's Syndrome?

    (A) Hypoglycemia
    (B) Hypertension
    (C) Hyperglycemia
    (D) Hypokalemia

137. What are the electrophysiologic effects of diltiazem on the myocardial cells?

    (A) Binding to calcium channels in their resting active state
    (B) Binding to T-type calcium channels
    (C) Binding to L-type calcium channels
    (D) Inhibiting potassium efflux during cardiac repolarization

138. Which is an appropriate initial intervention to correct intraoperative bronchospasm?

    (A) Deepen the level of anesthesia with a volatile agent.
    (B) Give 10 mg morphine IV.
    (C) Administer intravenous corticosteroids.
    (D) Give Labetalol 10 mg IV.

139. What is the correct classification of asthma symptoms that limit daily activity and require daily use of a short acting beta agonist?

    (A) Mild persistent asthma
    (B) Severe persistent asthma
    (C) Moderate persistent asthma
    (D) Intermittent asthma

140. What are the two strongest predictors of postoperative pulmonary complications?

    (A) Operative site and well controlled asthma
    (B) Operative site and history of dyspnea
    (C) Obesity and operative site
    (D) History of dyspnea and abnormal chest exam

141. Which two interventions lessen air trapping in a COPD patient?

    Select (2) two
    (A) Increase respiratory rate
    (B) Decrease respiratory rate
    (C) Increase I:E ratio
    (D) Decrease I:E ratio

142. What is the leading cause of cor pulmonale?

    (A) Obesity
    (B) Asthma
    (C) Sleep apnea
    (D) COPD

143. Which statement is false concerning anesthetic management of OSA patients?

(A) Patients who use CPAP at home should be encouraged to bring device from home for use in PACU.

(B) The anesthetist should anticipate a difficult intubation.

(C) Increased doses of benzodiazepines and opioids may be needed preoperatively.

(D) The anesthetist should anticipate a reduced FRC.

144. What type of pulmonary disease demonstrates an FEV_1/FVC ratio that is normal with a reduction in vital capacity?

(A) Asthma

(B) COPD

(C) Emphysema

(D) Pulmonary fibrosis

145. What diagnosis of a patient could be made with a pulmonary function test that revealed a FEV_1/FVC ratio that is 0.6 of predicted valve?

(A) Pulmonary fibrosis

(B) COPD

(C) Pulmonary edema

(D) Aspiration pneumonia

146. What clinical feature of a pulmonary embolism is false?

(A) Hypoxemia

(B) Tachycardia

(C) Decreased pulmonary vascular resistance

(D) Hypocapnia

147. Which I:E ratio is most appropriate in a patient with severe restrictive disease?

(A) I:E of 1:4

(B) I:E of 1:2

(C) I:E of 1:1

(D) I:E of 1:3

148. Deficiency in which protease inhibitor is linked to early-onset emphysema?

(A) Beta-1 antitrypsin

(B) Alpha-2 antitrypsin

(C) Alpha-1 antitrypsin

(D) Beta-2 antitrypsin

149. What is the hallmark sign of aspiration pneumonitis?

(A) Hypertension

(B) Pulmonary edema

(C) Arterial hypoxemia

(D) Tachycardia

150. Which statements regarding emphysema are true?

(A) Emphysema is a restrictive lung disease

(B) Elevated hematocrit

(C) Copious sputum

(D) Hyperinflation of the lungs on chest X-ray

151. Which mechanical ventilation modalities would be most appropriate for a patient with COPD?

(A) Increasing respiratory rate and an I:E ratio of 1:1

(B) Decreasing respiratory rate and an I:E ratio of 1:1

(C) Increasing respiratory rate and an I:E ratio of 2:1

(D) Decreasing respiratory rate and an I:E ratio of 1:3

152. Which four criteria are consistent with the diagnosis of Adult Respiratory Distress Syndrome?

(A) Acute onset, PAO_2 to Fio_2 ratio <200 regardless of the level of peep applied, bilateral infiltrates on chest X-ray, and a PA wedge pressure less than or equal to 18 mmHg

(B) Acute onset, PAO_2 to Fio_2 ratio <200 regardless of the level of peep applied, normal chest X-ray, and a PA wedge pressure less than or equal to 18 mmHg

(C) Acute onset, PAO_2 to Fio_2 ratio <300 regardless of the level of peep applied, bilateral infiltrates on chest X-ray, and a PA wedge pressure less than or equal to 18 mmHg

(D) Slow onset, PAO_2 to Fio_2 ratio <200 regardless of the level of peep applied, bilateral infiltrates on chest X-ray, and a PA wedge pressure less than or equal to 18 mmHg

153. Which criteria are consistent with the diagnosis of pulmonary hypertension?

    (A) A mean pulmonary artery pressure 14 mmHg with a with a pulmonary capillary occlusion pressure of no more than 15 mmHg

    (B) A mean pulmonary artery pressure at least 25 mmHg with a with a pulmonary capillary occlusion pressure of no more than 15 mmHg

    (C) A mean pulmonary artery pressure at least 10 mmHg with a with a pulmonary capillary occlusion pressure of no more than 15 mmHg

    (D) A mean pulmonary artery pressure at least 12 mmHg with a with a pulmonary capillary occlusion pressure of no more than 15 mmHg

154. Which of the following statements about chronic bronchitis is true?

    (A) Patients with chronic bronchitis display hyperinflation on the chest X-ray.

    (B) Patients with chronic bronchitis display decreased elastic recoil.

    (C) Patients with chronic bronchitis display a normal hematocrit.

    (D) Patients with chronic bronchitis display an elevated $PaCO_2$.

155. How long should a patient discontinue smoking in order to decrease secretions and reduce pulmonary complications?

    (A) 1-2 weeks

    (B) 2-4 weeks

    (C) 3-5 days

    (D) 4-6 weeks

156. What is the acid-base interpretation for a patient with the following ABG, pH 7.29, $PaCO_2$ 52, HCO_3 24?

    (A) Uncompensated respiratory alkalosis

    (B) Compensated respiratory acidosis

    (C) Compensated respiratory alkalosis

    (D) Uncompensated respiratory acidosis

157. When giving neostigmine, what is the resultant muscarinic effect?

    (A) Bradycardia

    (B) Tachyarrhythmias

    (C) Improved contractility

    (D) Increased conduction

158. Which anticholinesterase crosses the blood-brain barrier?

    (A) Edrophonium

    (B) Neostigmine

    (C) Pyridostigmine

    (D) Physostigmine

159. Your patient's Train-of-Four is ¼. You decide to use neostigmine to reverse neuromuscular blockade. What drug combination and doses will you use?

    (A) Neostigmine 0.04 mg/kg and glycopyrrolate 0.2 mg per 1 mg of neostigmine

    (B) Neostigmine 0.08 mg/kg and glycopyrrolate 0.2 mg per 1 mg of neostigmine

    (C) Neostigmine 0.02 mg/kg and atropine 0.014 mg per 1 mg of neostigmine

    (D) Neostigmine 0.01 mg/kg and atropine 0.1 mg per 1 mg of neostigmine

160. What is the acid-base interpretation for a patient with the following ABG, pH 7.49, $PaCO_2$ 22, HCO_3 24?

    (A) Uncompensated respiratory alkalosis

    (B) Compensated respiratory acidosis

    (C) Compensated respiratory alkalosis

    (D) Uncompensated respiratory acidosis

161. Which cardiovascular effect would you expect when stimulating B_1 receptors?

    (A) Decreased heart rate

    (B) Decreased conduction

    (C) Increased heart rate

    (D) Decreased contractility

162. What statement is true regarding internal cardioverter defibrillators (ICD)?

(A) ICDs are indicated for left ventricular ejection fractions >35%.

(B) Placement of ICDs requires general anesthesia.

(C) ICDs are indicated for intraoperative ventricular fibrillation.

(D) ICDs are indicated for patients with an ejection fraction <35%.

163. How does B2 stimulation affect insulin levels?

(A) Increases insulin

(B) No change in insulin level

(C) Decreases insulin

(D) Alpha 1 decreases insulin

164. What is the acid-base state of a patient with the following ABG, pH 7.35, $PaCO_2$ 50, HCO_3 44?

(A) Uncompensated respiratory alkalosis

(B) Compensated respiratory acidosis

(C) Compensated respiratory alkalosis

(D) Uncompensated respiratory acidosis

165. What is the classification of metoclopramide?

(A) Antacid

(B) H_1-Receptor antagonist

(C) Gastrointestinal prokinetic

(D) H_2-Receptor antagonist

166. Which of the following physiological effects is not associated with serotonin?

(A) Arteriolar and venous vasoconstrictor

(B) Bronchoconstrictor

(C) Increase bleeding time

(D) Decreased peristalsis

167. Which of the following is a serotonin receptor antagonist?

(A) Droperidol

(B) Dexamethasone

(C) Aprepitant

(D) Dolasetron

168. Which ABG result is indicative of acute hyperventilation?

(A) pH 7.25, $PaCO_2$ 20, HCO_3 24

(B) pH 7.35, $PaCO_2$ 50, HCO_3 44

(C) pH 7.35, $PaCO_2$ 40, HCO_3 24

(D) pH 7.45, $PaCO_2$ 30, HCO_3 14

169. What is the physical structure of succinylcholine?

(A) Two joined acetylcholine molecules

(B) Benzylisoquinoline

(C) Steroid ring with two modified ACh molecules

(D) Monoquaternary steroid

170. Which of the following factors produces 4 to 8 hours of succinylcholine-induced neuromuscular blockade?

(A) Homozygous atypical enzyme

(B) Hyperthermia

(C) Heterozygous atypical enzyme

(D) Reduced pseudocholinesterase levels

171. During a general anesthesia case with mechanical ventilation the ABG results are: pH 7.29, $PaCO_2$ 52, HCO_3 24. What intervention is appropriate?

(A) Decrease respiratory rate.

(B) Decrease tidal volume.

(C) Give 150 mEq sodium bicarbonate.

(D) Increase respiratory rate.

172. What are the primary anesthetic goals for patients with second- and third-degree burns?

Select (2) two

(A) Pain management

(B) Restoring circulating volume

(C) Administration of crystalloids

(D) Administration of colloids

173. Hypoxic pulmonary vasoconstriction (HPV) will cause which action in the lungs?

(A) Increase blood flow to non-ventilated lung

(B) Decrease blood flow to ventilated lung

(C) Decrease blood flow to non-ventilated lung

(D) Increase ventilation to the non perfused lung

174. Calculate the oxygen content given the following values: Hb = 14; $PaCO_2$ = 60; SaO_2 = 90%?

    (A) 4 mL O_2
    (B) 14 mL O_2
    (C) 17 mL O_2
    (D) 40 mL O_2

175. The Haldane effect is best described by which statement below?

    (A) The Haldane effect explains why deoxygenated blood can carry more CO_2.
    (B) The Haldane effect explains the influence of pH, PCO_2, and PO_2 on the oxyhemoglobin dissociation curve.
    (C) The Haldane effect governs the diffusion of O_2 at the capillary level.
    (D) The Haldane effect accounts for the difference in lung volume at inspiration versus expiration.

176. A 22-year-old male emerges from a laparoscopic appendectomy under general endotracheal anesthesia still intubated. The patient is without an oral airway. During emergence, the patient sits up bucking with teeth clamped down occluding the endotracheal tube. He forcefully attempts to breathe. Which respiratory phenomenon could occur based on this scenario?

    (A) Pulmonary embolism
    (B) Pulmonary edema
    (C) Aspiration pneumonia
    (D) Acute asthma attack

177. In which lung region are the alveoli most compliant in an upright healthy person?

    (A) Apex
    (B) Middle
    (C) Base
    (D) Pleura

178. A ventilation:perfusion (V:Q) ratio of zero (0) may be seen in which disorder?

    (A) Pulmonary embolism
    (B) Low cardiac output
    (C) Emphysema
    (D) Mucous plug

179. In what form is the majority of CO_2 transported in the blood?

    (A) Carbonic acid
    (B) Bicarbonate
    (C) Dissolved
    (D) Attached to hemoglobin

180. What would be the expected P_{50} of a patient with increased levels of 2,3-diphosphoglycerate?

    (A) P_{50} of 22 mmHg
    (B) P_{50} of 26 mmHg
    (C) P_{50} of 30 mmHg
    (D) P_{50} of 38 mmHg

181. Which anticholinergic possesses the least antisialogogue effect?

    (A) Atropine
    (B) Glycopyrrolate
    (C) Scopolamine
    (D) Neostigmine

182. The patient presents for outpatient surgery with a history of asthma. When using glycopyrrolate, what do you expect?

    (A) Constriction of bronchial smooth muscle
    (B) Increased gastric acid secretion
    (C) Decreased body temperature
    (D) Relaxation of bronchial smooth muscle

183. What would be the expected P_{50} of a patient with a body temperature of 35.2° Celsius?

    (A) P_{50} of 30 mmHg
    (B) P_{50} of 26 mmHg
    (C) P_{50} of 20 mmHg
    (D) P_{50} of 18 mmHg

184. Which type of pneumocytes in the pulmonary epithelium contains surfactant?

    (A) Type I pneumocytes
    (B) Pulmonary alveolar macrophages
    (C) Type II pneumocytes
    (D) Mast cells

185. Which is the origin of the phrenic nerves?

 (A) T10
 (B) C2
 (C) C3-C5
 (D) T4-T6

186. What are the two lung volumes that comprise the functional residual capacity?

 (A) Residual volume and tidal volume
 (B) Tidal volume and expiratory reserve volume
 (C) Residual volume and inspiratory reserve volume
 (D) Residual volume and expiratory reserve volume

187. What is vital capacity?

 (A) Volume remaining after maximal exhalation
 (B) Maximal additional volume that can be inspired above tidal volume
 (C) Maximal volume that can be expired below tidal volume
 (D) Maximum volume of gas that can be expired following maximal inspiration

188. Prior to rapid sequence induction of general anesthesia you plan to administer ranitidine. When is the best time to administer the medication?

 (A) 0.5-1 hours preoperatively
 (B) 1.0-1.5 hours preoperatively
 (C) 1-2 hours preoperatively
 (D) 1.5-2.5 hours preoperatively

189. Which H_2 receptor antagonist affects the metabolism of warfarin?

 (A) Cimetidine
 (B) Ranitidine
 (C) Diphenhydramine
 (D) Hydroxyzine

190. Which drug affects the absorption of digoxin?

 (A) Cimetidine
 (B) Bicitra
 (C) Metoclopramide
 (D) Omeprazole

191. What is the normal ratio of the forced expiratory volume in the first second of exhalation to the total forced vital capacity?

 (A) Less than 60%
 (B) Greater than 50%
 (C) Greater than or equal to 80%
 (D) Greater than or equal to 20%

192. What is the functional residual capacity in the supine position?

 (A) 2,300 mL
 (B) 1,300 mL
 (C) 1,200 mL
 (D) 500 mL

193. Which structure classifies local anesthetics?

 (A) Lipophilic group
 (B) Benzene ring
 (C) Hydrophilic group
 (D) Intermediate chain

194. Lipid solubility is greatest with which local anesthetic?

 (A) Tetracaine
 (B) Procaine
 (C) Cocaine
 (D) Chloroprocaine

195. Which factor most influences the duration of action for local anesthetics?

 (A) pKa
 (B) Ionization
 (C) Lipid solubility
 (D) Minimum concentration

196. What two factors can shift the hemoglobin dissociation curve to the right?

Select (2) two
 (A) Acidosis
 (B) Hypoventilation
 (C) Hyperthermia
 (D) Decrease in 2,3,-DPG

197. What is the anatomic dead space in a 75-kg healthy adult patient?

 (A) 75 mL
 (B) 100 mL
 (C) 150 mL
 (D) 200 mL

198. What law applies when determining blood flow through an intravenous catheter?

 (A) Poiseuille's Law
 (B) Bernoulli's Principle
 (C) LaPlace's Law
 (D) van der Waal's force

199. During a general anesthetic fentanyl and versed are administered. The interaction of the drugs produces a greater effect than the sum of the two medications. What is the interaction called?

 (A) Addition
 (B) Synergism
 (C) Tolerance
 (D) Tachyphylaxis

200. Which of the following is not a Phase I reaction?

 (A) Oxidation
 (B) Reduction
 (C) Conjugation
 (D) Hydrolysis

201. Which inhalational agent's metabolism produces compound A?

 (A) Sevoflurane with low flow
 (B) Desflurane with low flow
 (C) Sevoflurane with high flow
 (D) Desflurane with high flow

202. How is propofol classified?

 (A) Alkylphenol
 (B) Barbituric acid
 (C) Phencyclidine
 (D) Carboxylated imidazole

203. What induction agent is least protein-bound?

 (A) Ketamine
 (B) Propofol
 (C) Methohexital
 (D) Etomidate

204. Clearance of which benzodiazepine is greatest?

 (A) Diazepam
 (B) Lorazepam
 (C) Midazolam
 (D) Zaleplon

205. Following administration of a beta-lactam antibiotic, the patient exhibits urticaria, hypotension, and arrhythmias. What is the most likely cause?

 (A) Tachyphylaxis reaction
 (B) Anaphylaxis reaction
 (C) Atopic reaction
 (D) Anaphylactoid reaction

206. Which would be best in the care of a patient in myxedema coma needing emergent surgery?

 (A) Propylthiouracil
 (B) Liothyronine
 (C) Thyroxine
 (D) Thyroid stimulating hormone

207. Which indicates primary hypothyroidism?

 (A) Decreased thyroid stimulating hormone with decreased triiodothyronine and thyroxine
 (B) Increased thyroid stimulating hormone with decreased triiodothyronine and thyroxine
 (C) Decreased thyroid stimulating hormone with increased triiodothyronine and thyroxine
 (D) Increased thyroid stimulating hormone with increased triiodothyronine and thyroxine

208. Which statement is true regarding phenytoin?

 (A) Chronic treatment with phenytoin leads to prolonged neuromuscular blockade.
 (B) Lower doses of neuromuscular blockers are required.
 (C) Elimination of neuromuscular blockers is decreased.
 (D) Higher doses of neuromuscular blockers are required.

209. Which antiemetic will you avoid for patients with Parkinson's disease?

(A) Dolasetron

(B) Metoclopramide

(C) Odansetron

(D) Diphenhydramine

210. During surgery for breast cancer, the patient receives isosulfan blue dye. What will you expect?

(A) Increased SaO_2

(B) Tachycardia

(C) Decreased SaO_2

(D) Cardiac arrhythmias

211. Which analgesic for labor is not associated with significant respiratory depression affecting the mother or fetus?

(A) Morphine

(B) Nalbuphine

(C) Fentanyl

(D) Demerol

212. Why are benzodiazepines avoided during labor and delivery?

(A) Pain on injection

(B) Prolonged neonatal respiratory depression

(C) High Apgar scores

(D) Nausea and vomiting

213. Which inhalational agent affects the blood pressure the least?

(A) Sevoflurane

(B) Halothane

(C) Isoflurane

(D) Desflurane

214. Which analgesic given to renal failure patients results in prolonged respiratory depression?

(A) Remifentanil

(B) Demerol

(C) Sufentanil

(D) Morphine

215. Which COX-2 selective agent is linked to hepatic failure?

(A) Acetaminophen

(B) Aspirin

(C) Ketorolac

(D) Celecoxib

216. Your patient suffers from chronic renal failure. Which nondepolarizer will you avoid?

(A) Vecuronium

(B) Rocuronium

(C) Mivacron

(D) Anectine

217. What is the mechanism of action for reversal of succinylcholine?

(A) Metabolism by acetylcholinesterase

(B) Hydrolyzed pseudocholinesterase

(C) Complex formation with steroidal nondepolarizers

(D) Chemical degradation by L-cysteine

218. The patient undergoing cataract extraction takes echothiophate for glaucoma. If given succinylcholine, what will you expect?

(A) Duration <5 minutes

(B) Duration <10 minutes

(C) Duration >10 minutes

(D) No effect on duration of action

219. You administered propofol 2 mg/kg, succinylcholine 1.5 mg/kg, and fentanyl 2 ug/kg to a 70-kg patient undergoing emergent appendectomy. Following the 45-minute case, you observe no respiratory effort. What is the best choice for this patient?

(A) Administer naloxone

(B) Maintain ventilatory support with sedation

(C) Administer neostigmine

(D) Check the ventilator settings

220. Considering hyperkalemia, rhabdomyolysis, and cardiac arrest which neuromuscular blocking agent will you avoid in children?

(A) Rocuronium

(B) Succinylcholine

(C) Atracurium

(D) Cisatracurium

221. Which medication blocks muscarinic receptors?

(A) Atropine

(B) Rocuronium

(C) Pyridostigmine

(D) Neostigmine

222. What part of the structure of glycopyrrolate is responsible for binding to acetylcholine receptors?

(A) Organic base

(B) Ester linkage

(C) Aromatic base

(D) Benzene ring

223. What manifestation occurs as a result of anticholinergic overdose?

(A) Tachycardia

(B) Oral secretions

(C) Bradycardia

(D) Cutaneous vasoconstriction

224. How is eutectic mixture of local anesthetics (EMLA) cream formulated?

(A) 1:1 mixture of 0.5% lidocaine and 0.5% prilocaine

(B) 2:1 mixture of 1.5% lidocaine and 2.5% prilocaine

(C) 1:1 mixture of 0.75% benzocaine and 0.5% lidocaine

(D) 2:1 mixture of 0.75% benzocaine and 1.5% lidocaine

225. During an inguinal hernia repair, the surgeon asks how much bupivacaine is allowed for local infiltration. What is the correct maximum dose?

(A) 12 mg/kg

(B) 8 mg/kg

(C) 4.5 mg/kg

(D) 3 mg/kg

226. How does the duration of epidural ropivacaine differ from lidocaine?

(A) The duration of lidocaine is shorter than ropivacaine.

(B) The duration of lidocaine and ropivacaine is similar.

(C) The duration of lidocaine is longer than ropivacaine.

(D) Ropivacaine is similar to all amides.

227. Which local anesthetic is metabolized by pseudocholinesterase?

(A) Lidocaine

(B) Bupivacaine

(C) Ropivacaine

(D) Tetracaine

228. Prolonged neurological deficits have been associated with which local anesthetic?

(A) Epidural chloroprocaine

(B) EMLA

(C) Topical chloroprocaine

(D) Intrathecal lidocaine

229. What part of the body houses the greatest concentration of histamine?

(A) Parietal cells

(B) Circulating basophils and mast cells

(C) Gastric mucosa

(D) Peripheral tissues

230. Which cardiovascular effect occurs when administering diphenhydramine?

(A) Hypertension

(B) Peripheral arteriolar constriction

(C) Coronary vasoconstriction

(D) Hypotension

231. When administering promethazine, how long will sedative effects last?

(A) 3-6 hours

(B) 4-12 hours

(C) 8-24 hours

(D) 24 hours

232. Which of the following medications is potentiated by hydroxyzine?

    (A) Midazolam
    (B) Claritin
    (C) Fexofenadine
    (D) Metoclopramide

233. You include dexmedetomidine as an adjunct to general anesthesia. Which drug requirements will most likely decrease?

    (A) Vecuronium
    (B) Propofol
    (C) Ephedrine
    (D) Methoxamine

234. What is the primary receptor for phenylephrine?

    (A) B_1
    (B) A_1
    (C) B_2
    (D) A_2

235. How do direct and indirect adrenergic agonists differ?

    (A) Indirect agonists bind to the receptor.
    (B) Ephedrine binds to the receptor.
    (C) Direct agonists bind to the receptor.
    (D) Phenylephrine increases neurotransmitter activity.

236. What is the primary effect of phenylephrine?

    (A) Peripheral vasoconstriction
    (B) Decreased vascular resistance
    (C) Increased heart rate
    (D) Increased cardiac output

237. Which of the following halogenated agents potentiates the effects of epinephrine the most?

    (A) Desflurane
    (B) Sevoflurane
    (C) Isoflurane
    (D) Halothane

238. You plan to administer ephedrine for hypotension following spinal anesthesia. What do you expect?

    (A) Decreased heart rate
    (B) Decreased cardiac output
    (C) Increased heart rate
    (D) Short duration of action

239. How is ephedrine classified?

    (A) Indirect beta$_1$, beta$_2$ agonist
    (B) Direct beta agonist
    (C) Direct alpha agonist
    (D) Indirect alpha$_1$, beta$_1$, beta$_2$ agonist

240. What cardiac effect do you expect following administration of norepinephrine?

    (A) Decreased heart rate
    (B) Decreased mean arterial pressure
    (C) Increased heart rate
    (D) Decreased peripheral vascular resistance

241. You are planning to use clonidine during a general anesthetic. Primary receptor selectivity for clonidine includes with of the following?

    (A) Alpha$_2$
    (B) Beta$_1$
    (C) Beta$_2$
    (D) Alpha$_1$

242. Your patient is taking phenelzine. What is your primary concern when administering epinephrine to this patient?

    (A) Profound increase in heart rate
    (B) Lowered heart rate
    (C) Increased heart rate
    (D) Profound decrease in heart rate

243. You are administering an infusion of dopamine (0.5-3 µg/kg/min). What do you anticipate?

    (A) B_1 stimulation
    (B) DA_1 stimulation
    (C) Alpha$_1$ stimulation
    (D) B_2 stimulation

244. A patient scheduled for an open bowel resection presents with congestive heart failure and well-documented coronary artery disease. You note the patient's heart rate is 98. Which of the following adrenergic agonists would be the best choice for this patient?

(A) Dobutamine

(B) Esmolol

(C) Phentolamine

(D) Norepinephrine

245. A patient presents for removal of a pheochromocytoma. Preoperatively, which medication is most useful?

(A) Phenoxybenzamine

(B) Labetolol

(C) Esmolol

(D) Norepinephrine

246. During metabolism of nitrates (nitroglycerin and sodium nitroprusside) what substance is released?

(A) Guanylyl cyclase

(B) cGMP

(C) Nitric oxide

(D) Nitrate

247. You are infusing sodium nitroprusside at 3 ug/kg/min. What condition is likely to result?

(A) Cyanide toxicity

(B) Adsorption of polyvinylchloride

(C) Increased afterload

(D) Cerebral vessel constriction

248. During esophageal surgery, the endotracheal tube catches fire. What will you do first?

(A) Call for help.

(B) Remove the endotracheal tube.

(C) Stop the gas flow and remove the endotracheal tube.

(D) Remove the surgical drapes.

249. The patient with rheumatoid arthritis complains of long-term throbbing joint pain. Which fibers are activated?

(A) Efferent A and C fibers

(B) Alpha and beta efferent fibers

(C) Afferent A and C fibers

(D) Alpha and beta afferent fibers

250. Why is the primary metabolite of tramadol significant?

(A) Greater potency than the parent drug

(B) Shorter elimination half-life than the parent drug

(C) Respiratory depression is not reversible with naloxone

(D) Safety profile when using MAO inhibitors

251. Following general anesthesia for right should arthroscopy, the patient complains of pain. The patient's history includes congestive heart failure. Which analgesic will you avoid?

(A) Butorphanol

(B) Morphine

(C) Demerol

(D) Nalbuphine

252. Which two drugs would you avoid in an asthmatic patient?

Select (2) two

(A) Volatile anesthetics

(B) Labetalol

(C) Morphine

(D) Lidocaine

253. You decide to give butorphanol 2 mg to the patient postoperatively. What is the equipotent dose of morphine?

(A) 100 mg

(B) 8 mg

(C) 10 mg

(D) 80 mg

254. Your patient has a history of asthma. Which opioid will you avoid?

    (A) Fentanyl
    (B) Morphine
    (C) Remifentanil
    (D) Tramadol

255. How is remifentanil metabolized?

    (A) Hepatic cytochrome P
    (B) Hydrolysis by esterase enzymes
    (C) Hepatic conjugation
    (D) Conjugation with glucuronic acid

256. How does digoxin control atrial arrhythmias?

    (A) Enhancing vagal tone
    (B) Addition of calcium
    (C) Decreased intracellular sodium
    (D) Decreasing vagal tone

257. Your patient is undergoing a cholecystectomy with general endotracheal anesthesia. The patient takes digoxin for chronic congestive heart failure. What is the first sign of digitalis toxicity under anesthesia?

    (A) Bradycardia
    (B) Hypotension
    (C) Arrhythmias
    (D) Hypertension

258. What medication is indicated for treatment of ventricular fibrillation?

    (A) Vasopressin
    (B) Verapamil
    (C) Ibutilide
    (D) Adenosine

259. Why is terbutaline preferred for the treatment of asthma over isoetharine?

    (A) Isoetharine's B_1 adrenergic activity is less than terbutaline.
    (B) Either bronchodilator is acceptable.
    (C) Terbutaline's B_1 adrenergic activity is less than isoetharine.
    (D) Isoetharine's B_2 activity is greater than terbutaline.

260. During the preoperative interview you learn the patient takes daily lithium. How will lithium affect drugs used for general anesthesia?

    (A) Shorten the duration of action of vecuronium.
    (B) Increase the MAC of isoflurane.
    (C) Increase the duration of action of vecuronium.
    (D) No interaction with lithium exists for drugs used during general anesthesia.

261. In reviewing the patient's record, you note daily use of lithium and hydrochlorothiazide. What do you expect?

    (A) Hypernatremia
    (B) Therapeutic lithium levels
    (C) Decrease lithium levels
    (D) Hyponatremia

262. You are called for an emergency exploratory laparoscopy. The patient was involved in a motor vehicle accident and appears intoxicated. What do you expect?

    (A) Increased requirements for fentanyl
    (B) Decreased requirements for midazolam
    (C) Increased requirements for sodium pentothal
    (D) Decreased requirements for amphetamines

263. Why do patients who take tranylcypromine need to avoid eating cheese?

    (A) Hypotensive crisis due to tyramine
    (B) Decreased agitation
    (C) Hypertensive crisis due to tyramine
    (D) Jaundice

264. Which narcotic will you avoid in patients taking MAO inhibitors?

    (A) Demerol
    (B) Fentanyl
    (C) Morphine
    (D) Sufentanil

265. Which of the follow medications does not prolong the QT interval?

    (A) Fluoxetine
    (B) Sertraline
    (C) Azithromycin
    (D) Gentamicin

266. When treating hypotension for a patient taking dox-epin, what will you use?

   (A) Neosynephrine 10 ug IV
   (B) Ephedrine 5 mg IV
   (C) Neosynephrine 100 ug IV
   (D) Ephedrine 10 mg IV

267. Your patient is taking Amitriptyline. What will you tell your patient about taking this drug?

   (A) Continue taking Amitriptyline preoperatively.
   (B) Stop taking amitryptyline 24 hours before surgery.
   (C) Stop taking Amitryptyline 1 week before surgery.
   D) Stop taking Amitriptyline 2 weeks before surgery.

268. Contractions weaken despite use of oxytocin. Prosta-glandin is administered. What do you expect?

   (A) Constipation
   (B) Hypotension
   (C) Headache
   (D) Bronchodilation

269. The patient is scheduled for a cesarean section. You plan to use sevoflurane. How will this choice affect the uterus?

   (A) Increase uterine constriction
   (B) Decrease uterine bleeding
   (C) Increase uterine relaxation
   (D) Inhalational agents have no effect on the uterus.

270. Dantrolene was administered for malignant hyper-thermia. What is the most serious complication?

   (A) Respiratory insufficiency
   (B) Aspiration pneumonia
   (C) Hepatic dysfunction
   (D) Generalized muscle weakness

271. What is the result of an excess of glucocorticoids?

   (A) Cushing's syndrome
   (B) Addison's disease
   (C) Conn syndrome
   (D) Pheochromocytoma

272. What is the most effective treatment for moderate to severe Parkinson's disease?

   (A) Levodopa
   (B) Non-ergot derivatives
   (C) Levodopa with a decarboxylase inhibitor
   (D) Dopamine receptor agonists

273. The patient is scheduled for a thoracotomy. Upon review of the patient's medical history you note lovas-tatin as part of the medical management. What will you tell the patient preoperatively?

   (A) Take the statin as directed prior to surgery.
   (B) Stop the statin immediately.
   (C) Stop the statin 1 week prior to surgery.
   (D) Stop the statin 2 weeks prior to surgery.

274. What is the percent of total body water in the intra-cellular compartment?

   (A) 25%
   (B) 8%
   (C) 100%
   (D) 67%

275. What is the major extracellular cation?

   (A) Sodium
   (B) Potassium
   (C) Magnesium
   (D) Chloride

276. What substance poorly penetrates through the capil-lary endothelium?

   (A) Oxygen
   (B) Water
   (C) Lipid-soluble substances
   (D) Plasma proteins

277. At what value do serious complications of hyponatre-mia manifest?

   (A) 150 mEq/L
   (B) 145 mEq/L
   (C) 130 mEq/L
   (D) 120 mEq/L

278. The patient presents for surgery and you note a potassium level of 6 mEq/L. You choose to administer calcium gluconate. Which drug interaction is most concerning for this patient when administering potassium?

(A) Digoxin
(B) Furosemide
(C) Kayexalate
(D) Sodium polystyrene sulfonate

279. The patient presents with hypercalcemia secondary to a malignancy. What is the most effective means for lower serum calcium?

(A) A loop diuretic followed by rehydration
(B) Bisphosphonate
(C) Rehydration followed by a loop diuretic
(D) Etidronate

280. What target range is required for therapeutic effects of heparin?

(A) ACT 200-400 sec
(B) aPTT 1.5-2.5 times the control value
(C) ACT 100-200 sec
(D) aPTT 2.5-3.5 times the control value

281. Which statement is false regarding low molecular weight heparins (LMWHs)?

(A) LMWHs prevent formation of prothrombinase.
(B) Thrombolytic doses do not significantly cross the placenta.
(C) Bioavailability is greater with LMWHs as compared to heparin.
(D) Protamine is the antidote of choice for LMWHs.

282. The patient is taking subcutaneous unfractionated heparin. When is the best time to administer a spinal anesthetic?

(A) 4-6 hours after heparin administration
(B) 2-4 hours after heparin administration
(C) 12-24 hours after heparin administration
(D) 6-8 hours after heparin administration

283. What test is used to measure the effect of warfarin on blood coagulation?

(A) aPTT
(B) ACT
(C) AT
(D) INR

284. How does renal impairment affect insulin requirements?

(A) Insulin requirements decrease.
(B) No relationship exists between insulin requirements and renal impairment.
(C) Insulin requirements increase.
(D) The kidneys break down insulin to a greater extent.

285. What oral hypoglycemic is relatively contraindicated for patients with renal impairment?

(A) Glyburide
(B) Glipizide
(C) Tolbutamide
(D) Metformin

286. A patient with preexisting hypertension is undergoing an exploratory laparotomy. The blood pressure increases intraoperatively. What will you do first?

(A) Give esmolol
(B) Increase the concentration of isoflurane
(C) Give labetalol
(D) Decrease the concentration of isoflurane

287. A patient states they take nitroglycerin for angina. What statement is true regarding nitroglycerin's effect on the heart?

(A) Decreases preload
(B) Increases afterload
(C) Increases preload
(D) Decreases coronary vasodilatation

288. What patient history represents the greatest risk for cardiac complications?

(A) Recent angina
(B) Coronary artery disease involving two vessels
(C) History of MI 1 year ago
(D) Coronary artery disease involving three vessels

289. What characterizes a second-degree burn?

Select (3) three

(A) Penetrate epidermis

(B) Blisters form

(C) Replace fluids for burns >20% of the total body surface area

(D) Full thickness

(E) Requires debridement

290. An adult male who weighs 100 kg is burned over 50% of his body. Using the Parkland formula, calculate the fluid requirements for the first 24 hours.

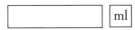 ml

291. Which of the following medications decrease the production of aqueous humor in glaucoma patients?

Select (2) two

(A) Pilocarpine

(B) Timolol

(C) Acetazolamide

(D) Echothiophate

292. What signs and symptoms are associated with acute opioid intoxication?

Select (2) two

(A) Tachypnea

(B) Hypotension

(C) Dilated pupils

(D) Pinpoint pupils

293. How does chronic alcohol ingestion affect anesthetic requirements including central nervous system hypnotics?

(A) Decreases requirements

(B) Increases requirements

(C) No effect on anesthetic requirements

(D) No affect with central nervous system hypnotics

294. Which of the following statements regarding cigarette smoking is true?

Select (3) three

(A) Carbon monoxide's affinity for hemoglobin is 300 times greater than oxygen.

(B) Carboxyhemoglobin returns to normal following one night without smoking.

(C) Smoking cessation within 12 to 48 hours of surgery decreases circulating catecholamines.

(D) Nicotine causes hypotension and tachycardia.

(E) Oxygen transport to tissues is increased.

295. During the preoperative interview the patient admits to the use of anabolic steroids. What implications for anesthesia are most concerning?

Select (2) two

(A) Impaired liver function

(B) Myocardial infarction

(C) Behavioral disturbances

(D) Atherosclerosis

296. The patient has a history of porphyria. What drugs will you avoid?

Select (2) two

(A) Methohexital

(B) Propofol

(C) Thiopental

(D) Nitrous oxide

297. Which risk factors exist for latex allergy?

Select (3) three

(A) Allergy to passion fruit

(B) Greater than five surgical procedures

(C) Spina bifida

(D) Greater than nine surgical procedures

(E) Acute exposure to latex

298. What statements are true regarding trauma-induced coagulopathy?

Select (2) two

(A) Tissue hyperperfusion results in coagulopathy.

(B) Thrombomodulin and activated protein C are released from the endothelium.

(C) Tissue hypoperfusion results in coagulopathy.

(D) Thrombomodulin binds to protein C.

299. Which statement is false regarding epidural hematomas?

   (A) Typically associated with skull fractures
   (B) Patient may present conscious and then lapse into an unconscious state.
   (C) When supratentorial hematomas exceed 30 mL volume, surgical decompression is used
   (D) Typically associated with blunt force injury

300. What condition results from a deficiency of complement 1 esterase inhibitor?

   (A) Angioedema
   (B) Neutropenia
   (C) Chronic granulomatous disease
   (D) Chediak-Higashi syndrome

301. What statements are true regarding allergic reactions?

   Select (3) three
   (A) Anaphylaxis is a Type I hypersensitivity reaction.
   (B) Type II hypersensitivity include transfusion reactions.
   (C) Anaphylactic reactions result due to an interaction with IgE.
   (D) Angioedema is a Type II hypersensitivity reaction.
   (E) Anaphylactoid reactions result due to an interaction with IgE.

302. Which classification of anesthetic agents is most commonly linked to anaphylactic reactions?

   (A) Thiobarbiturates
   (B) Narcotics
   (C) Benzodiazepines
   (D) Muscle relaxants

303. What statements about HIV and AIDS are true?

   Select (3) three
   (A) AIDS is caused by a retrovirus.
   (B) Seroconversion occurs 2-3 months following transmission of the HIV virus.
   (C) Highly active antiretroviral therapy (HAART) stops HIV replication.
   (D) Seroconversion occurs 2-3 weeks following transmission of the HIV virus.
   (E) There is no contraindication for the use of spinal anesthesia.

304. What signs and symptoms are linked to the pathophysiology of septic shock?

   Select (3) three
   (A) Hypervolemia
   (B) Bounding pulse
   (C) Wide pulse pressure
   (D) Bradycardia
   (E) Hypotension

305. What is the recommended minimum liter flow to avoid renal injury when using sevoflurane?

   (A) 1 L/min
   (B) 2 L/min
   (C) 3 L/min
   (D) 4 L/min

306. What percent of the total cardiac output flows through the kidneys?

   (A) 10-15%
   (B) 20-25%
   (C) 30-35%
   (D) 40-45%

307. What is the normal glomerular filtration rate (GFR)?

   (A) 440 mL/min
   (B) 660 mL/min
   (C) 1,200 mL/min
   (D) 120 mL/min

308. What drugs are associated with acute kidney injury?

   Select (2) two
   (A) Halothane
   (B) Demerol
   (C) Radiocontrast agents
   (D) NSAIDs

309. What narcotic metabolites are most likely to accumulate in patients with renal dysfunction?

   (A) Fentanyl
   (B) Demerol
   (C) Remifentanil
   (D) Morphine

310. What condition is most likely to cause complications during extracorporeal shock wave lithotripsy (ESWL)?

    (A) Renal calculi <4-mm
    (B) Cardiac arrhythmias
    (C) Ecchymosis
    (D) Skin blistering

311. What is the normal hepatic blood flow?

    (A) 15-20%
    (B) 25-30%
    (C) 20-25%
    (D) 30-35%

312. Which coagulation factor is not produced in the liver?

    (A) Factor V
    (B) Factor I
    (C) Factor VIII
    (D) Factor II

313. What factors cause a vitamin K deficiency?

    (A) VI, IX, X
    (B) VII, IX, X
    (C) VIII, IX, X
    (D) VII, IX, VI

314. What albumin level is associated with chronic liver disease?

    (A) 3.5 g/dL
    (B) 4.0 g/dL
    (C) 4.5 g/dL
    (D) 2.5 g/dL

315. Which of the following is false regarding prothrombin time (PT)?

    (A) The normal PT range is 11-14 seconds.
    (B) Measures factors V, VII, X, finbrinogen, and prothrombin.
    (C) Assists in the evaluation of chronic and acute liver disease.
    (D) PT is decreased in vitamin K deficiency.

316. What are the characteristics of hepatitis B?

    Select (3) three
    (A) Incubation period 20-37 days
    (B) Fecal-oral transmission
    (C) Incubation period 60-110 days
    (D) Percutaneous or body fluids
    (E) Development of chronic liver disease in 80-90% of children
    (F) No progression to chronic liver disease

317. What are the risk factors for halothane hepatitis?

    Select (3) three
    (A) >40 years
    (B) Male gender
    (C) Female gender
    (D) Obesity
    (E) Smoking

318. When evaluating a patient with cirrhosis, what laboratory findings are expected?

    Select (3) three
    (A) Increased bilirubin
    (B) Increased albumin
    (C) Increased prothrombin time
    (D) Decreased albumin
    (E) Hyponatremia

319. The intoxicated patient arrives for an emergent exploratory laparotomy following a motor vehicle accident. What statement is true regarding this scenario?

    (A) Anesthetic requirements are increased.
    (B) Alcohol increases MAC.
    (C) Alcohol decreases GABA receptor activity.
    (D) Alcohol inhibits NMDA receptors.

320. Which statements are true regarding the pneumatic tourniquet?

Select (3) three

(A) Hypertension occurs when the tourniquet is released.

(B) Tissue hypoxia occurs within 2 minutes of application.

(C) Hypotension occurs when the tourniquet is released.

(D) Metabolic acidosis occurs after tourniquet release.

(E) Core body temperature increases upon tourniquet release.

321. A 65-year-old patient presents for an open reduction and internal fixation following a hip fracture. The patient is short of breath, confused and you notice petechiae on the chest. What is the most likely cause?

(A) Fat embolism syndrome

(B) Mentation changes due to aging

(C) Deep vein thrombosis

(D) Thromboembolism

322. Which congenital cardiac malformations may benefit from a modified Blalock-Taussig shunt procedure?

Select (2) two

(A) Tetralogy of Fallot

(B) Truncus arteriosus

(C) Tricuspid atresia

(D) Transposition of the great vessels

323. What is the National Asthma Education and Prevention Program Expert Panel Report 3 definition of asthma?

(A) A chronic inflammatory disorder of the airways

(B) Preventable and treatable disease state characterized by airflow limitation that is not fully reversible

(C) Mechanical obstruction to breathing that occurs during sleep

(D) Right heart failure secondary to pulmonary pathology

324. How is the clinical diagnosis of chronic bronchitis made?

(A) Presence of a productive cough on most days of three consecutive months for a least two consecutive years

(B) Presence of an occasional productive cough for two consecutive months for at least 1 year

(C) Presence of a productive cough on most days of three consecutive weeks for a least two consecutive months

(D) Presence of a productive cough on three consecutive days for a least two consecutive weeks

325. Which congenital cardiac malformation includes a right-to-left intracardiac shunt?

(A) Tetralogy of Fallot

(B) Atrial septal defect

(C) Ventricular septal defect

(D) Patent ductus arteriosus

326. Which diseases place the patient at increased risk for developing cor pulmonale?

Select (3) three

(A) Adenotonsillar hypertrophy

(B) Chronic obstructive pulmonary disease

(C) Obesity

(D) Eaton-Lambert syndrome

327. What is indicated by an apnea/hypopnea index of 42 occurrences per hour?

(A) Normal result

(B) Mild obstructive sleep apnea

(C) Moderate sleep apnea

(D) Severe sleep apnea

328. What is the most common cause of obstructive sleep apnea?

(A) Ondine's curse

(B) Obesity

(C) Muscular dystrophy

(D) Central apnea

329. Which structure is most commonly occluded in obstructive hydrocephalus?

(A) Choroid plexus
(B) Foramen of Monro
(C) Aqueduct of Sylvius
(D) Foramen of Magendie

330. Which state should be avoided during the anesthetic care of a patient with multiple sclerosis?

(A) Hyperthermia
(B) Hyperoxia
(C) Hypercapnia
(D) Hypertension

331. What causes weakness in myasthenia gravis?

(A) Autoimmune damage to nerve axons
(B) Damage to presynaptic calcium channels
(C) Damage to postsynaptic cholinergic receptors
(D) Autoimmune damage to type I muscle fibers

332. What would be the effect on muscle strength if a patient with myasthenia gravis were treated with an anticholinesterase?

(A) No change
(B) Decreased strength
(C) Increased strength

333. Is an aneurysm in the brain more likely to occur in a larger vessel or a smaller vessel? Why?

(A) Equally likely in either a large or small vessel because blood pressure is constant
(B) More likely in a larger vessel due to increased diameter
(C) More likely in a smaller vessel due to increased resistance
(D) More likely in a smaller vessel due to decreased flow

334. Which level of spinal cord injury is most associated with autonomic hyperreflexia?

(A) T5-T8
(B) T10-L1
(C) L1-L4
(D) L4-S1

335. What is the most important cervical radiographic finding in a patient with rheumatoid arthritis?

(A) Cervical stenosis
(B) Cervical spondylosis
(C) Atlantoaxial subluxation
(D) Lordosis

336. What is the most common form of muscular dystrophy?

(A) Becker
(B) Limb-girdle
(C) Myotonic
(D) Duchenne

337. Which statement is true regarding Duchenne muscular dystrophy?

(A) The disease is X-linked and occurs more frequently in girls.
(B) The disease occurs equally in boys and girls and is diagnosed in early childhood.
(C) The disease is X-linked and symptoms occur only in boys.
(D) The disease primarily manifests as contractures of the large joints.

338. What is the anesthetic implication of a patient taking tricyclic antidepressants who is scheduled to receive general anesthesia?

(A) Meperidine will produce skeletal muscle rigidity and hyperpyrexia.
(B) Tricyclic antidepressants should be discontinued 2 weeks before surgery.
(C) MAC requirements may be increased for inhaled anesthetics.
(D) Ephedrine is preferred agent to treat post-induction hypotension.

339. Which characteristic is not shared by malignant hyperthermia and neuroleptic malignant syndrome?

(A) Generalized muscular rigidity
(B) Flaccid paralysis after vecuronium administration
(C) Effectively treated with dantrolene
(D) Hyperthermia

340. A patient is taking a MAO inhibitor. What anesthetic agent can be safely used in this patient?

(A) Phenylephrine
(B) Ketamine
(C) Bupivacaine with epinephrine
(D) Pancuronium

341. A 25-year old, 50 kg, otherwise healthy patient complains of nausea and demonstrates vomiting, refractory to ondansetron and dexamethasone therapy. Which dose of droperidol will achieve a safe therapeutic response?

(A) 1.25 mg IV
(B) 0.625 mg/kg IV
(C) 0.5 mg IV
(D) 12.5 mg IV

342. Which statement about phenytoin is correct?

(A) Chronic phenytoin therapy requires higher dose requirements of vecuronium.
(B) Chronic phenytoin therapy requires lower dose requirements of vecuronium.
(C) Chronic phenytoin therapy requires higher dose requirements of succinylcholine.
(D) Chronic phenytoin therapy requires lower dose requirements of succinylcholine.

343. Which statement about gabapentin is false?

(A) Gabapentin is not bound to plasma proteins.
(B) Gabapentin is an effective monotherapy for partial seizures.
(C) Gabapentin is unable to cross blood-brain barrier.
(D) Gabapentin undergoes no metabolism.

344. For which pathophysiologic state would gabapentin not be prescribed for management?

(A) Postherpetic neuralgia
(B) Diabetic neuropathy
(C) Acute postoperative pain adjuvant
(D) Status epilepticus

345. Which neuromuscular disease is associated with increased resistance to succinylcholine?

(A) Myasthenic syndrome
(B) Myasthenia gravis
(C) Myotonic dystrophy
(D) Muscular dystrophy

346. What is the initial dose of dantrolene for a 74-kg man in acute malignant hyperthermia crisis?

(A) 150 mg
(B) 185 mg
(C) 200 mg
(D) 215 mg

347. Which are early signs of malignant hyperthermia?

Select (3) three
(A) Increased end-tidal carbon dioxide
(B) Increased heart rate
(C) Increased temperature
(D) Masseter rigidity

348. Which disease is least likely to be associated with malignant hyperthermia?

(A) King syndrome
(B) Central-core disease
(C) Multi-minicore myopathy
(D) Duchenne muscular dystrophy

349. Which would be expected in a patient with Graves' disease?

(A) Increased thyroid stimulating hormone with decreased thyroid hormone.
(B) Increased thyroid stimulating hormone with increased thyroid hormone.
(C) Decreased thyroid stimulating hormone with decreased thyroid hormone.
(D) Decreased thyroid stimulating hormone with increased thyroid hormone.

350. Which diagnosis indicates adrenal insufficiency?

(A) Addison's disease
(B) Conn syndrome
(C) Cushing's disease
(D) Mendelsohn syndrome

351. Which is secreted from the posterior pituitary?

    (A) Antidiuretic hormone
    (B) Adrenocorticotropic hormone
    (C) Prolactin
    (D) Thyroid stimulating hormone

352. What causes acromegaly?

    (A) Hypersecretion of adrenocorticotropic hormone
    (B) Hypersecretion of thyroid stimulating hormone
    (C) Hypersecretion of growth hormone
    (D) Hypersecretion of prolactin

353. What condition results from hypersecretion of growth hormone in a child?

    (A) Acromegaly
    (B) Dwarfism
    (C) Osteomalacia
    (D) Gigantism

354. Which common anesthetic medications should be avoided during the induction of a patient diagnosed with acute intermittent porphyria?

    Select (2) two
    (A) Thiopental
    (B) Propofol
    (C) Etomidate
    (D) Fentanyl

355. Which correctly describes acute intermittent porphyria?

    (A) Accumulation of delta-aminolevulinic acid and porphobilinogen secondary to porphobilinogen deaminase deficiency.
    (B) Accumulation of protoporphyrin secondary to protoporphyrinogen oxidase deficiency.
    (C) Accumulation of delta-aminolevulinic acid and protoporphyrin secondary to ferrochelatase deficiency.
    (D) Accumulation of delta-aminolevulinic acid and coproporphyrinogen secondary to coproporphyrinogen oxidase deficiency.

356. Which are secreted by tumors in carcinoid syndrome?

    Select (3) three
    (A) Octreotide
    (B) Serotonin
    (C) Kallikrein
    (D) Histamine

357. What is the most likely location of a carcinoid tumor?

    (A) Kidney
    (B) Lung
    (C) Ovary
    (D) Appendix

358. What is the typical progression of Guillain-Barré syndrome?

    (A) Descending paralysis
    (B) Unilateral hemiparesis
    (C) Ascending paralysis
    (D) Concurrent upper and lower extremity weakness

359. Which neuromuscular blocking agent is most appropriate for use in severe cirrhosis?

    (A) Cisatracurium
    (B) Rocuronium
    (C) Vecuronium
    (D) Pancuronium

360. Which drugs will be prolonged in the glaucoma patient treated with echothiophate?

    Select (2) two
    (A) Cocaine
    (B) Succinylcholine
    (C) Glycopyrrolate
    (D) Chloroprocaine

361. What causes Eaton-Lambert syndrome?

    (A) Autoimmune destruction of calcium channels
    (B) Atypical pseudocholinesterase
    (C) Autoimmune destruction of cholinergic receptors
    (D) Autoimmune destruction of thyroid tissue

362. Which abnormality is associated with syringomyelia?

(A) Craniosynostosis

(B) Crouzon syndrome

(C) Arnold-Chiari malformation

(D) Apert syndrome

363. Which causes Zollinger-Ellison syndrome?

(A) Gastrinoma

(B) Pheochromocytoma

(C) Pituitary adenoma

(D) Osteosarcoma

364. A patient's cardiac assessment reveals a functional capacity of four metabolic equivalents. What activity can she most likely perform?

(A) Walk one to two blocks on level ground

(B) Singles tennis

(C) Cross-country skiing

(D) Swimming

Answers and Explanations: Basic Sciences

1. What results when alpha-1 receptors are activated?

   (A) Presynaptic nerve terminals are stimulated.

   (B) Adenylate cyclase activity is inhibited.

   (C) Negative feedback loop inhibits norepinephrine release.

   (D) Intracellular calcium ion concentration increases.

   Rationale: Alpha-1 receptors activate postsynaptic adrenoceptors resulting in increased intracellular calcium. Alpha-2 receptors are located presynaptically. Adenylate cyclase activity is inhibited when alpha-2 receptors are activated. When stimulating alpha-2 receptors, calcium ion concentration decreases creating a negative feedback loop that inhibits norepinephrine release.

   Ref: Butterworth, J.F., Mackey, D.C., & Wasnick, J.D. (2013). Ch 14 *Morgan & Mikhail's Clinical Anesthesiology* (5th ed.). New York, NY: McGraw-Hill.

2. Which initial intervention is correct if pulmonary embolism is suspected?

   (A) Discontinue intravenous fluids

   (B) Increase FiO_2

   (C) Extubate the patient

   (D) Discontinue inotropic support

   Rationale: Increase intravenous fluids, keep the patient intubated, provide inotropic support, and increase FiO_2.

   Ref: Butterworth, J.F., Mackey, D.C., & Wasnick, J.D. (2013). Ch 24 *Morgan & Mikhail's Clinical Anesthesiology* (5th ed.). New York, NY: McGraw-Hill.

   Nagelhout, J.J., & Plaus, K.L. (2014). Ch 26 *Nurse Anesthesia* (5th ed.). St. Louis, MO: Elsevier.

3. Which anticholinergic increases heart rate the most?

   (A) Scopolamine

   (B) Glycopyrrolate

   (C) Atropine

   (D) Pyridostigmine

   Rationale: While all anticholinergics increase heart rate, scopolamine exerts the least effect followed by glycopyrrolate. Pyridostigmine is a cholinesterase inhibitor.

   Ref: Butterworth, J.F., Mackey, D.C., & Wasnick, J.D. (2013). Ch 13 *Morgan & Mikhail's Clinical Anesthesiology* (5th ed.). New York, NY: McGraw-Hill.

4. What is the normal V/Q ratio?

   (A) 1

   (B) 0.8

   (C) 2

   (D) 0.5

   Rationale: Normally, ventilation (V) is approximately 4 L/min, whereas pulmonary blood flow (Q) is approximately 5 L/min. Therefore, the ventilation-perfusion ratio (V/Q) for the whole lung is 0.8.

   Ref: Butterworth, J.F., Mackey, D.C., & Wasnick, J.D. (2013). Ch 23 *Morgan & Mikhail's Clinical Anesthesiology* (5th ed.). New York, NY: McGraw-Hill.

   Nagelhout, J.J., & Plaus, K.L. (2014). Ch 26 *Nurse Anesthesia* (5th ed.). St. Louis, MO: Elsevier.

5. What is the underlying pathology of cor pulmonale?

   (A) Pulmonary hypertension

   (B) Decreased pulmonary vascular resistance

   (C) Systemic hypertension

   (D) Orthostatic hypotension

   Rationale: The underlying pathology of cor pulmonale is pulmonary hypertension.

   Ref: Butterworth, J.F., Mackey, D.C., & Wasnick, J.D. (2013). Ch 24 *Morgan & Mikhail's Clinical Anesthesiology* (5th ed.). New York, NY: McGraw-Hill.

   Nagelhout, J.J., & Plaus, K.L. (2014). Ch 26 *Nurse Anesthesia* (5th ed.). St. Louis, MO: Elsevier.

6. What is the blood-to-gas partition coefficient of halothane?

   (A) 0.47
   (B) 0.65
   (C) 1.4
   (D) 2.4

   Rationale: The blood to gas partition coefficient of nitrous oxide is 0.47; sevoflurane is 0.65; and isoflurane is 1.4.

TABLE 1-1. Partition coefficients of volatile anesthetics at 37°C.[1]

Agent	Blood/Gas	Brain/Blood	Muscle/Blood	Fat/Blood
Nitrous oxide	0.47	1.1	1.2	2.3
Halothane	2.4	2.9	3.5	60
Isoflurane	1.4	2.6	4.0	45
Desflurane	0.42	1.3	2.0	27
Sevoflurane	0.65	1.7	3.1	48

[1]These values are averages derived from multiple studies and should be used for comparison purposes, not as exact numbers.

   Ref: Butterworth, J.F., Mackey, D.C., & Wasnick, J.D. (2013). Ch 8 *Morgan & Mikhail's Clinical Anesthesiology* (5th ed.). New York, NY: McGraw-Hill.

7. Which inhalational agent is a halogenated alkane?

   (A) Halothane
   (B) Nitrous oxide
   (C) Desflurane
   (D) Sevoflurane

   Rationale: Nitrous oxide is an inorganic anesthetic gas. Desflurane and sevoflurane are halogenated with fluorine.

   Ref: Butterworth, J.F., Mackey, D.C., & Wasnick, J.D. (2013). Ch 8 *Morgan & Mikhail's Clinical Anesthesiology* (5th ed.). New York, NY: McGraw-Hill.

8. How would you classify a patient with repeated blood pressure measurements ranging from 160/100 to 179/109?

   (A) High normal
   (B) Stage 1 hypertension
   (C) Stage 2 hypertension
   (D) Stage 3 hypertension

   Rationale: Stage two or moderate hypertension is defined as systolic pressure between 160 to 179 mmHg and diastolic pressure between 100 to 109 mmHg.

   Ref: Butterworth, J.F., Mackey, D.C., & Wasnick, J.D. (2013). Ch 21 *Morgan & Mikhail's Clinical Anesthesiology* (5th ed.). New York, NY: McGraw-Hill.
   Nagelhout, J.J., & Plaus, K.L. (2014). Ch 19 *Nurse Anesthesia* (5th ed.). St. Louis, MO: Elsevier.

9. Which condition is not associated with precipitating unstable angina?

   (A) Polycythemia
   (B) Anemia
   (C) Thyrotoxicosis
   (D) Emotional stress

   Rationale: Unstable angina can be precipitated by anemia, thyrotoxicosis, emotional stress, or anything that causes myocardial ischemia due to an increased oxygen demand.

   Ref: Butterworth, J.F., Mackey, D.C., & Wasnick, J.D. (2013). Ch 21 *Morgan & Mikhail's Clinical Anesthesiology* (5th ed.). New York, NY: McGraw-Hill.
   Hines, R.L., & Marschall, K.E. (2012). Ch 1 *Stoelting's Anesthesia and Co-existing Disease* (6th ed.). Philadelphia, PA: Elsevier.

10. Which neuromuscular blocking drug is contraindicated during the care of a patient with Guillain-Barré syndrome?

    (A) Succinylcholine
    (B) Rocuronium
    (C) Atracurium
    (D) Pancuronium

    Rationale: The risk of severe hyperkalemia with succinylcholine is a contraindication.

    Ref: Butterworth, J.F., Mackey, D.C., & Wasnick, J.D. (2013). Ch 28 *Morgan & Mikhail's Clinical Anesthesiology* (5th ed.). New York, NY: McGraw-Hill.
    Miller, R.D., Eriksson, L.I., Fleisher, L.A., Wiener-Kronish, J.P., & Young, W.L. (Eds.) (2010). Ch 37 *Miller's Anesthesia* (7th ed.). Philadelphia, PA: Elsevier.

11. Which two lung pathologies are forms of COPD?

    Select (2) two
    (A) Asthma
    (B) Chronic bronchitis
    (C) Aspiration pneumonitis
    (D) Emphysema

    Rationale: Emphysema and chronic bronchitis provide the prototype of pathological changes in COPD.

Ref: Butterworth, J.F., Mackey, D.C., & Wasnick, J.D. (2013). Ch 24 *Morgan & Mikhail's Clinical Anesthesiology* (5th ed.). New York, NY: McGraw-Hill.

Nagelhout, J.J., & Plaus, K.L. (2014). Ch 26 *Nurse Anesthesia* (5th ed.). St. Louis, MO: Elsevier.

12. Which is a normal functional residual capacity?

    (A) 500 mL
    (B) 1,200 mL
    (C) 2,300 mL
    (D) 1,100 mL

    Rationale: A) is tidal volume, B) residual volume, and D) is expiratory reserve volume. Functional residual capacity is a combination of maximal volume that can be expired below tidal volume and the volume remaining after maximal exhalation.

    Ref: Butterworth, J.F., Mackey, D.C., & Wasnick, J.D. (2013). Ch 23 *Morgan & Mikhail's Clinical Anesthesiology* (5th ed.). New York, NY: McGraw-Hill.

    Nagelhout, J.J., & Plaus, K.L. (2014). Ch 26 *Nurse Anesthesia* (5th ed.). St. Louis, MO: Elsevier.

13. What are the **three** most common used pharmacological agents for treating ischemic heart disease?

    (A) Nitrates, alpha-blockers, and ACE-inhibitors
    (B) Nitrates, beta-blockers, and calcium channel blockers
    (C) Beta-blockers, calcium channel blockers, and ACE-inhibitors
    (D) Calcium channel blockers, nitrates, and ARBs

    Rationale: Nitrates, beta-blockers, and calcium channel blockers are the most commonly used pharmacological agents for treating ischemic heart disease.

    Ref: Butterworth, J.F., Mackey, D.C., & Wasnick, J.D. (2013). Ch 21 *Morgan & Mikhail's Clinical Anesthesiology* (5th ed.). New York, NY: McGraw-Hill.

    Hines, R.L., & Marschall, K.E. (2012). Ch 1 *Stoelting's Anesthesia and Co-existing Disease* (6th ed.). Philadelphia, PA: Elsevier.

14. Which narcotic does not cause histamine release?

    (A) Fentanyl
    (B) Morphine
    (C) Hydromorphone
    (D) Meperidine

Rationale: Lowered systemic vascular resistance results from bolus doses of morphine, hydromorphone and meperidine. Fentanyl administration may result in vagus mediated bradycardia.

Ref: Butterworth, J.F., Mackey, D.C., & Wasnick, J.D. (2013). Ch 10 *Morgan & Mikhail's Clinical Anesthesiology* (5th ed.). New York, NY: McGraw-Hill.

15. Which of the following occurs following administration of morphine?

    (A) Increased hypoxic drive
    (B) Decreased apneic threshold
    (C) Decreased hypoxic drive
    (D) Decreased $PaCO_2$

    Rationale: When administering narcotics, the hypoxic drive decreases as the $PaCO_2$ increases along with the apneic threshold.

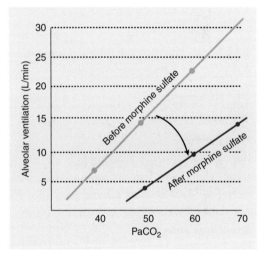

FIG. 1-1. Opioids depress ventilation. This is graphically (displayed by a shift of the CO_2 curve downward am d to the right.

Ref: Butterworth, J.F., Mackey, D.C., & Wasnick J.D. (2013). Ch 10 *Morgan & Mikhail's Clinical Anesthesiology* (5th ed.). New York, NY: McGraw-Hill.

16. The patient is shivering in the post–anesthesia care unit. Which intravenous medication will you use?

    (A) Meperidine 10 to 25 mg
    (B) Fentanyl 25 μg
    (C) Morphine 5 mg
    (D) Hyromorphone 5 mg

    Rationale: Compared to other narcotics, meperidine 10 to 25 mg IV decreases shivering in postoperative patients.

    Ref: Butterworth, J.F., Mackey, D.C., & Wasnick, J.D. (2013). Ch 10 *Morgan & Mikhail's Clinical Anesthesiology* (5th ed.). New York, NY: McGraw-Hill.

17. A patient with mitral stenosis is asymptomatic with occasional mild symptoms with exertion. Which mitral valve area is associated with these symptoms?

    (A) 0.2-0.5 cm²
    (B) 0.5-1.0 cm²
    (C) 1.5-2.0 cm²
    (D) 2.0-2.5 cm²

    Rationale: Patients with valve areas between 1.5 and 2.0 cm² are usually asymptomatic or have only mild symptoms with exertion. Critical mitral stenosis is associated with valve are 0.5-1.0 cm² or less. Mitral stenosis is usually diagnosed when the valve area is 1.5 cm² or less.

    Ref: Butterworth, J.F., Mackey, D.C., & Wasnick, J.D. (2013). Ch 21 *Morgan & Mikhail's Clinical Anesthesiology* (5th ed.). New York, NY: McGraw-Hill.

    Hines, R.L., & Marschall, K.E. (2012). Ch 2 *Stoelting's Anesthesia and Co-existing Disease* (6th ed.). Philadelphia, PA: Elsevier.

18. Which term describes full drug activation of a receptor?

    (A) Antagonist
    (B) Partial agonist
    (C) Agonist
    (D) Noncompetitive antagonist

    Rationale: Drugs that are agonists fully activate a receptor. Partial agonists activate parts of a receptor. Antagonists bind, but do not activate receptors. Noncompetitive antagonists irreversibly bind to a receptor.

    Ref: Nagelhout, J.J., & Plaus, K.L. (2014). Ch 5 *Nurse Anesthesia* (5th ed.). St. Louis, MO: Elsevier.

    Miller, R.D., & Pardo, M.C. (2011). Ch 5 *Basics of Anesthesia* (6th ed.). Philadelphia, PA: Elsevier.

19. A 60-year-old female with mitral stenosis has the following post induction vital signs: HR 125, BP 70/45 followed by sudden supraventricular tachycardia (SVT). What will you do first?

    (A) Cardioversion
    (B) Ephedrine
    (C) Phenylephrine
    (D) Vasopressin

    Rationale: Marked hemodynamic deterioration in a patient with mitral stenosis from sudden SVT is cause for immediate cardioversion.

Ref: Butterworth, J.F., Mackey, D.C., & Wasnick, J.D. (2013). Ch 21 *Morgan & Mikhail's Clinical Anesthesiology* (5th ed.). New York, NY: McGraw-Hill.

Hines, R.L., & Marschall, K.E. (2012). Ch 2 *Stoelting's Anesthesia and Co-existing Disease* (6th ed.). Philadelphia, PA: Elsevier.

20. Which adrenergic agonist affects the heart rate the greatest?

    (A) Norepinephrine
    (B) Dobutamine
    (C) Ephedrine
    (D) Isoproterenol

    Rationale: Heart rate is affected least by phenylephrine and norepinephrine (decreased); and ephedrine (increased). Administering isoproterenol increases heart rate the greatest.

    Ref: Butterworth, J.F., Mackey, D.C., & Wasnick, J.D. (2013). Ch 14 *Morgan & Mikhail's Clinical Anesthesiology* (5th ed.). New York, NY: McGraw-Hill.

21. What is the onset of analgesia following administration of epidural morphine 5 mg?

    (A) 30-60 minutes
    (B) 15-30 minutes
    (C) 5-15 minutes
    (D) >60 minutes

    Rationale: The onset of epidural morphine is 30 to 60 minutes. The duration of analgesia is 12 to 24 hours. Larger doses of epidural morphine are needed for analgesia. However, delayed respiratory depression may result.

    Ref: Butterworth, J.F., Mackey, D.C., & Wasnick, J.D. (2013). Ch 41 *Morgan & Mikhail's Clinical Anesthesiology* (5th ed.). New York, NY: McGraw-Hill.

22. Which of the following local anesthetics and dosages are used for cesarean section with spinal anesthesia?

    (A) Lidocaine (100 mg)
    (B) Tetracaine (14 mg)
    (C) Bupivacaine (12 mg)
    (D) Mepivacaine (16 mg)

    Rationale: The dose of spinal lidocaine for cesarean section is 50 to 60 mg; bupivacaine (10 to 15 mg); and tetracaine (7 to 10 mg). Mepivacaine is not administered for spinal anesthesia for cesarean section.

Ref: Butterworth, J.F., Mackey, D.C., & Wasnick, J.D. (2013). Ch 41 *Morgan & Mikhail's Clinical Anesthesiology* (5th ed.). New York, NY: McGraw-Hill.

23. Which anticholinergic is classified as a quaternary amine?

    (A) Scopolamine

    (B) Atropine

    (C) Neostigmine

    (D) Glycopyrrolate

    Rationale: Atropine and scopolamine are classified as tertiary amines. Neostigmine contains a quaternary ammonium.

    Ref: Butterworth, J.F., Mackey, D.C., & Wasnick, J.D. (2013). Ch 13 *Morgan & Mikhail's Clinical Anesthesiology* (5th ed.). New York, NY: McGraw-Hill.

24. Which anticholinergic cannot cross the blood-brain barrier?

    (A) Glycopyrrolate

    (B) Atropine

    (C) Scopolamine

    (D) Scopolamine and atropine

    Rationale: Tertiary amines atropine and scopolamine easily cross the blood-brain barrier. Quaternary amines (glycopyrrolate) are unable to cross the blood-brain barrier.

    Ref: Butterworth, J.F., Mackey, D.C., & Wasnick, J.D. (2013). Ch 13 *Morgan & Mikhail's Clinical Anesthesiology* (5th ed.). New York, NY: McGraw-Hill.

25. Which variable increases Minimum Alveolar Concentration (MAC)?

    (A) Hypernatremia

    (B) Hyperthermia

    (C) Acute intoxication

    (D) Ketamine

    Rationale: Hyperthermia, acute intoxication, and ketamine decrease MAC. Hypernatremia increases MAC.

    Ref: Butterworth, J.F., Mackey, D.C., & Wasnick, J.D. (2013). Ch 8 *Morgan & Mikhail's Clinical Anesthesiology* (5th ed.). New York, NY: McGraw-Hill.

TABLE 1-2. Factors affecting MAC.[1]

Variable	Effect on MAC	Comments	Variable	Effect on MAC	Comments
Temperature			Electrolytes		
Hypothermia	↓		Hypercalcemia	↓	
Hyperthermia	↓	↑ if >42°C	Hypernatremia	↑	Caused by altered CSF[2]
Age			Hyponatremia	↓	Caused by altered CSF
Young	↑		Pregnancy	↓	MAC decreased by
Elderly	↓			↓	one-third at 8 weeks'
Alcohol					gestation; normal by
Acute intoxication	↓				72 h postpartum
Chronic abuse	↑				
Anemia			Drugs		
Hematocrit <10%	↓		Local anesthetics	↓	Except cocaine
PaO$_2$			Opioids	↓	
<40 mm Hg	↓		Ketamine	↓	
PaCO$_2$	↑	Caused by ↓pH in CSF	Barbiturates	↓	
>95 mm Hg			Benzodiazepines Verapamil	↓	
Thyroid			Lithium	↓	
Hyperthyroid	No change		Sympatholytics		
Hypothyroid	No change		Methyldopa	↓	
Blood pressure			Clonidine	↓	
Mean arterial pressure	↓		Dexmedetomidine	↓	
<40 mm Hg			Sympathomimetics	↓	
			Amphetamine		
			Chronic	↓	
			Acute	↑	
			Cocaine	↑	
			Ephedrine	↑	

[1]These conclusions are based on human and animal studies.
[2]CSF, cerebrospinal fluid.

26. Which factors will exacerbate mitral regurgitation?

    (A) Tachycardia and acute increases in afterload.
    (B) Tachycardia and acute decreases in afterload.
    (C) Bradycardia and acute increases in afterload.
    (D) Bradycardia and acute decreases in afterload.

    Rationale: Although the anesthetic management will be tailored according to the severity of the mitral regurgitation, in general, factors such as slow heart rate and acute increases in afterload should be avoided in order to prevent exacerbation of disease. A normal to slightly fast heart rate as well as afterload reduction will improve forward flow.
    Ref: Butterworth, J.F., Mackey, D.C., & Wasnick, J.D. (2013). Ch 21 *Morgan & Mikhail's Clinical Anesthesiology* (5th ed.). New York, NY: McGraw-Hill.
    Hines, R.L., & Marschall, K.E. (2012). Ch 2 *Stoelting's Anesthesia and Co-existing Disease* (6th ed.). Philadelphia, PA: Elsevier.

27. Which volumes are included in vital capacity?

    (A) Tidal volume and residual volume
    (B) Residual volume and expiratory reserve volume
    (C) Expiratory reserve volume and inspiratory capacity volume
    (D) Inspiratory capacity volume and residual volume

    Rationale: Expiratory reserve volume and inspiratory capacity volume comprise vital capacity.
    Ref: Butterworth, J.F., Mackey, D.C., & Wasnick, J.D. (2013). Ch 23 *Morgan & Mikhail's Clinical Anesthesiology* (5th ed.). New York, NY: McGraw-Hill.
    Nagelhout, J.J., & Plaus, K.L. (2014). Ch 26 *Nurse Anesthesia* (5th ed.). St. Louis, MO: Elsevier.

28. Your patient's hemodynamic profile is as follows: HR = 100 beats/minute, cardiac output (CO) = 5.0 L/min, end-diastolic volume (EDV)= 100 mL. **Calculate the ejection fraction and write the answer in the box below:**

    | 50 | % |

    Rationale:

    STEP 1: $EF = \dfrac{EDV - ESV}{EDV} = \dfrac{SV}{EDV}$

    STEP 2: Must realize that SV is not given but can be calculated from: $CO = HR \times SV$

    STEP 3:

    $EF = \dfrac{CO/HR}{EDV} = \dfrac{5000 \text{ mL}/100}{100} = \dfrac{50}{100} = \dfrac{1}{2} = .50$

    STEP 4: Convert to % by multiplying $\times 100 = 50\%$
    Ref: Butterworth, J.F., Mackey, D.C., & Wasnick, J.D. (2013). Ch 20 *Morgan & Mikhail's Clinical Anesthesiology* (5th ed.). New York, NY: McGraw-Hill.
    Nagelhout, J.J., & Plaus, K.L. (2014). Ch 23 *Nurse Anesthesia* (5th ed.). St. Louis, MO: Elsevier.

29. What classic triad of symptoms is associated with aortic stenosis with a valve area <1 cm²?

    (A) Hypotension, dyspnea on exertion, and pulmonary congestion
    (B) Hoarseness, chest pain, and pulmonary emboli
    (C) Chest pains, arrhythmias, and embolic events
    (D) Dyspnea on exertion, angina, and exertional syncope

    Rationale: Patients with advanced aortic stenosis have a classic triad of symptoms: dyspnea on exertion (usually associated with congestive heart failure), angina, and exertional syncope. **A** is associated with mitral regurgitation. **B** is associated with mitral stenosis. **C** is associated with mitral valve prolapse.
    Ref: Butterworth, J.F., Mackey, D.C., & Wasnick, J.D. (2013). Ch 21 *Morgan & Mikhail's Clinical Anesthesiology* (5th ed.). New York, NY: McGraw-Hill.
    Nagelhout, J.J., & Plaus, K.L. (2014). Ch 23 *Nurse Anesthesia* (5th ed.). St. Louis, MO: Elsevier.

30. How does the elimination half-time of remifentanil differ from alfentanil?

    (A) Elimination half-time if longer for remifentanil.
    (B) Elimination half-time is shorter for alfentanil.
    (C) Elimination half-time is similar for alfentanil and remifentanil.
    (D) Elimination half-time is shorter for remifentanil.

    Rationale: Ester hydrolysis results in shorter elimination half-life for remifentanil as compared to all other opioids.

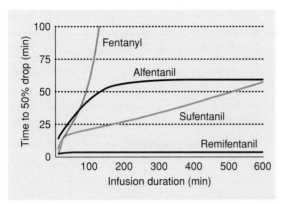

FIG. 1-2. In contrast to other opioids, the time necessary to achieve a 50% decrease in the plasma concentration of remifentanil (**its context-sensitive half-time**) is very short and is not influenced by the duration of the infusion. (Reproduced, with permission, from Egan TD: The pharmacokinetics of the new short-acting opioid remifentanil [GI87084B] in healthy adult male volunteers. Anesthesiology 1993,79:881.)

Ref: Butterworth, J.F., Mackey, D.C., & Wasnick, J.D. (2013). Ch 10 *Morgan & Mikhail's Clinical Anesthesiology* (5th ed.). New York, NY: McGraw-Hill.

31. One goal during a general anesthetic is decrease the neuroendocrine stress response to surgical stimulation. Which medication will be helpful?

    (A) Vecuronium
    (B) Midazolam
    (C) Lidocaine
    (D) Fentanyl

    Rationale: Narcotics in large doses help decrease release of catecholamines, cortisol, and antidiuretichormone. Muscle relaxants, benzodiazepines, and local anesthetics do not produce similar effects.
    Ref: Butterworth, J.F., Mackey, D.C., & Wasnick, J.D. (2013). Ch 10 *Morgan & Mikhail's Clinical Anesthesiology* (5th ed.). New York, NY: McGraw-Hill.

32. You administered meperidine IV. Immediately following administration the patient developed profound hypotension, hyperpyrexia and respiratory arrest. What drug interaction do you suspect?

    (A) Interaction with monoamine oxidase inhibitors (MAOs)
    (B) Interaction with erythromycin
    (C) Interaction with sodium pentothol
    (D) Interaction with etomidate

    Rationale: Patients receiving MAO inhibitors should not receive meperidine. In addition to hypotension, hypertension, hyperpyrexia, and respiratory arrest, coma may result. Interaction of alfentanil and

erythromycin may lead to respiratory depression and prolonged somnolence. Meperidine and other narcotics combined with central nervous system depressants foster synergism that affects the respiratory and cardiac systems.
Ref: Butterworth, J.F., Mackey, D.C., & Wasnick, J.D. (2013). Ch 10 *Morgan & Mikhail's Clinical Anesthesiology* (5th ed.). New York, NY: McGraw-Hill.

33. What is the normal aortic valve area?

    (A) 0.5-1.0 cm^2
    (B) 1.0-1.5 cm^2
    (C) 1.5-2.5 cm^2
    (D) 2.5-3.5 cm^2

    Rationale: The normal aortic valve has an area of 2.5 to 3.5 cm^2.
    Ref: Nagelhout, J.J., & Plaus, K.L. (2014). Ch 23 *Nurse Anesthesia* (5th ed.). St. Louis, MO: Elsevier.
    Hines, R.L., & Marschall, K.E. (2012). Ch 2 *Stoelting's Anesthesia and Co-existing Disease* (6th ed.). Philadelphia, PA: Elsevier.

34. For which severity of aortic stenosis is spinal anesthesia contraindicated?

    (A) 0.5-1.0 cm^2
    (B) 1.0-1.5 cm^2
    (C) 1.5-2.5 cm^2
    (D) 2.5-3.5 cm^2

    Rationale: An aortic valve area of 0.7 cm^2 is associated with sudden death. In general, neuraxial anesthesia is used cautiously with spinal anesthesia being relatively contraindicated due to the sympathectomy-induced drop in SVR.
    Ref: Butterworth, J.F., Mackey, D.C., & Wasnick, J.D. (2013). Ch 21 *Morgan & Mikhail's Clinical Anesthesiology* (5th ed.). New York, NY: McGraw-Hill.
    Nagelhout, J.J., & Plaus, K.L. (2014). Ch 23 *Nurse Anesthesia* (5th ed.). St. Louis, MO: Elsevier.

35. Which agent results in an increased heart rate during inhalational anesthesia?

    (A) Desflurane 0.75 MAC
    (B) Sevoflurane >1.5 MAC
    (C) Desflurane 0.5 MAC
    (D) Sevoflurane <1 MAC

    Rationale: Heart rate increases linearly with dose. There is a minimal increase in heart rate with desflurane when

TABLE 1-3. Clinical pharmacology of inhalational anesthetics.

	Nitrous Oxide	Halothane	Isoflurane	Desflurane	Sevoflurane
Cardiovascular					
Blood pressure	N/C[1]	↓↓	↓↓	↓↓	↓
Heart rate	N/C	↓	↑	N/C or ↑	N/C
Systemic vascular resistance	N/C	N/C	↓↓	↓↓	↓
Cardiac output[2]	N/C	↓	N/C	N/C or ↓	↓
Respiratory					
Tidal volume	↓	↓↓	↓↓	↓	↓
Respiratory rate	↑	↑↑	↑	↑	↑
Paco$_2$					
Resting	N/C	↑	↑	↑↑	↑
Challenge	↑	↑	↑	↑↑	↑
Cerebral					
Blood flow	↑	↑↑	↑	↑	↑
Intracranial pressure	↑	↑↑	↑	↑	↑
Cerebral metabolic rate	↑	↓	↓↓	↓↓	↓↓
Seizures	↓	↓	↓	↓	↓
Neuromuscular					
Nondepolarizing blockade [3]	↑	↑↑	↑↑↑	↑↑↑	↑↑
Renal					
Renal blood flow	↓↓	↓↓	↓↓	↓	↓
Glomerular filtration rate	↓↓	↓↓	↓↓	↓	↓
Urinary output	↓↓	↓↓	↓↓	↓	↓
Hepatic					
Blood flow	↓	↓↓	↓	↓	↓
Metabolism [4]	0.004%	15% to 20%	0.2%	<0.1%	5%

[1]N/C, no change.
[2]Controlled ventilation.
[3]Depolarizing blockage is probably also prolonged by these agents, but this is usually not clinically significant.
[4]Percentage of absorbed anesthetic undergoing metabolism.

using less than 1 MAC. The heart rate increases with Sevoflurane at 1.5 MAC or greater.

Ref: Butterworth, J.F., Mackey, D.C., & Wasnick, J.D. (2013). Ch 8 *Morgan & Mikhail's Clinical Anesthesiology* (5th ed.). New York, NY: McGraw-Hill.

Miller, R.D., & Pardo, M.C. (2011). Chapter 8 *Basics of Anesthesia* (6th ed.). Philadelphia, PA: Elsevier.

36. The anesthetic plan includes an inhalational induction. Which inhalational agent is the least desirable for a patient with chronic bronchitis and a 50-pack/year history of smoking?

   (A) Desflurane
   (B) Sevoflurane
   (C) Halothane
   (D) Nitrous oxide

Rationale: Irritation of the airway is common with desflurane and isoflurane. These inhalational agents

are pungent. Less pungency exists with nitrous oxide, sevoflurane, halothane, and therefore, less airway irritation.

Ref: Butterworth, J.F., Mackey, D.C., & Wasnick, J.D. (2013). Ch 5 *Morgan & Mikhail's Clinical Anesthesiology* (5th ed.). New York, NY: McGraw-Hill.

Miller, R.D., & Pardo, M.C. (2011). Chapter 8 *Basics of Anesthesia* (6th ed.). Philadelphia, PA: Elsevier.

37. Which local anesthetic is metabolized by *0*-toluidine?

   (A) Nesacaine
   (B) Cocaine
   (C) Prilocaine
   (D) Mepivacaine

Rationale: Prilocaine is the only amide local anesthetic not metabolized by P-450 microsomal enzymes. Ester local anesthetics nesacaine is metabolized by pseudocholinesterase whereas N-methylation and ester hydrolysis is responsible for cocaine metabolism. Mepivacaine is metabolized by P-450 microsomal enzymes.

Ref: Butterworth, J.F., Mackey, D.C., & Wasnick, J.D. (2013). Ch 16 *Morgan & Mikhail's Clinical Anesthesiology* (5th ed.). New York, NY: McGraw-Hill.

38. Which local anesthetic is linked to methemoglobinemia?

(A) Prilocaine

(B) EMLA

(C) Lidocaine

(D) Cocaine

Rationale: Methemoglobinemia is caused by prilocaine's metabolic pathway that includes *o*-toluidine. EMLA cream is associated with skin blanching, erythema, and edema. Cauda equine syndrome has been associated with lidocaine. Cardiac symptoms include profound arrhythmias and hypertension.

Ref: Butterworth, J.F., Mackey, D.C., & Wasnick, J.D. (2013). Ch 16 *Morgan & Mikhail's Clinical Anesthesiology* (5th ed.). New York, NY: McGraw-Hill.

39. Which risk factor contributes to myocardial ischemia in a patient with aortic regurgitation?

(A) Heart rate 40-50 beats/minute

(B) Heart rate 50-70 beats /minute

(C) Heart rate 80-100 beats/minute

(D) Heart rate 110-120 beats/minute

Rationale: One anesthetic goal of managing a patient with aortic regurgitation is to maintain the heart rate toward the upper limits of normal (i.e., c. 80 to 100 beats/minute). A heart rate that is too slow or an increase in systemic vascular resistance will increase the regurgitant volume (A and B). Tachycardia, on the other hand, will contribute to myocardial ischemia in a patient with aortic regurgitation.

Ref: Butterworth, J.F., Mackey, D.C., & Wasnick, J.D. (2013). Ch 21 *Morgan & Mikhail's Clinical Anesthesiology* (5th ed.). New York, NY: McGraw-Hill.

Nagelhout, J.J., & Plaus, K.L. (2014). Ch 23 *Nurse Anesthesia* (5th ed.). St. Louis, MO: Elsevier.

40. Prior to general anesthesia the patient reports taking daily imipramine. What is your most serious concern for this patient?

(A) Dry mouth

(B) Sedation

(C) Orthostatic hypotension

(D) Sympathomimetic activity

Rationale: Dry mouth, sedation, orthostatic hypotension, prolonged QT interval, dry mouth, blurred vision, and urinary retention are side effects linked to tricyclic antidepressants-TCAs (imipramine). The most serious concern for patients taking TCAs is sympathomimetic activity resulting in hypertensive crisis and cardiac arrhythmias.

Ref: Butterworth, J.F., Mackey, D.C., & Wasnick, J.D. (2013). Ch 28 *Morgan & Mikhail's Clinical Anesthesiology* (5th ed.). New York, NY: McGraw-Hill.

Nagelhout, J.J., & Plaus, K.L. (2014). Ch 19 & 51 *Nurse Anesthesia* (5th ed.). St. Louis, MO: Elsevier.

41. Where is the primary location of hepatic microsomal enzymes?

(A) Hepatic smooth endoplasmic reticulum

(B) Kidneys

(C) Gastrointestinal system

(D) Small intestine

Rationale: The primary location of hepatic microsomal enzyme activity is the hepatic smooth endoplasmic reticulum. Microsomal enzymes are also located in the kidneys and gastrointestinal system to a lesser extent. The majority of reactions in the small intestine involve P450 enzymes.

Ref: Butterworth, J.F., Mackey, D.C., & Wasnick, J.D. (2013). Ch 5 *Morgan & Mikhail's Clinical Anesthesiology* (5th ed.). New York, NY: McGraw-Hill.

Stoelting, R.K. & Hillier, S.C. (2006). Ch 5 *Pharmacology and Physiology in Anesthetic Practice* (4th ed.). Philadelphia, PA: Elsevier.

42. In which valvular disease is the pulmonary capillary wedge pressure (PCWP) an overestimation of the left ventricular end-diastolic pressure (LVEDP)?

(A) Mitral stenosis

(B) Mitral regurgitation

(C) Aortic stenosis

(D) Aortic regurgitation

Rationale: Because of the abnormal transvalvular gradient in mitral stenosis, the PCWP overestimates the LVEDP.

Ref: Butterworth, J.F., Mackey, D.C., & Wasnick, J.D. (2013). Ch 5 *Morgan & Mikhail's Clinical Anesthesiology* (5th ed.). New York, NY: McGraw-Hill.

Nagelhout, J.J., & Plaus, K.L. (2014). Ch 23 *Nurse Anesthesia* (5th ed.). St. Louis, MO: Elsevier.

43. Which of the following medications block alpha- and beta receptors?

(A) Phentolamine

(B) Isoproterenol

(C) Propranolol

(D) Labetalol

Rationale: Alpha$_1$, beta$_1$, and beta$_2$ receptors are blocked by labetalol. A competitive block is produced by phentolamine (alpha$_1$ and alpha$_2$ receptors). Isoproterenol is a selective beta blocker whereas propranolol is a nonselective beta$_1$ and beta$_2$ receptor blocker.

Ref: Butterworth, J.F., Mackey, D.C., & Wasnick, J.D. (2013). Ch 14 *Morgan & Mikhail's Clinical Anesthesiology* (5th ed.). New York, NY: McGraw-Hill.

44. The patient arrives in the operating room following a motor vehicle accident. Forty percent of the body is burned. When is it permissible to use succinylcholine?

Select (2) two

(A) Within 8 hours of injury.

(B) Within 48 hours of injury.

(C) After 48 hours of injury.

(D) No succinylcholine is used for patients with burns.

Rationale: Succinylcholine may be used for burn patients within 48 hours of injury. Significant elevation of potassium occurs when succinylcholine is administered after 48 hours.

Ref: Butterworth, J.F., Mackey, D.C., & Wasnick, J.D. (2013). Ch 39 *Morgan & Mikhail's Clinical Anesthesiology* (5th ed.). New York, NY: McGraw-Hill.

45. What variables are needed to calculate systemic vascular resistance (SVR)?

(A) Body surface area, cardiac output, and central venous pressure

(B) Mean arterial pressure, heart rate, and pulmonary capillary wedge pressure

(C) Mean arterial pressure, cardiac output, and pulmonary capillary wedge pressure

(D) Mean arterial pressure, cardiac output, and central venous pressure

Rationale: SVR = 80 x [MAP-CVP]/CO.

Ref: Butterworth, J.F., Mackey, D.C., & Wasnick, J.D. (2013). Ch 20 *Morgan & Mikhail's Clinical Anesthesiology* (5th ed.). New York, NY: McGraw-Hill.

Nagelhout, J.J., & Plaus, K.L. (2014). Ch 24 *Nurse Anesthesia* (5th ed.). St. Louis, MO: Elsevier.

46. The patient is scheduled for a tympanoplasty. Which inhalational agent will you avoid?

(A) Sevoflurane

(B) Nitrous oxide

(C) Desflurane

(D) Isoflurane

Rationale: When using nitrous oxide, air-filled cavities expand. The blood-gas partition coefficient of nitrous oxide is 0.46. The rapid movement of gas into air-filled cavities is 34 times greater than nitrogen. In this case, the middle ear is subject to increased pressures.

Ref: Butterworth, J.F., Mackey, D.C., & Wasnick, J.D. (2013). Ch 5 *Morgan & Mikhail's Clinical Anesthesiology* (5th ed.). New York, NY: McGraw-Hill.

Miller, R.D., & Pardo, M.C. (2011). Chapter 8 *Basics of Anesthesia* (6th ed.). Philadelphia, PA: Elsevier.

47. Which agent increases the cerebral metabolic rate for oxygen (CMRO$_2$)?

(A) Halothane

(B) Isoflurane

(C) Sevoflurane

(D) Nitrous oxide

Rationale: Cerebral vasodilatation and increased cerebral blood flow are linked to nitrous oxide administration without volatile anesthetics. Isoflurane, sevoflurane, desflurane, and halothane decrease CMRO$_2$.

Ref: Butterworth, J.F., Mackey, D.C., & Wasnick, J.D. (2013). Ch 8 *Morgan & Mikhail's Clinical Anesthesiology* (5th ed.). New York, NY: McGraw Hill.

48. Which hemodynamic event will decrease coronary perfusion pressure the most?

(A) Decreased systolic blood pressure

(B) Decrease in left ventricular end-diastolic pressure (LVEDP)

(C) Increase in pulmonary capillary wedge pressure (PCWP)

(D) Increase in diastolic blood pressure

Rationale: Coronary perfusion pressure = arterial diastolic pressure minus the LVEDP. Any decreases in aortic pressure or increases in ventricular end-diastolic pressure will reduce coronary perfusion pressure. Since PCWP is an indirect measure of LVEDP, an increase in PCWP will decrease coronary perfusion pressure.

Ref: Butterworth, J.F., Mackey, D.C., & Wasnick, J.D. (2013). Ch 20 *Morgan & Mikhail's Clinical Anesthesiology* (5th ed.). New York, NY: McGraw-Hill.

Nagelhout, J.J., & Plaus, K.L. (2014). Ch 23 *Nurse Anesthesia* (5th ed.). St. Louis, MO: Elsevier.

49. Which antibiotic is classified as a beta-lactam?

    (A) Penicillin
    (B) Gentamicin
    (C) Erythromycin
    (D) Ciprofloxacin

    Rationale: Gentamicin is an aminoglycoside, erythromycin a macrolide, and ciprofloxacin is classified as a fluoroquinolone.

    Ref: Stoelting, R.K., & Hillier, SC. (2006). Ch 28 *Pharmacology and Physiology in Anesthetic Practice* (4th ed.). Philadelphia, PA: Elsevier.

50. To avoid hypotension and possible cardiac arrest what is the best method for administering IV vancomycin?

    (A) >60 minutes
    (B) <30 minutes
    (C) >20 minutes
    (D) <10 minutes

    Rationale: Rapidly infused vancomycin (<30 minutes) results in life-threatening hypotension. Patient's experience head to toe erythema often termed "red man" syndrome.

    Ref: Stoelting, R.K., & Hillier, S.C. (2006). Ch 28 *Pharmacology and Physiology in Anesthetic Practice* (4th ed.). Philadelphia, PA: Elsevier.

51. What is the most common cause of myocardial remodeling?

    (A) Congenital heart disease
    (B) Myocardial ischemic injury
    (C) Chronic lung disease
    (D) Cardiomyopathy

    Rationale: Ischemic injury is the most common cause of myocardial remodeling and encompasses both hypertrophy and dilation of the left ventricle.

    Ref: Butterworth, J.F., Mackey, D.C., & Wasnick, J.D. (2013). Ch 20 *Morgan & Mikhail's Clinical Anesthesiology* (5th ed.). New York, NY: McGraw-Hill.

    Hines, R.L., & Marschall, K.E. (2012). Ch 6 *Stoelting's Anesthesia and Co-existing Disease* (6th ed.). Philadelphia, PA: Elsevier.

52. A 55-year-old male with congestive heart failure, with a status of post–cardiac transplantation is now undergoing elective surgery for hernia repair. Thirty minutes into the case, his heart rate drops to 28. What medication will you give for bradycardia?

    (A) Atropine
    (B) Ephedrine
    (C) Isoproterenol
    (D) Dexmedetomidine

    Rationale: When the denervated heart post–cardiac transplantation is bradycardic, a direct-acting beta-adrenergic agonist such a isoproterenol or epinephrine must be given in order to achieve an increase in heart rate.

    Ref: Nagelhout, J.J., & Plaus, K.L. (2014). Ch 24 *Nurse Anesthesia* (5th ed.). St. Louis, MO: Elsevier.

    Hines, R.L., & Marschall, K.E. (2012). Ch 6 *Stoelting's Anesthesia and Co-existing Disease* (6th ed.). Philadelphia, PA: Elsevier.

53. The patient with renal disease is scheduled for an exploratory laparotomy. What muscle relaxant is the best choice for this patient?

    (A) Vecuronium
    (B) Pancuronium
    (C) Rocuronium
    (D) Cisatracurium

    Rationale: Ester hydrolysis and Hofmann elimination make cisatracurium the best choice for muscle relaxation for patients with renal disease. Rocuronium and vecuronium elimination is mainly hepatic. However, 20% of vecuronium is eliminated renally. Prolonged neuromuscular relaxation is linked to rocuronium. Both drugs may be used for patients with renal disease. Pancuronium depends on primary renal elimination.

TABLE 1-4. Drugs with a potential for significant accumulation in patients with renal impairment.

Muscle relaxants	Antiarrhythmics
Pancuronium	Bretylium
Anticholinergics	Disopyramide
Atropine	Encainide (genetically
Glycopyrrolate	determined)
Metoclopramide	Procainamide
H₂-receptor antagonists	Tocainide
Cimetidine	**Bronchodilators**
Ranitidine	Terbutaline
Digitalis	**Psychiatric**
Diuretics	Lithium
Calcium channel antagonists	**Antibiotics**
Diltiazem	Aminoglycosides
Nifedipine	Cephalosporins
ß-Adrenergic blockers	Penicillins
Atenolol	Tetracycline
Nadolol	Vancomycin
Pindolol	**Anticonvulsants**
Propranolol	Carbamazepine
Antihypertensives	Ethosuximide
Captopril	Primidone
Clonidine	
Enalapril	
Hydralazine	
Lisinopril	
Nitroprusside (thiocyanate)	

Ref: Butterworth, J.F., Mackey, D.C., & Wasnick, J.D. (2013). Ch 30 *Morgan & Mikhail's Clinical Anesthesiology* (5th ed.). New York, NY: McGraw-Hill.
Hines, R.L., & Marschall, K.E. (2012). Ch 17 *Stoelting's Anesthesia and Co-Exiting Disease* (6th ed.). Philadelphia, PA: Elsevier.

54. The patient's glomerular filtration rate is 20 mL/min. What condition most likely exists?

    (A) Acute glomerulonephritis
    (B) Uremia
    (C) Renal calculi
    (D) Acute kidney failure

    Rationale: When a patient's GFR falls below 25 mL/min uremia exists. Chronic glomerulonephritis, diabetic nephropathy, hypertensive nephrosclerosis, and polycystic kidney disease characterize uremia.
    Ref: Butterworth, J.F., Mackey, D.C., & Wasnick, J.D. (2013). Ch 30 *Morgan & Mikhail's Clinical Anesthesiology* (5th ed.). New York, NY: McGraw-Hill.
    Hines, R.L., & Marschall, K.E. (2012). Ch 17 *Stoelting's Anesthesia and Co-Exiting Disease* (6th ed.). Philadelphia, PA: Elsevier.

55. What arterial line waveform might you observe in a patient with severe aortic regurgitation?

    (A) Pulsus paradoxus
    (B) Pulsus alternans
    (C) Pulsus bisferiens
    (D) Anacrotic pulse

    Rationale: Pulsus bisferiens may be present in patients with moderate to severe aortic insufficiency as a result of rapid ejection of a large stroke volume.
    Ref: Butterworth, J.F., Mackey, D.C., & Wasnick, J.D. (2013). Ch 24 *Morgan & Mikhail's Clinical Anesthesiology* (5th ed.). New York, NY: McGraw-Hill.
    Nagelhout, J.J., & Plaus, K.L. (2014). Ch 23 *Nurse Anesthesia* (5th ed.). St. Louis, MO: Elsevier.

56. Which characteristic describes a typical patient with diastolic heart failure?

    (A) Left ventricular ejection fraction less than 40%
    (B) Dilated left ventricular cavity size
    (C) Persistent atrial fibrillation
    (D) Fourth heart sound

    Rationale: Fourth heart sound is a characteristic finding in diastolic heart failure. The other characteristics are typical for systolic heart failure.
    Ref: Nagelhout, J.J., & Plaus, K.L. (2014). Ch 24 *Nurse Anesthesia* (5th ed.). St. Louis, MO: Elsevier.
    Hines, R.L., & Marschall, K.E. (2012). Ch 6 *Stoelting's Anesthesia and Co-existing Disease* (6th ed.). Philadelphia, PA: Elsevier.

57. How does the mechanism of action of methylxanthines affect patients with asthma?

    (A) Blocks degranulation of mast cells
    (B) Bronchodilates via B₂ receptors
    (C) Bronchodilates via B₁ receptors
    (D) Inhibits phosphodiesterase

    Rationale: Commonly used methylxanthines such as theopylline and aminophylline bronchodilate asthmatic patients by inhibiting phosphodiesterase. In addition, catecholamine release, histamine blockade and stimulation of the diaphragm promote stability in asthmatic conditions.

TABLE 1-5. A comparison of commonly used bronchodilators.[1]

Agent	Adrenergic Activity	
	β_1	β_2
Albuterol (Ventolin)	+	+++
Bitolterol (Tornalate)	+	++++
Epinephrine	++++	++
Fenoterol (Berotec)	+	+++
Formoterol (Foradil)	+	++++
Isoetharine (Bronkosol)	++	+++
Isoproterenol (Isuprel)	++++	—
Metaproterenol (Alupent)	+	+
Pirbuterol (Maxair)	+	++++
Salmeterol (Serevent)	+	++++
Terbutaline (Brethaire)	+	+++

[1] + Indicates level of activity.

Ref: Butterworth, J.F., Mackey, D.C., & Wasnick, J.D. (2013). Ch 24 *Morgan & Mikhail's Clinical Anesthesiology* (5th ed.). New York, NY: McGraw-Hill.

58. A 42-year-old female with multiple sclerosis is scheduled for major surgery with general anesthesia. She has been taking corticosteroid therapy. Which approximate equivalent dose achieves the anti-inflammatory potency of prednisone 50 mg?

(A) 8 mg dexamethasone

(B) 100 mg methylprednisolone

(C) 25 mg prednisolone

(D) 300 mg cortisone

Rationale: A is correct: 50 mg prednisone = 8 mg dexamethasone (4:25 potency ratio, i.e., 1/6 the dose) B is incorrect: 50 mg prednisone = 40 mg methylprednisone (4:5 potency ratio, i.e., 4/5 of dose) C incorrect: 50 mg prednisone = 50 mg prednisolone (1:1 potency ratio, equivalent doses) D incorrect: 50 mg prednisone = 250 mg cortisone (4: 0.8 potency ratio, i.e., 5x the dose)

Ref: Stoelting, R., & Hillier, S. (2006). Ch 23 *Pharmacology & Physiology in Anesthetic Practice* (4th ed.). Philadelphia, PA: Lippincott Williams &Wilkins.

Nagelhout, J.J., & Plaus, K.L. (2014). Ch 33 *Nurse Anesthesia* (5th ed.). St. Louis, MO: Elsevier.

59. A patient with rheumatoid arthritis has been receiving long-term corticosteroid therapy and infliximab. Which statement best describes the major anesthetic implication for this drug regimen?

(A) Avoiding anesthetic drugs that are excreted via kidneys

(B) Administering PO dose of infliximab via NGT intraoperatively

(C) Paying meticulous attention to sterile techniques

(D) Monitoring intraoperative labs for hypoglycemia

Rationale: Both long-term steroid therapy and infliximab predispose patients to infection. A is incorrect because there is not such a contraindication with steroids and TNF-antagonists. B is incorrect because there are only IV formulations of infliximab. D is incorrect because long-term steroid effects are associated with hyperglycemia, not hypoglycemia

Ref: Stoelting, R., & Hillier, S. (2006). Ch 23 *Pharmacology & Physiology in Anesthetic Practice* (4th ed.). Philadelphia, PA: Lippincott Williams & Wilkins.

Nagelhout, J.J., & Plaus K.L. (2014). Ch 32 *Nurse Anesthesia* (5th ed.). St. Louis, MO: Elsevier.

60. A patient with a prosthetic heart valve presents for a scheduled total abdominal hysterectomy with a heparin infusion. How far in advance of surgery will you recommend this heparin be discontinued?

(A) 2-4 hours

(B) 4-6 hours

(C) 24 hours

(D) 48 hours

Rationale: Heparin should be discontinued 4 to 6 hours prior to surgery and then restarted postoperatively when the risk of bleeding has diminished.

Ref: Butterworth, J.F., Mackey, D.C., & Wasnick, J.D. (2013). Ch 21 *Morgan & Mikhail's Clinical Anesthesiology* (5th ed.). New York, NY: McGraw-Hill.

Hines, R.L., & Marschall, K.E. (2012). Ch 2 *Stoelting's Anesthesia and Co-existing Disease* (6th ed.). Philadelphia, PA: Elsevier.

61. What is the predicted FEV_1/FVC ratio for a patient whose history includes a 55-pack/year history of smoking with wheezing on auscultation?

(A) FEV_1/FVC ratio of >0.7

(B) FEV_1/FVC ratio equal to 0.8

(C) FEV_1/FVC ratio of >0.9

(D) FEV_1/FVC ratio of <0.7

Rationale: The combination of greater than 55-pack/year history, wheezing on auscultation, and patient self-reported wheezing almost assures FEV_1/FVC ratio of <0.7.

Ref: Nagelhout, J.J., & Plaus, K.L. (2014). Ch 26 *Nurse Anesthesia* (5th ed.). St. Louis, MO: Elsevier.

62. Where do local anesthetics exert their primary mechanism of action?

 (A) Sodium channel alpha subunit
 (B) Calcium channel
 (C) Vanilloid 1 channel
 (D) Potassium channel

Rationale: While local anesthetics may bind to calcium, potassium, and vanilloid 1, the primary mechanism of action is exerted at the alpha subunit of the sodium channel.

Ref: Butterworth, J.F., Mackey, D.C., & Wasnick, J.D. (2013). Ch 16 *Morgan & Mikhail's Clinical Anesthesiology* (5th ed.). New York, NY: Lange Medical Books McGraw-Hill.

63. Which neuromuscular blocker is considered an acetylcholine (ACh) receptor agonist?

 (A) Vecuronium
 (B) Rocuronium
 (C) Cisatracurium
 (D) Succinylcholine

Rationale: Depolarizing muscle relaxants (succinylcholine) mimic acetylcholine.

Nondepolarizing muscle relaxants (vecuronium, rocuronium, and cisatracurium) are competitive antagonists binding ACh receptors.

Ref: Butterworth, J.F., Mackey, D.C., & Wasnick, J.D. (2013). Ch 11 *Morgan & Mikhail's Clinical Anesthesiology* (5th ed.). New York, NY: McGraw-Hill.

64. When administering neuromuscular blockers to patients with myasthenia gravis, what do you expect?

 (A) Up-regulation
 (B) Profound response to succinylcholine
 (C) Down-regulation
 (D) Decreased sensitivity to vecuronium

Rationale: Up-regulation occurs when more receptors are depolarized and then results in a profound response to depolarizing muscle relaxants. Down-regulation occurs when there are less acetylcholine receptors as in myasthenia gravis. Sensitivity to nondepolarizers is increased. There is a resistance to depolarizers.

Ref: Butterworth, J.F., Mackey, D.C., & Wasnick, J.D. (2013). Ch 11 *Morgan & Mikhail's Clinical Anesthesiology* (5th ed.). New York, NY: McGraw-Hill.

65. Which fibers are most sensitive to local anesthetics?

 (A) A-alpha fibers
 (B) Small unmyelinated C fibers
 (C) A-gamma
 (D) C fibers

Rationale: A-alpha fibers are less sensitive to local anesthetics as compared to A-gamma fibers. C fibers including small unmyelinated C fibers resist local anesthetic action.

Ref: Butterworth, J.F., Mackey, D.C., & Wasnick, J.D. (2013). Ch 16 *Morgan & Mikhail's Clinical Anesthesiology* (5th ed.). New York, NY: McGraw-Hill.

TABLE 1-6. Nerve fiber classification.[1]

Fiber Type	Modality Served	Diameter (mm)	Conduction (m/s)	Myelinated?
Aα	Motor efferent	12–20	70–120	Yes
Aα	Proprioception	12–20	70–120	Yes
Aβ	Touch, pressure	5–12	30–70	Yes
Aγ	Motor efferent (muscle spindle)	3–6	15–30	Yes
Aδ	Pain			
	Temperature	2–5	12–30	Yes
	Touch			
B	Preganglionic autonomic fibers	<3	3–14	Some
C Dorsal root	Pain, temperature	0.4–1.2	0.5–2	No
C Sympathetic	Postganglionic sympathetic fibers	0.3–1.3	0.7–2.3	No

[1]An alternative numerical system is sometimes used to classify sensory fibers.

66. Which ratio of the forced expiratory volume in the first second of exhalation (FEV$_1$) to the total forced vital capacity (FVC) would signify the greatest degree of obstruction?

    (A) FEV$_1$/FVC ratio of 80%
    (B) FEV$_1$/FVC ratio of 40%
    (C) FEV$_1$/FVC ratio of 20%
    (D) FEV$_1$/FVC ratio of 60%

    Rationale: The normal ratio of the forced expiratory volume in the first second of exhalation to the total forced vital capacity is greater to or equal to 80%.

    Ref: Butterworth, J.F., Mackey, D.C., & Wasnick, J.D. (2013). Ch 23 *Morgan & Mikhail's Clinical Anesthesiology* (5th ed.). New York, NY: McGraw-Hill.

    Nagelhout, J.J., & Plaus, K.L. (2014). Ch 26 *Nurse Anesthesia* (5th ed.). St. Louis, MO: Elsevier.

67. What compensatory mechanism is commonly seen with aortic regurgitation?

    (A) Eccentric hypertrophy
    (B) Dilated annulus of aortic valve
    (C) Concentric hypertrophy
    (D) Elevated brain natriuretic peptide

    Rationale: A volume-overloaded ventricle will cause the sarcomeres to replicate in series resulting in eccentric hypertrophy. Eccentric hypertrophy is commonly seen in aortic regurgitation.

    Ref: Butterworth, J.F., Mackey, D.C., & Wasnick, J.D. (2013). Ch 20 *Morgan & Mikhail's Clinical Anesthesiology* (5th ed.). New York, NY: McGraw-Hill.

    Nagelhout, J.J., & Plaus, K.L. (2014). Ch 23 *Nurse Anesthesia* (5th ed.). St. Louis, MO: Elsevier.

68. Which pharmacological agent is contraindicated in the patient with Wolff-Parkinson-White (WPW) syndrome exhibiting atrial fibrillation?

    (A) Atropine
    (B) Diltiazem
    (C) Verapamil
    (D) Metoprolol

    Rationale: Verapamil is contraindicated in this population because of the risk of accelerating a ventricular response. Atropine can be used cautiously, though not contraindicated. Glycopyrrolate would be a more suitable alternative to atropine.

    Ref: Butterworth, J.F., Mackey, D.C., & Wasnick, J.D. (2013). Ch 20 *Morgan & Mikhail's Clinical Anesthesiology* (5th ed.). New York, NY: McGraw-Hill.

Nagelhout, J.J., & Plaus, K.L. (2014). Ch 13 *Nurse Anesthesia* (5th ed.). St. Louis, MO: Elsevier.

69. Your patient has mitral valve prolapse. What is the most common arrhythmia associated with this disease?

    (A) Paroxysmal supraventricular tachycardia
    (B) Atrial fibrillation
    (C) Premature ventricular contraction
    (D) Junctional tachycardia

    Rationale: Paroxysmal SVT is the most commonly encountered sustained arrhythmia in patients with mitral valve prolapse.

    Ref: Butterworth, J.F., Mackey, D.C., & Wasnick, J.D. (2013). Ch 21 *Morgan & Mikhail's Clinical Anesthesiology* (5th ed.). New York, NY: McGraw-Hill.

    Nagelhout, J.J., & Plaus, K.L. (2014). Ch 23 *Nurse Anesthesia* (5th ed.). St. Louis, MO: Elsevier.

70. From where do the cardiac sympathetic fibers originate?

    (A) T1-T4
    (B) T2-T4
    (C) T3-T6
    (D) T4-T8

    Rationale: The cardiac sympathetic fibers, also known as the cardioaccelerator fibers, originate from the cells in the intermediolateral columns of the higher thoracic segments of the spinal cord and synapse at the first through fifth thoracic paravertebral ganglia, or T1-T4.

    Ref: Butterworth, J.F., Mackey, D.C., & Wasnick, J.D. (2013). Ch 20 *Morgan & Mikhail's Clinical Anesthesiology* (5th ed.). New York, NY: McGraw-Hill.

    Nagelhout, J.J., & Plaus, K.L. (2014). Ch 23 *Nurse Anesthesia* (5th ed.). St. Louis, MO: Elsevier.

71. Which statement about coronary blood flow is incorrect?

    (A) At rest, approximately 4-5% of the cardiac output passes through the coronary vessels.
    (B) The left ventricle is perfused almost entirely during diastole.
    (C) The right ventricle is perfused during systole and diastole.
    (D) Increases in the aortic pressure can reduce coronary perfusion pressure.

Rationale: All are correct except for D. Coronary perfusion pressure is determined by the difference between aortic pressure and left ventricular end-diastolic pressure (LVEDP). Any decrease in aortic pressure or increase in LVEDP will reduce coronary perfusion pressure.

Ref: Butterworth, J.F., Mackey, D.C., & Wasnick, J.D. (2013). Ch 20 *Morgan & Mikhail's Clinical Anesthesiology* (5th ed.). New York, NY: McGraw-Hill.

Nagelhout, J.J., & Plaus, K.L. (2014). Ch 23 *Nurse Anesthesia* (5th ed.). St. Louis, MO: Elsevier.

72. What is indicated by a V/Q ratio that is equal to infinity?

    (A) Dead space
    (B) Shunting
    (C) Normal V/Q ratio
    (D) Inadequate ventilation

    Rationale: V/Q is where V is ventilation and Q is perfusion relationship. If perfusion is 0 than the V/Q ratio is infinity.

    Ref: Butterworth, J.F., Mackey, D.C., & Wasnick, J.D. (2013). Ch 23 *Morgan & Mikhail's Clinical Anesthesiology* (5th ed.). New York, NY: McGraw-Hill.

    Nagelhout, J.J., & Plaus, K.L. (2014). Ch 26 *Nurse Anesthesia* (5th ed.). St. Louis, MO: Elsevier.

73. As compared to other anticholinergics, what are scopolamine's sedative effects?

    (A) Less than atropine
    (B) Greater than glycopyrrolate
    (C) Same as atropine
    (D) Same as atropine and glycopyrrolate

    Rationale: The sedative effect of anticholinergics is greatest with scopolamine. Glycopyrrolate possesses no sedative effects. Sedation is minimal with atropine.

    Ref: Butterworth, J.F., Mackey, D.C., & Wasnick, J.D. (2013). Ch 13 *Morgan & Mikhail's Clinical Anesthesiology* (5th ed.). New York, NY: McGraw-Hill.

74. Who studied the relationship between volume and temperature when pressure remains constant?

    (A) Boyle
    (B) Charles
    (C) Gay-Lussac
    (D) Dalton

Rationale: Boyle examined the relationship of pressure and volume with constant temperature.

Gay-Lussac examined pressure and temperature when volume is constant. Dalton's Law shares that the sum of individual gas pressures is equal to the total pressure.

Ref: Nagelhout, J.J., & Plaus, K.L. (2014). Ch 14 *Nurse Anesthesia* (5th ed.). St. Louis, MO: Elsevier.

75. Which factor most negatively affects myocardial oxygen consumption?

    (A) Cardiac volume work
    (B) Electrical activity
    (C) Heart rate
    (D) Wall stress

    Rationale: There are many factors that increase myocardial oxygen demand: heart rate, pressure work, contractility, wall stress, volume work, and electrical activity. Pressure work and heart rate increase myocardial oxygen consumption the most. Of the options above, heart rate is the most important factor that negatively affects myocardial oxygen consumption.

    Ref: Butterworth, J.F., Mackey, D.C., & Wasnick, J.D. (2013). Ch 20 *Morgan & Mikhail's Clinical Anesthesiology* (5th ed.). New York, NY: McGraw-Hill.

    Nagelhout, J.J., & Plaus, K.L. (2014). Ch 23 *Nurse Anesthesia* (5th ed.). St. Louis, MO: Elsevier.

76. What is the functional residual capacity for an adult patient in the supine position following induction of general anesthesia?

    (A) 500 mL
    (B) 800 mL
    (C) 1,300 mL
    (D) 2,300 mL

    Rationale: The supine position reduces the functional residual capacity by 800 to 1,000 mL, and induction of general anesthesia further reduces the functional residual capacity by another 500 mL.

    Ref: Butterworth, J.F., Mackey, D.C., & Wasnick, J.D. (2013). Ch 23 *Morgan & Mikhail's Clinical Anesthesiology* (5th ed.). New York, NY: McGraw-Hill.

    Nagelhout, J.J., & Plaus, K.L. (2014). Ch 26 *Nurse Anesthesia* (5th ed.). St. Louis, MO: Elsevier.

77. What is the normal coronary blood flow at rest?

(A) 175-200 mL/min

(B) 200-225 mL/min

(C) 225-250 mL/min

(D) 250-275 mL/min

Rationale: At rest, approximate 4% to 5% of the cardiac output, or 225 to 250 mL/min of blood passes the coronary vessels at rest.

Ref: Butterworth, J.F., Mackey, D.C., & Wasnick, J.D. (2013). Ch 20 *Morgan & Mikhail's Clinical Anesthesiology* (5th ed.). New York, NY: McGraw-Hill.

Nagelhout, J.J., & Plaus, K.L. (2014). Ch 23 *Nurse Anesthesia* (5th ed.). St. Louis, MO: Elsevier.

78. If a 64-kg woman receives a standard initial dose of dantrolene during malignant hyperthermia crisis, how many grams of mannitol have been administered?

(A) 12

(B) 16

(C) 20

(D) 24

Rationale: Standard initial dose is 2.5 mg/kg, or 160 mg in this case. Each vial contains 20 mg of dantrolene; 8 vials would be needed. Each vial contains 3 grams of mannitol. Eight vials x 3 g each = 24 grams of mannitol.

Ref: Butterworth, J.F., Mackey, D.C., & Wasnick, J.D. (2013). Ch 52 *Morgan & Mikhail's Clinical Anesthesiology* (5th ed.). New York, NY: McGraw-Hill.

Longnecker, D.E., Brown, D.L., Newman, M.F., & Zapol, W.M. (Eds.) (2012). Ch 87 *Anesthesiology* (5th ed.). New York, NY: McGraw-Hill.

79. Which statement about protamine is incorrect?

(A) A hypotensive reaction can be treated with incremental doses of phenylephrine.

(B) Administering protamine over 10-15 minutes will decrease risk of hypotension reaction.

(C) The normal dose is 10 mg of protamine for every 100 units of heparin.

(D) 50-100 mg supplementary doses can be administered to reverse residual anticoagulation.

Rationale: All are correct, except C. The typical dose is 1 to 1.3 mg of protamine per 100 units of heparin.

Ref: Butterworth, J.F., Mackey, D.C., & Wasnick, J.D. (2013). Ch 20 *Morgan & Mikhail's Clinical Anesthesiology* (5th ed.). New York, NY: McGraw-Hill.

Nagelhout, J.J., & Plaus, K.L. (2014). Ch 23 *Nurse Anesthesia* (5th ed.). St. Louis, MO: Elsevier.

80. What two pathologies can increase alveolar dead space?

Select (2) two

(A) Mucus plug

(B) Pulmonary embolism

(C) Decreased cardiac output

(D) Hypoventilation

Rationale: Alveolar dead space is defined as ventilation without perfusion.

Ref: Butterworth, J.F., Mackey, D.C., & Wasnick, J.D. (2013). Ch 23 *Morgan & Mikhail's Clinical Anesthesiology* (5th ed.). New York, NY: McGraw-Hill.

Nagelhout, J.J., & Plaus, K.L. (2014). Ch 26 *Nurse Anesthesia* (5th ed.). St. Louis, MO: Elsevier.

81. How is residual volume defined?

(A) Maximum volume of air expired from resting end-expiratory level

(B) Maximum volume of air inspired from the resting end-inspiratory level

(C) Normal breath

(D) Volume remaining after maximal exhalation

Rationale: Residual volume is the air that remains in the lungs after a maximal exhalation, which is about 1,200 mL in an average adult.

Ref: Butterworth, J.F., Mackey, D.C., & Wasnick, J.D. (2013). Ch 23 *Morgan & Mikhail's Clinical Anesthesiology* (5th ed.). New York, NY: McGraw-Hill.

Nagelhout, J.J., & Plaus, K.L. (2014). Ch 26 *Nurse Anesthesia* (5th ed.). St. Louis, MO: Elsevier.

82. Which patient does not pose an increased risk for an allergic reaction to protamine sulfate?

(A) A patient who has a history of two previous cardiac catheterizations.

(B) A patient who is currently undergoing aortic valve replacement.

(C) A diabetic patient on maintenance NPH insulin therapy.

(D) A patient who is maintained on a weekly hemodialysis regimen.

Rationale: There is an increased incidence of reactions to protamine in patients sensitized to protamine from previous cardiac catheterization, hemodialysis, cardiac surgery, or exposure to neutral protamine Hagedorn (NPH) insulin. A patient who is undergoing their aortic valve replacement for the first time is not an increased risk.

Ref: Butterworth, J.F., Mackey, D.C., & Wasnick, J.D. (2013). Ch 22 *Morgan & Mikhail's Clinical Anesthesiology* (5th ed.). New York, NY: McGraw-Hill.

Barash, P.G., Cullen, B.F., Stoelting, R.K., Calahan, M.K., and Stock, M.C. (2009). Ch 41 *Clinical Anesthesia* (6th ed.). Philadelphia, PA: Lippincott Williams & Wilkins.

83. Compared to neostigmine, what is the onset of action of pyridostigmine?

    (A) Longer than neostigmine
    (B) Same as neostigmine
    (C) Slower than neostigmine
    (D) Clinically inconsequential

    Rationale: The onset of action of pyridostigmine (10 to 15 minutes) is slower than neostigmine (5 minutes).

    Ref: Butterworth, J.F., Mackey, D.C., & Wasnick J.D. (2013). Ch 12 *Morgan & Mikhail's Clinical Anesthesiology* (5th ed.). New York, NY: McGraw-Hill.

84. Which condition potentiates neuromuscular blockade?

    (A) Hypomagnesaemia
    (B) Hypercalcemia
    (C) Hyperkalemia
    (D) Hypothermia

    Rationale: Factors potentiating neuromuscular blockade include: hypothermia, respiratory acidosis, hypomagnesaemia, hypocalcemia, hypokalemia. In addition, volatile anesthetics, dantrolene, verapamil, furosemide, lidocaine, and antibiotics (aminoglycosides, polymiyxin B, neomycin, tetracycline, and clindamycin) potentiate neuromuscular blockade.

    Ref: Butterworth, J.F., Mackey, D.C., & Wasnick J.D. (2013). Ch 12 *Morgan & Mikhail's Clinical Anesthesiology* (5th ed.). New York, NY: McGraw-Hill.

85. What is the result of acetylcholine acting on the muscarinic receptor (M2) in the sinoatrial node?

    Select (3) three

    (A) Positive dromotropic effects
    (B) Negative dromotropic effects
    (C) Positive chronotropic effects
    (D) Negative chronotropic effects
    (E) Positive inotropic effects
    (F) Negative inotropic effects

    Rationale: Acetylcholine acting on the cardiac muscarinic receptors (M2) will produce negative chronotropic, negative dromotropic, and negative inotropic effects.

    Ref: Butterworth, J.F., Mackey, D.C., & Wasnick, J.D. (2013). Ch 20 *Morgan & Mikhail's Clinical Anesthesiology* (5th ed.). New York, NY: McGraw-Hill.

    Nagelhout, J.J., & Plaus, K.L. (2014). Ch 23 *Nurse Anesthesia* (5th ed.). St. Louis, MO: Elsevier.

86. Which paradoxical cardiac wall motion, when diagnosed with transesophageal echocardiography (TEE) is indicative of myocardial infarction?

    (A) Dyskinesia
    (B) Hypokinesia
    (C) Akinesia
    (D) Hyperkinesia

    Rationale: Dyskinesia, paradoxical movement, is the hallmark of myocardial infarction. Akinesia is absence of motion (not paradoxical motion) but can be associated with myocardial infarction. Hypokinesia describes less vigorous contractions than normal. Hyperkinesia is not an associated term with TEE abnormal wall motion.

    Ref: Butterworth, J.F., Mackey, D.C., & Wasnick, J.D. (2013). Ch 20 *Morgan & Mikhail's Clinical Anesthesiology* (5th ed.). New York, NY: McGraw-Hill.

    Nagelhout, J.J., & Plaus, K.L. (2014). Ch 16 *Nurse Anesthesia* (5th ed.). St. Louis, MO: Elsevier.

87. You plan a standard induction for an 80-kg patient scheduled for cholecystectomy. What induction dose of cisatracurium will you use?

    (A) 16 mg
    (B) 8 mg
    (C) 1.6 mg
    (D) 0.8 mg

    Rationale: The intubating dose of cisatracurium is 0.2 mg/kg.

TABLE 1-7. Clinical characteristics of nondepolarizing muscle relaxants.

Drug	ED$_{95}$ for Adductor Pollicis During Nitrous Oxide/Oxygen/ Intravenous Anesthesia (mg/kg)	Intubation Dose (mg/kg)	Onset of Action for Intubating Dose (min)	Duration of Intubating Dose (min)	Maintenance Dosing by Boluses (mg/kg)	Maintenance Dosing by Infusion (μg/kg/min)
Succinylcholine	0.5	1.0	0.5	5–10	0.15	2–15 mg/min
Gantacurium[1]	0.19	0.2	1–2	4–10	N/A	—
Rocuronium	0.3	0.8	1.5	35–75	0.15	9–12
Mivacurium[2]	0.08	0.2	2.5–3.0	15–20	0.05	4–15
Atracurium	0.2	0.5	2.5–3.0	30–5	0.1	5–12
Cisatracurium	0.05	0.2	2.0–3.0	40–75	0.02	1–2
Vecuronium	0.05	0.12	2.0–3.0	45–90	0.01	1–2
Pancuronium	0.07	0.12	2.0–3.0	60–120	0.01	—
Pipecuronium[2]	0.05	0.1	2.0–3.0	80–120	0.01	—
Doxacurium[2]	0.025	0.07	4.0–5.0	90–150	0.05	—

[1]Not commercially available in the United States.
[2]No longer available in the United States.

Ref: Butterworth, J.F., Mackey, D.C., & Wasnick J.D. (2013). Ch 11 *Morgan & Mikhail's Clinical Anesthesiology* (5th ed.). New York, NY: McGraw-Hill.

88. Following topical administration of a local anesthetic you note erythema, skin blanching, and edema. Which local anesthetic did you apply?

    (A) Chloroprocaine
    (B) Tetracaine
    (C) Ropivacaine
    (D) EMLA

Rationale: Chloroprocaine and ropivacaine are not administered topically. Tetracaine is topically administered to the eye.
Ref: Butterworth, J.F., Mackey, D.C., & Wasnick J.D. (2013). Ch 16 *Morgan & Mikhail's Clinical Anesthesiology* (5th ed.). New York, NY: McGraw-Hill.

89. Which rate of systemic absorption of local anesthetics is true?

    (A) Intravenous > tracheal > intercostal > paracervical > epidural > brachial plexus > sciatic > subcutaneous
    (B) Tracheal > intercostal > intravenous > paracervical > epidural > brachial plexus > sciatic > subcutaneous
    (C) Intravenous < tracheal < intercostal < paracervical < epidural < brachial plexus < sciatic < subcutaneous
    (D) Tracheal < intercostal < intravenous < paracervical < epidural < brachial plexus < sciatic < subcutaneous

Rationale: One factor that determines systemic absorption of local anesthetics is the site of the injection. The intravenous route has the greatest absorption of local anesthetic.
Ref: Butterworth, J.F., Mackey, D.C., & Wasnick, J.D. (2013). Ch 16 *Morgan & Mikhail's Clinical Anesthesiology* (5th ed.). New York, NY: McGraw-Hill.

90. What do you expect when adding epinephrine to local anesthetic?

    (A) Vasodilation at the site of injection
    (B) Increased absorption
    (C) Decreased duration of action
    (D) Vasoconstriction at the site of injection

Rationale: Adding epinephrine to local anesthetic solutions causes vasoconstriction at the site of injection. There is less absorption of the local anesthetic. An increased duration of action results.
Ref: Butterworth, J.F., Mackey, D.C., & Wasnick, J.D. (2013). Ch 16 *Morgan & Mikhail's Clinical Anesthesiology* (5th ed.). New York, NY: McGraw-Hill.

91. During surgery for a bowel obstruction, you note persistent tachycardia and hypertension. What neuromuscular blocker was most likely used?

    (A) Rocuronium
    (B) Cisatracurium
    (C) Atracurium
    (D) Pancuronium

Rationale: Vagal blockade and sympathetic stimulation result in tachycardia and hypertension when using pancuronium. No significant cardiac effects are associated with cisatracurium, atracurium, and rocuronium.

Ref: Butterworth, J.F., Mackey, D.C., & Wasnick J.D. (2013). Ch 11 *Morgan & Mikhail's Clinical Anesthesiology* (5th ed.). New York, NY: McGraw-Hill.

92. Which factor is a relative contraindication to pulmonary artery (PA) catheterization?

    (A) Left bundle branch block
    (B) Right bundle branch block
    (C) A patient in septic shock
    (D) A patient undergoing thoracic aortic aneurysm repair

    Rationale: Left bundle branch block is a relative contraindication to PA catheterization because of the concern for complete heart block. C and D are cases where PA catheterization should be strongly considered in order to measure cardiac index, preload, volume status, and mixed venous blood oxygenation.

    Ref: Butterworth, J.F., Mackey, D.C., & Wasnick, J.D. (2013). Ch 5 *Morgan & Mikhail's Clinical Anesthesiology* (5th ed.). New York, NY: McGraw-Hill.
    Barash, P.G., Cullen, B.F., Stoelting, R.K., Calahan, M.K., & Stock, M.C. (2009). Ch 16 *Clinical Anesthesia* (6th ed.). Philadelphia, PA: Lippincott Williams & Wilkins.

93. Which statement about the central venous waveform *a* wave is correct?

    (A) It is produced by the passive filling of the right atrium.
    (B) It is produced by right atrial contraction.
    (C) It is produced by the closure of the tricuspid valve.
    (D) It is produced by the venous return against a closed tricuspid valve.

    Rationale: The *a* wave is produced by atrial contraction.

    Ref: Butterworth, J.F., Mackey, D.C., & Wasnick, J.D. (2013). Ch 5 *Morgan & Mikhail's Clinical Anesthesiology* (5th ed.). New York, NY: McGraw-Hill.
    Nagelhout, J.J., & Plaus, K.L. (2014). Ch 16 *Nurse Anesthesia* (5th ed.). St. Louis, MO: Elsevier.

94. Which statement is false regarding nitric oxide (NO)?

    (A) NO regulates pulmonary vascular resistance.
    (B) NO inhibits platelet activation.
    (C) NO regulates systemic vascular resistance.
    (D) NO is an exogenous neurotransmitter.

Rationale: Nitric oxide (NO), an endogenous neurotransmitter, affects multiple body systems. NO regulates pulmonary and systemic vascular resistance. NO inhibits platelet aggregation. Multiple actions including immune function and nervous system effects are notable.

Ref: Butterworth, J.F., Mackey, D.C., & Wasnick, J.D. (2013). Ch 15 *Morgan & Mikhail's Clinical Anesthesiology* (5th ed.). New York, NY: McGraw-Hill.

95. The patient is taking gabapentin. In which patient would you decrease the dose?

    (A) Hepatic compromised patients
    (B) Cardiac compromised patients
    (C) Renal compromised patients
    (D) Respiratory compromised patients

    Rationale: Gabapentin is excreted unchanged in the kidneys. Dose requirements are lower for patients with renal disease. Gabapentin is not metabolized in the liver nor bound to plasma proteins.

    Ref: Nagelhout, J.J., & Plaus, K.L (2014). Ch 51 *Nurse Anesthesia* (5th ed.). Philadelphia, PA: Elsevier.

96. Which statement about monitoring the CVP waveform in a patient with atrial fibrillation is correct?

    (A) There are large *v* waves.
    (B) The *v* waves are absent.
    (C) There are giant "cannon" *a* waves.
    (D) The *a* waves are absent.

    Rationale: The *a* waves are absent in a patient with atrial fibrillation. Commonly, only the *v* waves are present.

    Ref: Butterworth, J.F., Mackey, D.C., & Wasnick, J.D. (2013). Ch 5 *Morgan & Mikhail's Clinical Anesthesiology* (5th ed.). New York, NY: McGraw-Hill.
    Nagelhout, J.J., & Plaus, K.L. (2014). Ch 16 *Nurse Anesthesia* (5th ed.). St. Louis, MO: Elsevier.

97. Which pathologic state will not cause giant "cannon" *a* waves on the CVP waveform?

    (A) Tricuspid stenosis
    (B) Tricuspid regurgitation
    (C) Mitral stenosis
    (D) Ventricular hypertrophy

    Rationale: All conditions will cause cannon *a* waves except tricuspid regurgitation, which will cause large *v* waves.

Ref: Butterworth, J.F., Mackey, D.C., & Wasnick, J.D. (2013). Ch 5 *Morgan & Mikhail's Clinical Anesthesiology* (5th ed.). New York, NY: Lange Medical Books McGraw-Hill.

Nagelhout, J.J., & Plaus, K.L. (2014). Ch 16 *Nurse Anesthesia* (5th ed.). St. Louis, MO: Elsevier.

98. The patient received streptokinase. When is surgery permitted?

(A) 3 days following administration

(B) 5 days following administration

(C) 7 days following administration

(D) 10 days following administration

Rationale: Patients receiving thrombolytic therapy should not be scheduled for surgery within 10 days of administration.

Ref: Miller, R.D., & Pardo, M.C. (2011). Ch 22 *Basics of Anesthesia* (6th ed.). Philadelphia, PA: Elsevier Saunders.

99. Where does acetazolamide exert its action?

(A) Proximal convoluted tubule

(B) Ascending loop of Henle

(C) Distal convoluted tubule

(D) Collecting ducts

Rationale: Carbonic anhydrase inhibitors including acetazolamide exert their action in the proximal convoluted tubule. Loop diuretics act in the ascending Loop of Henle; thiazide diuretics at the distal convoluted tubules and potassium sparing diuretics at the collecting ducts.

Ref: Butterworth, J.F., Mackey, D.C., & Wasnick, J.D. (2013). Ch 46 *Morgan & Mikhail's Clinical Anesthesiology* (5th ed.). New York, NY: McGraw-Hill.

Hemmings, H., & Egan, T. (2013). Ch 34 *Pharmacology and Physiology for Anesthesia: Foundations and Clinical Application.* Philadelphia, PA: Elsevier.

100. Which hemodynamic profile is consistent with pulmonary embolism?

	CVP	PCWP
(A)	High	High
(B)	High	Normal
(C)	High	Low
(D)	Normal	High

Rationale: A patient with pulmonary embolism will demonstrate an elevated central venous pressure and a normal pulmonary capillary wedge pressure.

Ref: Butterworth, J.F., Mackey, D.C., & Wasnick, J.D. (2013). Ch 24 *Morgan & Mikhail's Clinical Anesthesiology* (5th ed.). New York, NY: McGraw-Hill.

Nagelhout, J.J., & Plaus, K.L. (2014). Ch 16 *Nurse Anesthesia* (5th ed.). St. Louis, MO: Elsevier.

101. Which antibiotic would you avoid in patients with myasthenia gravis?

(A) Chloramphenicol

(B) Amphotericin B

(C) Ciprofloxacin

(D) Gentamicin

Rationale: Aminoglycosides that includes gentamicin result in skeletal muscle weakness.

Skeletal muscle weakness due to myasthenia gravis is aggravated by the aminoglycosides as compared to other antibiotic groups. Nondepolarizing neuromuscular blockers effects are prolonged.

Ref: Stoelting, R.K., & Hillier, SC. (2006). Ch 28 *Pharmacology and Physiology in Anesthetic Practice* (4th ed.). Philadelphia, PA: Saunders.

102. Which chemotherapeutic agent is strongly associated with pulmonary fibrosis?

(A) 5-FU

(B) Cyclophosphamide

(C) Doxorubicin

(D) Bleomycin

Rationale: Bleomycin is strongly associated with pulmonary fibrosis, pulmonary hypertension, and pulmonary toxicity. 5-FU is commonly associated with cerebellar ataxia, cardiac toxicity, gastritis, and myelosuppression. Cyclophosphamide side effects include encephalopathy, hemorrhagic cystitis, myelosuppression, cardiac symptoms, and pulmonary fibrosis. Doxorubicin is strongly associated with cardiotoxicity.

Ref: Hines, R.L., & Marschall, K.E. (2012). Ch 23 *Stoelting's Anesthesia and Co-Exiting Disease* (6th ed.). Philadelphia, PA: Saunders.

103. Which hemodynamic profile reflects chronic left ventricular failure?

	CVP	PCWP
(A)	High	High
(B)	High	Normal
(C)	High	Low
(D)	Normal	High

Rationale: A patient with chronic left ventricular failure will demonstrate an elevated central venous pressure (CVP) and an elevated pulmonary capillary wedge pressure (PCWP). In acute left ventricular failure, the CVP will be normal and the PCWP will be elevated.
Ref: Butterworth, J.F., Mackey, D.C., & Wasnick, J.D. (2013). Ch 5 *Morgan & Mikhail's Clinical Anesthesiology* (5th ed.). New York, NY: McGraw-Hill.
Nagelhout, J.J., & Plaus, K.L. (2014). Ch 16 *Nurse Anesthesia* (5th ed.). St. Louis, MO: Elsevier.

104. In which west zone must the tip of the pulmonary artery catheter lie in order for the pulmonary artery wedge pressure (PAWP) measurement to be accurate?

    (A) 1
    (B) II
    (C) III
    (D) IV

    Rationale: The goal for placement of a PA catheter is west zone III because the bulk of pulmonary blood flow lies within this lung region. Zone III allows for direct physiologic communication between the right heart and pulmonary pressures with the left heart pressures.
    Ref: Nagelhout, J.J., & Plaus, K.L. (2014). Ch 16 *Nurse Anesthesia* (5th ed.). St. Louis, MO: Elsevier.
    Miller, R., Fleisher, L., Wiener-Krunish, J., Young, W., & Eriksson, L. Ch 40 *Miller's Anesthesia* (7th ed.). St. Louis, MO: Elsevier.

105. How do codeine and morphine differ?

    (A) Codeine undergoes O-demethylation.
    (B) Codeine is less antitussive than morphine.
    (C) Codeine undergoes 2 glucuronide conjugation.
    (D) Codeine's equipotent dose is 1.5 mg.

    Rationale: Codeine is an effective antitussive, but is less potent than morphine. Morphine undergoes 2 glucuronide conjugation resulting in morphine-6-glucuronide. Codeine's equipotent dose to morphine is 75 mg.
    Ref: Nagelhout, J.J., & Plaus, K.L. (2014). Ch 5 *Nurse Anesthesia* (5th ed.). St. Louis, MO: Elsevier.
    Brunton, L.L., Chabner, B.A., & Knollmann, B.C. (Eds) (2010). Ch 18 *Goodman & Gilman's The Pharmacological Basis of Therapeutics* (12th ed.). New York, NY: McGraw-Hill.

106. What is the characteristic pulmonary artery catheter (PAC) pressure waveform that tells you the catheter has entered the pulmonary artery?

    (A) A sharp, upstroke/down stroke waveform with the highest point reaching the 10 mmHg point.
    (B) A brisk upstroke followed by a steep down stroke returning to mean central venous pressure levels.
    (C) A brisk upstroke followed by a notched, sloping down stroke with acute rise in diastolic pressure.
    (D) An undulating waveform that occurs near the 10 mmHg point.

    Rationale: The acute rise in diastolic pressure is characteristic of PAP waveform compared to the lower diastolic pressure reading of the right ventricle. *A* describes the RA waveform; *B* describes the RV and *D* describes the PAOP.
    Ref: Butterworth, J.F., Mackey, D.C., & Wasnick, J.D. (2013). Ch 5 *Morgan & Mikhail's Clinical Anesthesiology* (5th ed.). New York, NY: McGraw-Hill.
    Nagelhout, J.J., & Plaus, K.L. (2014). Ch 16 *Nurse Anesthesia* (5th ed.). St. Louis, MO: Elsevier.

107. Which statement about correlation of the CVP waveform and the EKG waveform is incorrect?

    (A) The *a* wave follows the P wave on the ECG.
    (B) The *c* wave immediately follows the start of the QRS complex on ECG.
    (C) The *v* wave appears shortly after the start of the T wave on the ECG.
    (D) The *y* descent occurs during the QRS complex on the ECG.

    Rationale: All are correct except D. The *y* descent of the CVP waveform corresponds to the opening of the tricuspid valve during diastole and therefore is observed immediately following the *v* wave on CVP and shortly after the T wave on the ECG.
    Ref: Butterworth, J.F., Mackey, D.C., & Wasnick, J.D. (2013). Ch 5 *Morgan & Mikhail's Clinical Anesthesiology* (5th ed.). New York, NY: McGraw-Hill.
    Nagelhout, J.J., & Plaus, K.L. (2014). Ch 16 *Nurse Anesthesia* (5th ed.). St. Louis, MO: Elsevier.

108. During induction of anesthesia you note the inability to ventilate the patient. The chest wall appears rigid. Which medication did you administer?

    (A) Sufentanil
    (B) Versed

(C) Etomidate

(D) Methohexital

Rationale: The fentanyl family is known to produce chest wall rigidity (Fentanyl, sufenta, alfenta, and remifentanil). All narcotics may produce chest wall rigidity in high doses.

Ref: Butterworth, J.F., Mackey, D.C., & Wasnick, J.D. (2013). Ch 10 *Morgan & Mikhail's Clinical Anesthesiology* (5th ed.). New York, NY: McGraw-Hill.

109. Which of the following is inhibited by opioids?

(A) Coupling to G proteins

(B) Binding to agonists

(C) Voltage gated sodium channels

(D) Activation of adenylyl cyclase

Rationale: The mechanisms of action of opioids include coupling to G proteins, binding to agonists and inhibition of adenylyl cyclase. Inhibition of calcium, not sodium channels is inhibited by opioids.

Ref: Butterworth, J.F., Mackey, D.C., & Wasnick, J.D. (2013). Ch 10 *Morgan & Mikhail's Clinical Anesthesiology* (5th ed.). New York, NY: McGraw-Hill.

110. How do COX-1 and COX-2 enzymes differ?

(A) COX 1 responds to inflammation.

(B) COX-1 inhibition increases thrombosis.

(C) COX-2 inhibition increases heart attack risk.

(D) COX-1 sites attract large molecules.

Rationale: Large molecules are preferential to COX-2 receptors. COX-2 inhibition may result in thrombosis, stroke, and myocardial infarction. COX-1 inhibition decreases thrombosis. Inflammatory response prompts production of COX-2.

Ref: Butterworth, J.F., Mackey, D.C., & Wasnick, J.D. (2013). Ch 10 *Morgan & Mikhail's Clinical Anesthesiology* (5th ed.). New York, NY: McGraw-Hill.

111. If amiodarone is not available, what antiarrhythmic will you use to treat unsuccessful defibrillation?

(A) Lidocaine

(B) Diltiazem

(C) Dobutamine

(D) Magnesium

Rationale: Lidocaine is used as a second-line therapy for PVCs and V-Tach that is unresponsive to defibrillation. Diltiazem improves atrial fibrillation or flutter. Dobutamine is indicated for the treatment of

systolic heart failure while magnesium is given for Torsades de pointes with prolonged QT interval.

Ref: Butterworth, J.F., Mackey, D.C., & Wasnick, J.D. (2013). Ch 55 *Morgan & Mikhail's Clinical Anesthesiology* (5th ed.). New York, NY: McGraw-Hill.

112. What is the mechanism of action of aspirin?

(A) Irreversible inhibition of COX-2

(B) Low binding to plasma proteins

(C) Plasma esterase hydrolysis

(D) Irreversible inhibition of COX-1

Rationale: Aspirin prevents thrombosis and is useful in treatment for myocardial infarction by irreversibly inhibiting COX-1. COX inhibitors are highly bound to plasma proteins and undergo hepatic biotransformation.

Ref: Butterworth, J.F., Mackey, D.C., & Wasnick, J.D. (2013). Ch 10 *Morgan & Mikhail's Clinical Anesthesiology* (5th ed.). New York, NY: McGraw-Hill.

113. Which central line site has the shortest distance to the junction of the vena cava and the right atrium?

(A) Left internal jugular

(B) Right internal jugular

(C) Subclavian vein

(D) Right median basilic vein

Rationale: The subclavian vein provides the shortest distance to the junction of the vena cava and the right atrium (approximately 10 cm) compared to other anatomic sites such as the internal jugular veins (15–20 cm); the femoral vein (40 cm); and the right basilica vein (40 cm).

Ref: Butterworth, J.F., Mackey, D.C., & Wasnick, J.D. (2013). Ch 5 *Morgan & Mikhail's Clinical Anesthesiology* (5th ed.). New York, NY: McGraw-Hill.

Nagelhout, J.J., & Plaus, K.L. (2014). Ch 16 *Nurse Anesthesia* (5th ed.). St. Louis, MO: Elsevier.

114. What is the hallmark sign of a catheter-induced pulmonary artery rupture?

(A) Hypotension

(B) Hypoxemia

(C) Hemoptysis

(D) Arrhythmias

Rationale: Hemoptysis is a common sign of PA rupture. Hypotension/hypoxemia would occur as a result of PA hemorrhage but it is nonspecific to PA rupture. Arrhythmias are unrelated to the PA rupture.

Ref: Butterworth, J.F., Mackey, D.C., & Wasnick, J.D. (2013). Ch 5 *Morgan & Mikhail's Clinical Anesthesiology* (5th ed.). New York, NY: McGraw-Hill.

Miller, R., Fleisher, L., Wiener-Krunish, J., Young, W., & Eriksson, L. Ch 40 *Miller's Anesthesia* (7th ed.). St. Louis, MO: Elsevier.

115. Which law of physics explains why an increase in left ventricular wall thickness will reduce ventricular wall tension?

(A) La Place's Law
(B) Ohm's Law
(C) Poiseuille's Law
(D) Fick's Law

Rationale: LaPlace's Law states that circumferential stress equals intraventricular pressure times ventricular radius divided by two times the thickness of the ventricular wall. Therefore, the larger the ventricular wall radius, the greater the wall tension. And conversely, an increase in ventricular wall thickness will reduce ventricular wall tension.

Ref: Butterworth, J.F., Mackey, D.C., & Wasnick, J.D. (2013). Ch 20 *Morgan & Mikhail's Clinical Anesthesiology* (5th ed.). New York, NY: McGraw-Hill.

Nagelhout, J.J., & Plaus, K.L. (2014). Ch 23 *Nurse Anesthesia* (5th ed.). St. Louis, MO: Elsevier.

116. Which cardiovascular reflex does not result in an efferent vagal response?

(A) Baroreceptor reflex
(B) Bainbridge reflex
(C) Valsalva maneuver
(D) Oculocardiac reflex

Rationale: Each reflex results in an efferent vagal response and subsequent decreased heart rate except the Bainbridge reflex (also known as the atrial stretch reflex). This reflex is caused by an increased venous return due to hypervolemia causing a stimulation of atrial stretch receptors. The stimulation of atrial stretch receptors results in an increased heart rate.

Ref: Butterworth, J.F., Mackey, D.C., & Wasnick, J.D. (2013). Ch 20 *Morgan & Mikhail's Clinical Anesthesiology* (5th ed.). New York, NY: McGraw-Hill.

Nagelhout, J.J., & Plaus, K.L. (2014). Ch 23 *Nurse Anesthesia* (5th ed.). St. Louis, MO: Elsevier.

117. Which herbal remedy does not delay awakening from anesthesia?

(A) Valerian
(B) Kava kava
(C) St. John's wort
(D) Garlic

Rationale: Valerian, Kava kava, and St. John's Wort interact with anesthetic drugs including benzodiazepines. The interaction may result in delayed emergence from anesthesia. Garlic potentiates the action of warfarin that may result in bleeding.

Ref: Nagelhout, J.J., & Plaus, K.L. (2014). Ch 19 *Nurse Anesthesia* (4th ed.). Philadelphia, PA: Elsevier.

Stoelting, R.K., & Hillier, S.C. (2006). Ch 34 *Pharmacology and Physiology in Anesthetic Practice* (5th ed.). Philadelphia, PA: Elsevier.

118. While floating a pulmonary artery catheter via the right internal jugular, the patient monitor shows a run of ventricular tachycardia. Which insertion depth is most likely to induce this arrhythmia?

(A) 15 cm
(B) 22 cm
(C) 28 cm
(D) 45 cm

Rationale: A PA catheter inserted through the right internal jugular vein will reach the right ventricle somewhere between 25 to 35 cm, depending on the size of the patient. Transient ectopy from irritation of the right ventricle by the balloon and catheter tip is common.

Ref: Butterworth, J.F., Mackey, D.C., & Wasnick, J.D. (2013). Ch 5 *Morgan & Mikhail's Clinical Anesthesiology* (5th ed.). New York, NY: McGraw-Hill.

Nagelhout, J.J., & Plaus, K.L. (2014). Ch 16 *Nurse Anesthesia* (5th ed.). St. Louis, MO: Elsevier.

119. At what dose is the onset of action of rocuronium similar to that of succinylcholine for rapid sequence intubation?

(A) 0.9-1.2 mg/kg
(B) 1.5-2.0 mg/kg
(C) 2.0-2.5 mg/kg
(D) >2.5 mg/kg

Rationale: The standard intubating dose of rocuronium is 0.8 mg/kg. Larger intubating doses (0.9-1.2 mg/kg) facilitates the onset of action to that approximating succinylcholine (0.5 min). The normal onset of action of rocuronium is 1.5 minutes. The larger dose of rocuronium makes it a viable choice for rapid sequence induction.

Ref: Butterworth, J.F., Mackey, D.C., & Wasnick, J.D. (2013). Ch 11 *Morgan & Mikhail's Clinical Anesthesiology* (5th ed.). New York, NY: McGraw-Hill.

120. What is the primary neurotransmitter of the parasympathetic nervous system?

(A) Norepinephrine

(B) Acetylcholine

(C) Acetylcoenzyme A

(D) Muscarine

Rationale: Parasympathetic nervous system (cholinergic) effects are due to acetylcholine. Adrenergic effects are due to the transmitter norepinephrine. Acetylcoenzyme A is significant in the synthesis and hydrolysis of acetylcholine. Muscarinic receptors represent one of two major divisions of the cholinergic receptors.

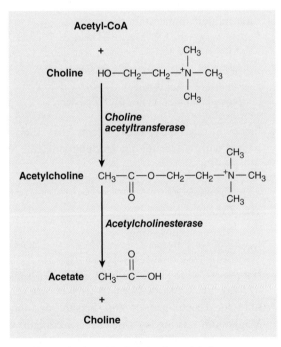

FIG. 1-3. The synthesis and hydrolysis of acetylcholine.

Ref: Butterworth, J.F., Mackey, D.C., & Wasnick J.D. (2013). Ch 12 *Morgan & Mikhail's Clinical Anesthesiology* (5th ed.). New York, NY: McGraw-Hill.

121. Which is correct about the CVP waveform in a patient with tricuspid regurgitation?

(A) Decreasing CVP pressure implies worsening right ventricular dysfunction.

(B) The *x* descent is usually absent.

(C) Giant, "cannon" *a*-waves are apparent.

(D) The *v*-waves become diminished.

Rationale: In the setting of tricuspid regurgitation, central venous pressure will increase, indicating a worsening right ventricular dysfunction. The *x* descent is absent and prominent *v* waves are usually present on the waveform.

Ref: Butterworth, J.F., Mackey, D.C., & Wasnick, J.D. (2013). Ch 21 *Morgan & Mikhail's Clinical Anesthesiology* (5th ed.). New York, NY: McGraw-Hill.

Nagelhout, J.J., & Plaus, K.L. (2014). Ch 23 *Nurse Anesthesia* (5th ed.). St. Louis, MO: Elsevier.

122. Which sympathomimetic amine structurally related to amphetamine may cause cardiac arrhythmias, myocardial infarction, and stroke?

(A) Echinacea

(B) Ma huang

(C) Ginkgo biloba

(D) Ginseng

Rationale: Ma Huang (ephedra) is a popular herbal formula. Ephedrine is the active form of ephedra responsible for the sympathomimetic effects. Ginseng may cause tachycardia and hypertension especially if combined with other stimulants. Side effects of ginkgo biloba include gastrointestinal discomfort, headache, dizziness, bleeding, and seizures. Use of echinacea may result in hypersensitivity reactions.

Ref: Nagelhout, J.J., and Plaus, K.L. (2014). Ch 19 *Nurse Anesthesia*, 5th Ed. Philadelphia, PA: Elsevier.

Stoelting, R.K. & Hillier, S.C. (2006). Ch 34 *Pharmacology and Physiology in Anesthetic Practice*, 4th Ed. Philadelphia, PA: Elsevier.

123. How does hydromorphone differ from morphine?

(A) Hydromorphone is more potent.

(B) Hydromorphone has a shorter duration of action.

(C) Hydormorphone is less potent.

(D) Hydromorphone is less lipid-soluble.

Rationale: Hydromorphone is 4 to 5 times more potent than morphine. Both drugs are lipid-soluble, but morphine is less lipid-soluble than hydromorphone. The duration of action of hydromorphone is the same as morphine.

Ref: Nagelhout, J.J. & Plaus, K.L. (2014). Ch 11 *Nurse Anesthesia* (5th ed.). St. Louis, MO: Elsevier.

Brunton, L.L., Chabner, B.A., & Knollmann, B.C. (Eds) (2010). Ch 18 *Goodman & Gilman's The Pharmacological Basis of Therapeutics* (12th ed.). New York, NY: McGraw-Hill.

124. What should be used to reconstitute a standard vial of dantrolene?

    (A) 60 mL normal saline
    (B) 100 mL normal saline
    (C) 60 mL sterile water
    (D) 100 mL sterile water

    Rationale: Each vial of dantrolene is reconstituted using 60 mL of sterile water.
    Ref: Butterworth, J.F., Mackey, D.C., & Wasnick, J.D. (2013). Ch 52 *Morgan & Mikhail's Clinical Anesthesiology* (5th ed.). New York, NY: McGraw-Hill.
    Hines, R.L., & Marschall, K.E. (Eds.) (2012). Ch 27 *Stoelting's Anesthesia and Co-Existing Disease* (6th ed.). Philadelphia, PA: Elsevier.

125. Preoperatively, you learn that the patient is taking warfarin. Which herbal remedy poses the potential for bleeding?

    (A) Ginkgo biloba
    (B) Evening primrose
    (C) Kola nut
    (D) Goldenseal

    Rationale: Ginkgo biloba is linked to bleeding and hemorrhage due to antiplatelet activity. Use of evening primrose may lead to nausea and vomiting. Kola nut interacts with stimulants and may result in irritability and insomnia. There are no known drug interactions with goldenseal, but the herbal remedy is known to cause hypertension and edema.
    Ref: Nagelhout, J.J., & Plaus, K.L. (2014). Ch 19 *Nurse Anesthesia* (5th ed.). Philadelphia, PA: Elsevier.
    Stoelting, R.K. & Hillier, SC. (2006). Ch 34 *Pharmacology and Physiology in Anesthetic Practice* (4th ed.). Philadelphia, PA: Elsevier.

126. Which antibiotic should not be administered during pregnancy?

    (A) Penicillin
    (B) Aminoglycosides
    (C) Tetracycline
    (D) Erythromycin

    Rationale: Each of the antibiotics is safe to administer during pregnancy except tetracycline. Tetracycline

is absorbed in teeth and bones resulting in brown, discolored teeth.
    Ref: Stoelting, R.K., & Hillier, S.C. (2006). Ch 28 *Pharmacology and Physiology in Anesthetic Practice* (4th ed.). Philadelphia, PA: Elsevier.

127. How is emphysema characterized?

    (A) Narrowing of small airways by inflammation and mucus.
    (B) Destruction of parenchyma that leads to loss of surface area, elastic recoil, and structural support to maintain the airway.
    (C) Antigen binding to immunoglobulin E on the surface of mast cells causes degranulation.
    (D) Reversible enlargement of the airways distal to terminal bronchioles with damage of the alveolar septa.

    Rationale: Emphysema is an obstructive disorder characterized by destruction of parenchyma that leads to loss of surface area, elastic recoil, and structural support to maintain the airway
    Ref: Butterworth, J.F., Mackey, D.C., & Wasnick, J.D. (2013). Ch 24 *Morgan & Mikhail's Clinical Anesthesiology* (5th ed.). New York, NY: McGraw-Hill.
    Nagelhout, J.J., & Plaus, K.L. (2014). Ch 26 *Nurse Anesthesia* (5th ed.). St. Louis, MO: Elsevier.

128. Preoperatively, the patient shares that they were treated with vincristine for Hodgkin's disease. What side effect would you expect?

    (A) Paresthesias
    (B) Coagulopathy
    (C) Magnesium wasting
    (D) Arthralgias

    Rationale: Peripheral neuropathy and paresthesias are strongly linked to vincristine. Asparaginase is responsible for coagulopathies and hepatic dysfunction. Magnesium wasting is a side effect of cisplatin while arthralgias are prominent for patients taking palitaxel.
    Ref: Hines, R.L., & Marschall, K.E. (Eds.) (2012). Ch 23 *Stoelting's Anesthesia and Co-Exiting Disease*, (6th ed.). Philadelphia, PA: Elsevier.

129. A 70-kg adult patient with mitral valve prolapse is scheduled for an exploratory laparotomy. If the patient has history of anaphylaxis to penicillin, what antibiotic prophylaxis will you administer?

    (A) Cefazolin 1 gram IV
    (B) Clindamycin 600 mg IV

(C) Ampicillin 2 grams IV

(D) Amoxicillin 2 grams IV

Rationale: Antibiotic prophylaxis is recommended for patients with mitral valve prolapse because of the potential for endocarditis. A penicillin-allergic adult patient can safely receive clindamycin 600 mg IV. The other options are contraindicated for the patient allergic to penicillin, including cephalosporins if the patient has a history of anaphylaxis, angioedema or urticaria.

Ref: Butterworth, J.F., Mackey, D.C., & Wasnick, J.D. (2013). Ch 21 *Morgan & Mikhail's Clinical Anesthesiology* (5th ed.). New York, NY: McGraw-Hill.

Nagelhout, J.J., & Plaus, K.L. (2014). Ch 23 *Nurse Anesthesia* (5th ed.). St. Louis, MO: Elsevier.

130. A 70-year-old female is undergoing a large bowel resection when the following hemodynamic profile is obtained: BP 100/80, cardiac output 6 L/min, and central venous pressure 3 mmHg. What is the systemic vascular resistance?

(A) 504 dynes/sec/cm^5

(B) 1,120 dynes/sec/cm^5

(C) 1,160 dynes/sec/cm^5

(D) 2,200 dynes/sec/cm^5

Rationale: The formula for calculating SVR is: SVR = [MAP − CVP] × 80 CO. In this question, the MAP can be calculated first by plugging into the formula:

$$MAP = SBP + 2DBP/3$$

The MAP is 87 mmHg. Next plug the numbers into the SVR formula to derive the SVR. SVR = [87 − 3] × 80/6 The final answer is 1,120 dynes/sec/cm^5

Ref: Butterworth, J.F., Mackey, D.C., & Wasnick, J.D. (2013). Ch 20 *Morgan & Mikhail's Clinical Anesthesiology* (5th ed.). New York, NY: McGraw-Hill.

Nagelhout, J.J., & Plaus, K.L. (2014). Ch 24 *Nurse Anesthesia* (5th ed.). St. Louis, MO: Elsevier.

131. What has been firmly established as the primary environmental risk factor associated with emphysema and bronchitis?

(A) Homozygous α_1-antitrypsin

(B) Cigarette smoking

(C) Antigen binding to immunoglobulin E

(D) Drug toxicity with bleomycin and nitrofurantoin

Rationale: Cigarette smoking has been firmly established as the primary environmental risk factor associated with emphysema and bronchitis.

Ref: Butterworth, J.F., Mackey, D.C., & Wasnick, J.D. (2013). Ch 24 *Morgan & Mikhail's Clinical Anesthesiology* (5th ed.). New York, NY: McGraw-Hill.

Nagelhout, J.J., & Plaus, K.L. (2014). Ch 26 *Nurse Anesthesia* (5th ed.). St. Louis, MO: Elsevier.

132. What is the most significant precipitating factor leading to obstructive sleep apnea (OSA)?

(A) History of stroke

(B) History of type II diabetes

(C) Obesity

(D) Hypertension

Rationale: Obesity is the most significant precipitating factor leading to obstructive sleep apnea (OSA).

Ref: Butterworth, J.F., Mackey, D.C., & Wasnick, J.D. (2013). Ch 44 *Morgan & Mikhail's Clinical Anesthesiology* (5th ed.). New York, NY: McGraw-Hill.

Nagelhout, J.J., & Plaus, K.L. (2014). Ch 26 *Nurse Anesthesia* (5th ed.). St. Louis, MO: Elsevier.

133. By what mechanism do local anesthetics depress cardiac contractility?

(A) By increasing Ca^{2+} influx and release into the myocardial cell.

(B) By decreasing Ca^{2+} influx and release into the myocardial cell.

(C) By enhancing the intracellular levels of cAMP of the myocardial cell.

(D) By enhancing the intracellular levels of cGMP of the myocardial cell.

Rationale: Local anesthetics depress cardiac contractility by reducing Ca^{2+} influx and release into the myocardial cell in a dose-dependent fashion.

Ref: Butterworth, J.F., Mackey, D.C., & Wasnick, J.D. (2013). Ch 20 *Morgan & Mikhail's Clinical Anesthesiology* (5th ed.). New York, NY: McGraw-Hill.

Nagelhout, J.J., & Plaus, K.L. (2014). Ch 23 *Nurse Anesthesia* (5th ed.). St. Louis, MO: Elsevier.

134. Which local anesthetic agent depresses cardiac contractility the least?

(A) Bupivacaine

(B) Tetracaine

(C) Ropivacaine

(D) Lidocaine

Rationale: The more potent local anesthetics for nerve block such as bupivicaine, ropivacaine, and tetracaine depress left ventricular contractility more significantly than the less potent local anesthetics such as lidocaine and chlorprocaine.

Ref: Butterworth, J.F., Mackey, D.C., & Wasnick, J.D. (2013). Ch 20 *Morgan & Mikhail's Clinical Anesthesiology* (5th ed.). New York, NY: McGraw-Hill.

Nagelhout, J.J., & Plaus, K.L. (2014). Ch 10 *Nurse Anesthesia* (5th ed.). St. Louis, MO: Elsevier.

135. A patient is scheduled for a general anesthetic. You plan to induce with propofol. What is the best dose for a 70-kg male?

(A) 350 mg
(B) 100 mg
(C) 250 mg
(D) 200 mg

Rationale: The induction dose of propofol is 1 to 2.5 mg/kg. The dose range for the 70-kg patient is 70 to 175 mg.

Ref: Butterworth, J.F., Mackey, D.C., & Wasnick, J.D. (2013). Ch 9 *Morgan & Mikhail's Clinical Anesthesiology* (5th ed.). New York, NY: McGraw-Hill.

Miller, R.D., & Pardo, M.C. (2011). Ch 9 *Basics of Anesthesia* (6th ed.). Philadelphia, PA: Elsevier.

136. What clinical sign is not consistent with Cushing Syndrome?

(A) Hypoglycemia
(B) Hypertension
(C) Hyperglycemia
(D) Hypokalemia

Rationale: Clinical signs consistent with Cushing Syndrome include: hyperglycemia, hypertension, hypokalemic metabolic alkalosis, hirsutism, osteoporosis, muscle weakness, mental status disorders, buffalo hump, weight gain, moon face, menstrual changes, and increased likelihood of infection.

Ref: Butterworth, J.F., Mackey, D.C., & Wasnick, J.D. (2013). Ch 34 *Morgan & Mikhail's Clinical Anesthesiology* (5th ed.). New York, NY: McGraw-Hill.

Nagelhout, J.J., & Plaus, K.L. (2014). Ch 33 *Nurse Anesthesia* (5th ed.). St. Louis, MO: Elsevier.

137. What are the electrophysiologic effects of diltiazem on the myocardial cells?

(A) Binding to calcium channels in their resting active state

(B) Binding to T-type calcium channels
(C) Binding to L-type calcium channels
(D) Inhibiting potassium efflux during cardiac repolarization

Rationale: Calcium channel blockers such as diltiazem block Ca^{2+} influx through L-type, but not T-type channels in a dose-dependent fashion.

Ref: Butterworth, J.F., Mackey, D.C., & Wasnick, J.D. (2013). Ch 20 *Morgan & Mikhail's Clinical Anesthesiology* (5th ed.). New York, NY: McGraw-Hill.

Nagelhout, J.J., & Plaus, K.L. (2014). Ch 10 *Nurse Anesthesia* (5th ed.). St. Louis, MO: Elsevier.

138. Which is an appropriate initial intervention to correct intraoperative bronchospasm?

(A) Deepen the level of anesthesia with a volatile agent.
(B) Give 10 mg morphine IV.
(C) Administer intravenous corticosteroids.
(D) Give labetalol 10 mg IV.

Rationale: Morphine can release histamine which could cause bronchoconstriction and Labetalol can produce bronchoconstriction related to the B2 blocking effects. Administer intravenous corticosteroids will not have an immediate effect. The potent inhalation agents produce bronchial relaxation and have all been successfully used in asthmatic patients.

Ref: Butterworth, J.F., Mackey, D.C., & Wasnick, J.D. (2013). Ch 23 *Morgan & Mikhail's Clinical Anesthesiology* (5th ed.). New York, NY: McGraw-Hill.

Nagelhout, J.J., & Plaus, K.L. (2014). Ch 26 *Nurse Anesthesia* (5th ed.). St. Louis, MO: Elsevier.

139. What is the correct classification of asthma symptoms that limit daily activity and require daily use of a short acting beta agonist?

(A) Mild persistent asthma
(B) Severe persistent asthma
(C) Moderate persistent asthma
(D) Intermittent asthma

Rationale: In intermittent asthma symptoms occur 0 to 2 days a week, an inhaler is used 0 to 2 days a week and there is no activity limitation. Symptoms occur 2 to 6 days a week in mild persistent asthma. An inhaler is used 3 to 6 days a week and there is minor activity limitation. Severe persistent asthma is characterized by continuous signs and symptoms. An inhaler is used several times a day. There is extremely limited activity. With moderate persistent asthma there is some activity limitations with daily symptoms. An inhaler is typically used daily.

Ref: Nagelhout, J.J., & Plaus, K.L. (2014). Ch 26 *Nurse Anesthesia* (5th ed.). St. Louis, MO: Elsevier.

140. What are the two strongest predictors of postoperative pulmonary complications?

(A) Operative site and well controlled asthma

(B) Operative site and history of dyspnea

(C) Obesity and operative site

(D) History of dyspnea and abnormal chest exam

Rationale: Obesity and well controlled asthma show good evidence against being a risk factor. Abnormal chest exam is supported by fair evidence for postoperative pulmonary complications. The two strongest predictors of postoperative pulmonary complications are operative site and history of dyspnea which correlate with the degree of preexisting pulmonary disease.

Ref: Butterworth, J.F., Mackey, D.C., & Wasnick, J.D. (2013). Ch 24 *Morgan & Mikhail's Clinical Anesthesiology* (5th ed.). New York, NY: McGraw-Hill.

141. Which two interventions lessen air trapping in a COPD patient?

Select (2) two

(A) Increase respiratory rate

(B) Decrease respiratory rate

(C) Increase I:E ratio

(D) Decrease I:E ratio

Rationale: Decreasing respiratory rate and decreasing I:E ratio will give the COPD patient more time to exhale and lessen air trapping.

Ref: Butterworth, J.F., Mackey, D.C., & Wasnick, J.D. (2013). Ch 24 *Morgan & Mikhail's Clinical Anesthesiology* (5th ed.). New York, NY: McGraw-Hill.

Nagelhout, J.J., & Plaus, K.L. (2014). Ch 26 *Nurse Anesthesia* (5th ed.). St. Louis, MO: Elsevier.

142. What is the leading cause of cor pulmonale?

(A) Obesity

(B) Asthma

(C) Sleep apnea

(D) COPD

Rationale: COPD is the leading cause of cor pulmonale superseding sleep apnea, obesity and, asthma.

Ref: Nagelhout, J.J., & Plaus, K.L. (2014). Ch 26 *Nurse Anesthesia* (5th ed.). St. Louis, MO: Elsevier.

143. Which statement is false concerning anesthetic management of OSA patients?

(A) Patients who use CPAP at home should be encouraged to bring device from home for use in PACU.

(B) The anesthetist should anticipate a difficult intubation.

(C) Increased doses of benzodiazepines and opioids may be needed preoperatively.

(D) The anesthetist should anticipate a reduced FRC.

Rationale: Preoperatively, sedative medications should be used cautiously. As a result of central nervous system sensitization, patients may be hypersensitive to effects of benzodiazepines and opioids.

Ref: Butterworth, J.F., Mackey, D.C., & Wasnick, J.D. (2013). Ch 44 *Morgan & Mikhail's Clinical Anesthesiology* (5th ed.). New York, NY: McGraw-Hill.

Nagelhout, J.J., & Plaus, K.L. (2014). Ch 26 *Nurse Anesthesia* (5th ed.). St. Louis, MO: Elsevier.

144. What type of pulmonary disease demonstrates an FEV_1/FVC ratio that is normal with a reduction in vital capacity?

(A) Asthma

(B) COPD

(C) Emphysema

(D) Pulmonary fibrosis

Rationale: FEV_1/FVC ratio that is normal with a reduction in vital capacity is diagnostic of restrictive pulmonary disease.

Ref: Butterworth, J.F., Mackey, D.C., & Wasnick, J.D. (2013). Ch 24 *Morgan & Mikhail's Clinical Anesthesiology* (5th ed.). New York, NY: McGraw-Hill.

Nagelhout, J.J., & Plaus, K.L. (2014). Ch 26 *Nurse Anesthesia* (5th ed.). St. Louis, MO: Elsevier.

145. What diagnosis of a patient could be made with a pulmonary function test that revealed a FEV_1/FVC ratio that is 0.6 of predicted valve?

(A) Pulmonary fibrosis

(B) COPD

(C) Pulmonary edema

(D) Aspiration pneumonia

Rationale: FEV_1/FVC ratio that is that is less than or equal to 0.7 is diagnostic of COPD.

Ref: Butterworth, J.F., Mackey, D.C., & Wasnick, J.D. (2013). Ch 24 *Morgan & Mikhail's Clinical Anesthesiology* (5th ed.). New York, NY: McGraw-Hill.

Nagelhout, J.J., & Plaus, K.L. (2014). Ch 26 *Nurse Anesthesia* (5th ed.). St. Louis, MO: Elsevier.

146. What clinical feature of a pulmonary embolism is false?

    (A) Hypoxemia

    (B) Tachycardia

    (C) Decreased pulmonary vascular resistance

    (D) Hypocapnia

    Rationale: There would be an increase in pulmonary vascular resistance. A, B, and D are all clinical features of a pulmonary embolism.

    Ref: Butterworth, J.F., Mackey, D.C., & Wasnick, J.D. (2013). Ch 24 *Morgan & Mikhail's Clinical Anesthesiology* (5th ed.). New York, NY: McGraw-Hill.

    Nagelhout, J.J., & Plaus, K.L. (2014). Ch 26 *Nurse Anesthesia* (5th ed.). St. Louis, MO: Elsevier.

147. Which I:E ratio is most appropriate in a patient with severe restrictive disease?

    (A) I:E of 1:4

    (B) I:E of 1:2

    (C) I:E of 1:1

    (D) I:E of 1:3

    Rationale: An I:E ratio of 1:1 may help to maximize the inspiratory time per tidal volume and minimize the peak and plateau ventilator pressures in patients with severe restrictive disease.

    Ref: Butterworth, J.F., Mackey, D.C., & Wasnick, J.D. (2013). Ch 24 *Morgan & Mikhail's Clinical Anesthesiology* (5th ed.). New York, NY: McGraw-Hill.

    Nagelhout, J.J., & Plaus, K.L. (2014). Ch 26 *Nurse Anesthesia* (5th ed.). St. Louis, MO: Elsevier.

148. Deficiency in which protease inhibitor is linked to early-onset emphysema?

    (A) Beta-1 antitrypsin

    (B) Alpha-2 antitrypsin

    (C) Alpha-1 antitrypsin

    (D) Beta-2 antitrypsin

    Rationale: Alpha-1 antitrypsin is a protease inhibitor that prevents excessive activity of proteolytic enzymes in the lungs.

149. What is the hallmark sign of aspiration pneumonitis?

    (A) Hypertension

    (B) Pulmonary edema

    (C) Arterial hypoxemia

    (D) Tachycardia

    Rationale: A, B, and D are conditions associated with aspiration pneumonitis. However, arterial hypoxemia is the hallmark clinical feature of aspiration pneumonitis.

    Ref: Butterworth, J.F., Mackey, D.C., & Wasnick, J.D. (2013). Ch 24 *Morgan & Mikhail's Clinical Anesthesiology* (5th ed.). New York, NY: McGraw-Hill.

    Nagelhout, J.J., & Plaus, K.L. (2014). Ch 26 *Nurse Anesthesia* (5th ed.). St. Louis, MO: Elsevier.

150. Which statements regarding emphysema are true?

    (A) Emphysema is a restrictive lung disease

    (B) Elevated hematocrit

    (C) Copious sputum

    (D) Hyperinflation of the lungs on chest X-ray

    Rationale: Emphysema is an obstructive lung disease with a normal hematocrit, minimal sputum and demonstrates hyperinflation of the lungs on chest X-ray.

    Ref: Butterworth, J.F., Mackey, D.C., & Wasnick, J.D. (2013). Ch 24 *Morgan & Mikhail's Clinical Anesthesiology* (5th ed.). New York, NY: McGraw-Hill.

    Nagelhout, J.J., & Plaus, K.L. (2014). Ch 26 *Nurse Anesthesia* (5th ed.). St. Louis, MO: Elsevier.

151. Which mechanical ventilation modalities would be most appropriate for a patient with COPD?

    (A) Increasing respiratory rate and an I:E ratio of 1:1

    (B) Decreasing respiratory rate and an I:E ratio of 1:1

    (C) Increasing respiratory rate and an I:E ratio of 2:1

    (D) Decreasing respiratory rate and an I:E ratio of 1:3

    Rationale: Decreasing respiratory rate and an I:E ratio of 1:3 allows more time for exhalation.

    Ref: Butterworth, J.F., Mackey, D.C., & Wasnick, J.D. (2013). Ch 24 *Morgan & Mikhail's Clinical Anesthesiology* (5th ed.). New York, NY: McGraw-Hill.

    Nagelhout, J.J., & Plaus, K.L. (2014). Ch 26 *Nurse Anesthesia* (5th ed.). St. Louis, MO: Elsevier.

152. Which four criteria are consistent with the diagnosis of Adult Respiratory Distress Syndrome?

(A) Acute onset, PAO_2 to Fio_2 ratio <200 regardless of the level of peep applied, bilateral infiltrates on chest X-ray, and a PA wedge pressure less than or equal to 18 mmHg

(B) Acute onset, PAO_2 to Fio_2 ratio <200 regardless of the level of peep applied, normal chest X-ray, and a PA wedge pressure less than or equal to 18 mmHg

(C) Acute onset, PAO_2 to Fio_2 ratio <300 regardless of the level of peep applied, bilateral infiltrates on chest X-ray, and a PA wedge pressure less than or equal to 18 mmHg

(D) Slow onset, PAO_2 to Fio_2 ratio <200 regardless of the level of peep applied, bilateral infiltrates on chest X-ray, and a PA wedge pressure less than or equal to 18 mmHg

Rationale: Acute onset, PAO_2 to Fio_2 ratio <200 regardless of the level of peep applied, bilateral infiltrates on chest X-ray, and a PA wedge pressure less than or equal to 18 mmHg is consistent with the diagnosis of Adult Respiratory Distress Syndrome.
Ref: Nagelhout, J.J., & Plaus, K.L. (2014). Ch 26 *Nurse Anesthesia* (5th ed.). St. Louis, MO: Elsevier.

153. Which criteria are consistent with the diagnosis of pulmonary hypertension?

(A) A mean pulmonary artery pressure 14 mmHg with a with a pulmonary capillary occlusion pressure of no more than 15 mmHg

(B) A mean pulmonary artery pressure at least 25 mmHg with a with a pulmonary capillary occlusion pressure of no more than 15 mmHg

(C) A mean pulmonary artery pressure at least 10 mmHg with a with a pulmonary capillary occlusion pressure of no more than 15 mmHg

(D) A mean pulmonary artery pressure at least 12 mmHg with a with a pulmonary capillary occlusion pressure of no more than 15 mmHg

Rationale: A mean pulmonary artery pressure at least 25 mmHg with a pulmonary capillary occlusion pressure of no more than 15 mmHg is consistent with the diagnosis of pulmonary hypertension.
Ref: Butterworth, J.F., Mackey, D.C., & Wasnick, J.D. (2013). Ch 24 *Morgan & Mikhail's Clinical Anesthesiology* (5th ed.). New York, NY: McGraw-Hill.

Nagelhout, J.J., & Plaus, K.L. (2014). Ch 26 *Nurse Anesthesia* (5th ed.). St. Louis, MO: Elsevier.

154. Which of the following statements about chronic bronchitis is true?

(A) Patients with chronic bronchitis display hyperinflation on the chest X-ray.

(B) Patients with chronic bronchitis display decreased elastic recoil.

(C) Patients with chronic bronchitis display a normal hematocrit.

(D) Patients with chronic bronchitis display an elevated $PaCO_2$.

Rationale: Choices A to C refer to patients with emphysema.
Ref: Butterworth, J.F., Mackey, D.C., & Wasnick, J.D. (2013). Ch 24 *Morgan & Mikhail's Clinical Anesthesiology* (5th ed.). New York, NY: McGraw-Hill.
Nagelhout, J.J., & Plaus, K.L. (2014). Ch 26 *Nurse Anesthesia* (5th ed.). St. Louis, MO: Elsevier.

155. How long should a patient discontinue smoking in order to decrease secretions and reduce pulmonary complications?

(A) 1-2 weeks

(B) 2-4 weeks

(C) 3-5 days

(D) 4-6 weeks

Rationale: A patient will get the optimal benefit if they discontinue smoking 4 to 6 weeks prior to surgery to decrease secretions and to reduce pulmonary complications.
Ref: Butterworth, J.F., Mackey, D.C., & Wasnick, J.D. (2013). Ch 24 *Morgan & Mikhail's Clinical Anesthesiology* (5th ed.). New York, NY: McGraw-Hill.

156. What is the acid-base interpretation for a patient with the following ABG, pH 7.29, $PaCO_2$ 52, HCO_3 24?

(A) Uncompensated respiratory alkalosis

(B) Compensated respiratory acidosis

(C) Compensated respiratory alkalosis

(D) Uncompensated respiratory acidosis

Rationale: An HCO_3 24 is normal so there is no compensation; pH 7.29, $PaCO_2$ 52 indicates respiratory acidosis.

Ref: Butterworth, J.F., Mackey, D.C., & Wasnick, J.D. (2013). Ch 50 *Morgan & Mikhail's Clinical Anesthesiology* (5th ed.). New York, NY: McGraw-Hill.

Nagelhout, J.J., & Plaus, K.L. (2014). Ch 26 *Nurse Anesthesia* (5th ed.). St. Louis, MO: Elsevier.

157. When giving neostigmine, what is the resultant muscarinic effect?

    (A) Bradycardia
    (B) Tachyarrhythmias
    (C) Improved contractility
    (D) Increased conduction

    Rationale: Cardiovascular muscarinic responses include lowered heart rate and brady arrhythmias. Decreased conduction and contractility are also muscarinic side effects.

TABLE 1-8. Muscarinic side effects of cholinesterase inhibitors.

Organ System	Muscarinic Side Effects
Cardiovascular	Decreased heart rate, bradyarrhythmias
Pulmonary	Bronchospasm, bronchial secretions
Cerebral	Diffuse excitation[1]
Gastrointestinal	Intestinal spasm, increased salivation
Genitourinary	Increased bladder tone
Ophthalmological	Pupillary constriction

[1]Applies only to physostigmine.

Ref: Butterworth, J.F., Mackey, D.C., & Wasnick, J.D. (2013). Ch 12 *Morgan & Mikhail's Clinical Anesthesiology* (5th ed.). New York, NY: McGraw-Hill.

158. Which anticholinesterase crosses the blood-brain barrier?

    (A) Edrophonium
    (B) Neostigmine
    (C) Pyridostigmine
    (D) Physostigmine

    Rationale: Physostigmine is a tertiary amine with no quaternary ammonium. Edrophonium, neostigmine and pyridostigmine contain quaternary ammonium. Quaternary ammonium limits entry of these anticholinesterases through the blood-brain barrier due to lipid insolubility.

Ref: Butterworth, J.F., Mackey, D.C., & Wasnick J.D. (2013). Ch 12 *Morgan & Mikhail's Clinical Anesthesiology* (5th ed.). New York, NY: McGraw-Hill.

159. Your patient's Train-of-Four is ¼. You decide to use neostigmine to reverse neuromuscular blockade. What drug combination and doses will you use?

    (A) Neostigmine 0.04 mg/kg and glycopyrrolate 0.2 mg per 1 mg of neostigmine
    (B) Neostigmine 0.08 mg/kg and glycopyrrolate 0.2 mg per 1 mg of neostigmine
    (C) Neostigmine 0.02 mg/kg and atropine 0.014 mg per 1 mg of neostigmine
    (D) Neostigmine 0.01 mg/kg and atropine 0.1 mg per 1 mg of neostigmine

    Rationale: The usual dose of neostigmine is 0.04 to 0.08 mg/kg. Glycopyrrolate is given prior to or with the anticholinesterase to minimize the muscarinic effects. There is less tachycardia when administering atropine. Higher doses of neostigmine are given for profound paralysis. Atropine is typically given with edrophonium as the onset of action is similar for both drugs.

Ref: Butterworth, J.F., Mackey, D.C., & Wasnick, J.D. (2013). Ch 12 *Morgan & Mikhail's Clinical Anesthesiology* (5th ed.). New York, NY: McGraw-Hill.

160. What is the acid-base interpretation for a patient with the following ABG, pH 7.49, $PaCO_2$ 22, HCO_3 24?

    (A) Uncompensated respiratory alkalosis
    (B) Compensated respiratory acidosis
    (C) Compensated respiratory alkalosis
    (D) Uncompensated respiratory acidosis

    Rationale: An HCO_3 24 is normal so there is no compensation; pH 7.49, $PaCO_2$ 22 indicates respiratory alkalosis.

Ref: Butterworth, J.F., Mackey, D.C., & Wasnick, J.D. (2013). Ch 50 *Morgan & Mikhail's Clinical Anesthesiology* (5th ed.). New York, NY: McGraw-Hill.

Nagelhout, J.J., & Plaus, K.L. (2014). Ch 26 *Nurse Anesthesia* (5th ed.). St. Louis, MO: Elsevier.

161. Which cardiovascular effect would you expect when stimulating B_1 receptors?

    (A) Decreased heart rate
    (B) Decreased conduction
    (C) Increased heart rate
    (D) Decreased contractility

    Rationale: Stimulation of myocardial B_1 receptors results in increased heart rate, conduction, and contractility.

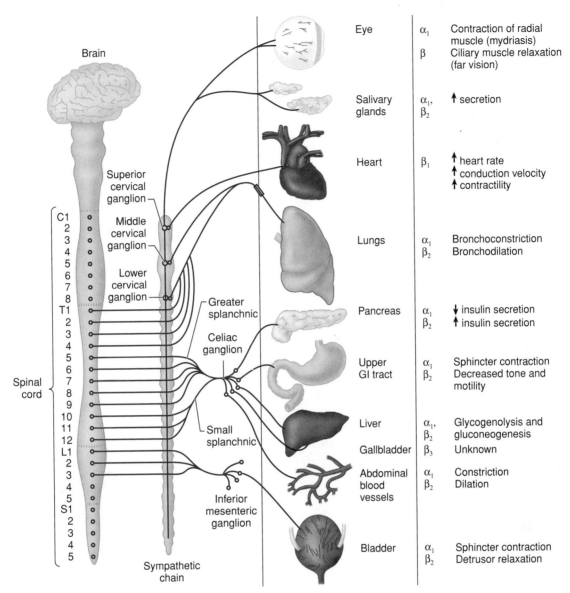

Eye	α_1	Contraction of radial muscle (mydriasis)
	β	Ciliary muscle relaxation (far vision)
Salivary glands	α_1, β_2	↑ secretion
Heart	β_1	↑ heart rate ↑ conduction velocity ↑ contractility
Lungs	α_1	Bronchoconstriction
	β_2	Bronchodilation
Pancreas	α_1	↓ insulin secretion
	β_2	↑ insulin secretion
Upper GI tract	α_1	Sphincter contraction
	β_2	Decreased tone and motility
Liver	α_1, β_2	Glycogenolysis and gluconeogenesis
Gallbladder	β_3	Unknown
Abdominal blood vessels	α_1	Constriction
	β_2	Dilation
Bladder	α_1	Sphincter contraction
	β_2	Detrusor relaxation

FIG. 1-4. The sympathetic nervous system Organ innervation, receptor type, and response to stimulation. The origin of the sympathetic chain is the thoracoabdominal (T1–L3) spinal cord, in contrast to the craniosacral distribution of the para sympathetic nervous system. Another anatomic difference is the greater distance from the sympathetic ganglion to the visceral structures.

Ref: Butterworth, J.F., Mackey, D.C., & Wasnick, J.D. (2013). Ch 14 *Morgan & Mikhail's Clinical Anesthesiology* (5th ed.). New York, NY: McGraw-Hill.

162. What statement is true regarding internal cardioverter defibrillators (ICD)?

   (A) ICDs are indicated for left ventricular ejection fractions >35%.

   (B) Placement of ICDs requires general anesthesia.

   (C) ICDs are indicated for intraoperative ventricular fibrillation.

   (D) ICDs are indicated for patients with an ejection fraction <35%.

Rationale: ICDs are indicated for patients with left ventricular function resulting from a myocardial infarction; ejection fraction <35%; and for those who survive cardiac death. Placement of ICDs may be performed using sedation or general anesthesia. Intraoperative ventricular fibrillation requires defibrillation and pharmacological intervention (amiodarone).

Ref: Butterworth, J.F., Mackey, D.C., & Wasnick, J.D. (2013). Ch 21 *Morgan & Mikhail's Clinical Anesthesiology* (5th ed.). New York, NY: McGraw-Hill.

163. How does B2 stimulation affect insulin levels?

(A) Increases insulin

(B) No change in insulin level

(C) Decreases insulin

(D) Alpha1 decreases insulin

Rationale: Insulin levels are increased due to B2 stimulation. Alpha1 stimulation decreases insulin secretion.

Ref: Butterworth, J.F., Mackey, D.C., & Wasnick, J.D. (2013). Ch 14 *Morgan & Mikhail's Clinical Anesthesiology* (5th ed.). New York, NY: McGraw-Hill.

164. What is the acid-base state of a patient with the following ABG, pH 7.35, PaCO$_2$ 50, HCO$_3$ 44?

(A) Uncompensated respiratory alkalosis

(B) Compensated respiratory acidosis

(C) Compensated respiratory alkalosis

(D) Uncompensated respiratory acidosis

Rationale: The HCO$_3$ is elevated so there is compensation; pH 7.35, PaCO$_2$ 50 indicates respiratory acidosis.

Ref: Butterworth, J.F., Mackey, D.C., & Wasnick, J.D. (2013). Ch 50 *Morgan & Mikhail's Clinical Anesthesiology* (5th ed.). New York, NY: McGraw-Hill.

Nagelhout, J.J., & Plaus, K.L. (2014). Ch 26 *Nurse Anesthesia* (5th ed.). St. Louis, MO: Elsevier.

165. What is the classification of metoclopramide?

(A) Antacid

(B) H$_1$-Receptor antagonist

(C) Gastrointestinal prokinetic

(D) H$_2$-receptor antagonist

Rationale: Metoclopramide is a prokinetic, speeding gastric emptying, lowering esophageal sphincter tone and lowering gastric volume. Gastrointestinal prokinetics do not alter gastric pH. Antacids alter the gastric pH. Histamine$_2$ receptor antagonists decrease gastric acid volume. H$_1$ receptor antagonists have no effect on gastric emptying.

TABLE 1-9. Properties of commonly used H$_1$-receptor antagonists.[1]

Drug	Route	Dose (mg)	Duration (h)	Sedation	Antiemesis
Diphenhydramine (Benadryl)	PO, IM, IV	25–50	3–6	+++	++
Dimenhydrinate (Dramamine)	PO, IM, IV	50–100	3–6	+++	++
Chlorpheniramine (Chlor-Trimeton)	PO IM, IV	2–12 5–20	4–8	++	0
Hydroxyzine (Atarax, Vistaril)	PO, IM	25–100	4–12	+++	++
Promethazine (Phenergan)	PO, IM, IV	12.5–50	4–12	+++	+++
Cetirizine (Zyrtec)	PO	5–10	24	+	
Cyproheptadine (Periactin)	PO	4	6–8	++	
Dimenhydrinate (Dramamine)	PO	50	6–12	++	
Fexofenadine (Allegra)	PO	30–60	12	0	
Meclizine (Antivert)	PO	12.5–50	8–24	+	
Loratadine (Claritin)	PO	10	24	0	

[1]0, no effect; ++, moderate activity; +++, marked activity.

TABLE 1-10. Pharmacology of aspiration pneumonia prophylaxis.[1]

Drug	Route	Dose	Onset	Duration	Acidity	Volume	LES Tone
Cimetidine (Tagamet)	PO IV	300–800 mg 300 mg	1–2 h	4–8 h	↓↓↓	↓↓	0
Ranitidine (Zantac)	PO IV	150–300 mg 50 mg	1–2 h	10–12 h	↓↓↓	↓↓	0
Famotidine (Pepcid)	PO IV	20–40 mg 20 mg	1–2 h	10–12 h	↓↓↓	↓↓	0
Nizatidine (Axid)	PO	150–300 mg	0.5–1 h	10–12 h	↓↓↓	↓↓	0
Nonparticulate antacids (Bicitra, Polycitra)	PO	15–30 mL	5–10 min	30–60 min	↓↓↓	↑	0
Metoclopramide (Reglan)	IV PO	10 mg 10–15 mg	1–3 min	1–2 h 30–60 min[2]	0	↓↓	↑↑

[1]0, no eff ect; ↓↓, moderate decrease; ↓↓↓, marked decrease; ↑, slight increase; ↑↑, moderate increase; LES, lower esophageal sphincter.
[2]Oral metoclopramide has a quite variable onset of action and duration of action.

Ref: Butterworth, J.F., Mackey, D.C., & Wasnick, J.D. (2013). Ch 17 *Morgan & Mikhail's Clinical Anesthesiology* (5th ed.). New York, NY: McGraw-Hill.

166. Which of the following physiological effects is not associated with serotonin?

   (A) Arteriolar and venous vasoconstrictor
   (B) Bronchoconstrictor
   (C) Increase bleeding time
   (D) Decreased peristalsis

Rationale: 5-hydroxytryptamine (5-HT), serotonin, vasoconstricts arterioles and veins, causes platelet aggregation and bronchoconstriction. Serotonin increases gastrointestinal peristalsis.
Ref: Butterworth, J.F., Mackey, D.C., & Wasnick, J.D. (2013). Ch 17 *Morgan & Mikhail's Clinical Anesthesiology* (5th ed.). New York, NY: McGraw-Hill.

167. Which of the following is a serotonin receptor antagonist?

   (A) Droperidol
   (B) Dexamethasone
   (C) Aprepitant
   (D) Dolasetron

Rationale: Droperidol is classified as a butyrophenone; dexmethasone a glucocorticoid; and Aprepitant a neurokinin-1 receptor antagonist. Serotonin receptor antagonists include ondansetron, granisetron and dolasetron.
Ref: Butterworth, J.F., Mackey, D.C., & Wasnick J.D. (2013). Ch 17 *Morgan & Mikhail's Clinical Anesthesiology* (5th ed.). New York, NY: McGraw-Hill.

168. Which ABG result is indicative of acute hyperventilation ?

   (A) pH 7.25, PaCO[2] 20, HCO3 24
   (B) pH 7.35, PaCO[2] 50, HCO3 44
   (C) pH 7.35, PaCO[2] 40, HCO3 24
   (D) pH 7.45, PaCO[2] 30, HCO3 14

Rationale: Uncompensated respiratory alkalosis would be reflected in acute hyperventilation.
Ref: Butterworth, J.F., Mackey, D.C., & Wasnick, J.D. (2013). Ch 50 *Morgan & Mikhail's Clinical Anesthesiology* (5th ed.). New York, NY: McGraw-Hill.
Nagelhout, J.J., & Plaus, K.L. (2014). Ch 26 *Nurse Anesthesia* (5th ed.). St. Louis, MO: Elsevier.

169. What is the physical structure of succinylcholine?

   (A) Two joined acetylcholine molecules
   (B) Benzylisoquinoline
   (C) Steroid ring with two modified ACh molecules
   (D) Monoquaternary steroid

Rationale: Atracurium is classified as a benzylisoquinoline. Two modified ACh molecules are separated by a steroid ring in pancuronium. Rocuronium's physical structure consists of a monoquaternary steroid.

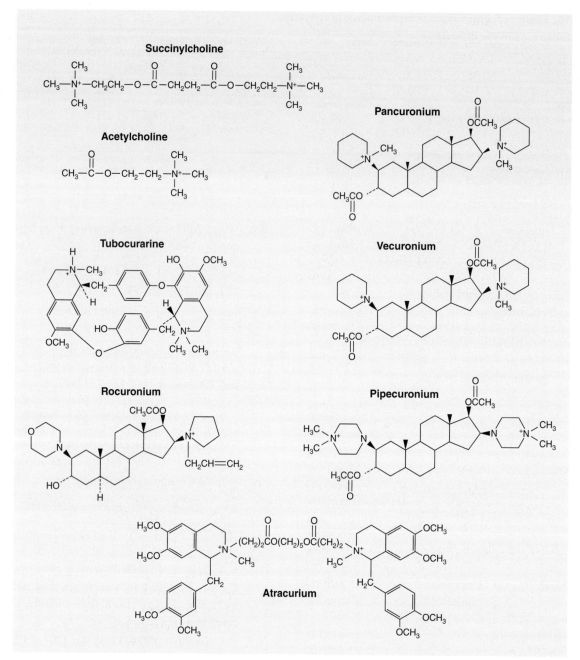

FIG. 1-5. Chemical structures of neuromuscular blocking agents.

Ref: Butterworth, J.F., Mackey, D.C., & Wasnick, J.D. (2013). Ch 11 *Morgan & Mikhail's Clinical Anesthesiology* (5th ed.). New York, NY: McGraw-Hill.

170. Which of the following factors produces 4 to 8 hours of succinylcholine-induced neuromuscular blockade?

(A) Homozygous atypical enzyme

(B) Hyperthermia

(C) Heterozygous atypical enzyme

(D) Reduced pseudocholinesterase levels

Rationale: Reduced pseudocholinesterase levels and heterozygous atypical enzyme may results in prolonged succinylcholine block (2–20 minutes and 20–30 minutes) respectively. Hypothermia, pregnancy, renal and liver failure as well as drugs may prolong succinylcholine neuromuscular blockade. Lengthy prolonged blocks (4–8 hours) are linked to homozygous atypical enzyme. This is commonly associated with the dibucaine resistant allele.

Ref: Butterworth, J.F., Mackey, D.C., & Wasnick, J.D. (2013). Ch 11 *Morgan & Mikhail's Clinical Anesthesiology* (5th ed.). New York, NY: McGraw-Hill.

171. During a general anesthesia case with mechanical ventilation the ABG results are: pH 7.29, $PaCO_2$ 52, HCO_3 24. What intervention is appropriate?

    (A) Decrease respiratory rate.
    (B) Decrease tidal volume.
    (C) Give 150 mEq sodium bicarbonate.
    (D) Increase respiratory rate.

    Rationale: The patient is in uncompensated respiratory acidosis likely due to hypoventilation. Increasing ventilation will reduce $PaCO_2$.

    Ref: Butterworth, J.F., Mackey, D.C., & Wasnick, J.D. (2013). Ch 50 *Morgan & Mikhail's Clinical Anesthesiology* (5th ed.). New York, NY: McGraw-Hill.

    Nagelhout, J.J., & Plaus, K.L. (2014). Ch 26 *Nurse Anesthesia* (5th ed.). St. Louis, MO: Elsevier.

172. What are the primary anesthetic goals for patients with second- and third-degree burns?

    Select (2) two
    (A) Pain management
    (B) Restoring circulating volume
    (C) Administration of crystalloids
    (D) Administration of colloids

    Rationale: Cardiac output declines rapidly for burn patients. Infusion of crystalloids improves survival. In burn patients kidney failure is associated with the use of hypertonic saline. Patient demise is linked to administration of blood products.

    Ref: Butterworth, J.F., Mackey, D.C., & Wasnick, J.D. (2013). Ch 39 *Morgan & Mikhail's Clinical Anesthesiology* (5th ed.). New York, NY: McGraw-Hill.

173. Hypoxic pulmonary vasoconstriction (HPV) will cause which action in the lungs?

    (A) Increase blood flow to non-ventilated lung
    (B) Decrease blood flow to ventilated lung
    (C) Decrease blood flow to non-ventilated lung
    (D) Increase ventilation to the nonperfused lung

    Rationale: Hypoxic Pulmonary Vasoconstriction (HPV) will cause decreased blood flow to non-ventilated lung.

Ref: Butterworth, J.F., Mackey, D.C., & Wasnick, J.D. (2013). Ch 25 *Morgan & Mikhail's Clinical Anesthesiology* (5th ed.). New York, NY: McGraw-Hill.

Nagelhout, J.J., & Plaus, K.L. (2014). Ch 26 *Nurse Anesthesia* (5th ed.). St. Louis, MO: Elsevier.

174. Calculate the oxygen content given the following values: Hgb = 14; $PaCO_2$ = 60; SaO_2 = 90%?

    (A) 4 mL O_2
    (B) 14 mL O_2
    (C) 17 mL O_2
    (D) 40 mL O_2

    Rationale: $CaO_2 = (1.36 \times Hgb \times \%$ arterial Hgb saturation$) + (PaO_2 \times 0.003)$

    Ref: Butterworth, J.F., Mackey, D.C., & Wasnick, J.D. (2013). Ch 23 *Morgan & Mikhail's Clinical Anesthesiology* (5th ed.). New York, NY: McGraw-Hill.

    Nagelhout, J.J., & Plaus, K.L. (2014). Ch 26 *Nurse Anesthesia* (5th ed.). St. Louis, MO: Elsevier.

175. The Haldane effect is best described by which statement below?

    (A) The Haldane effect explains why deoxygenated blood can carry more CO^2.
    (B) The Haldane effect explains the influence of pH, PCO_2, and PO_2 on the oxyhemoglobin dissociation curve.
    (C) The Haldane effect governs the diffusion of O_2 at the capillary level.
    (D) The Haldane effect accounts for the difference in lung volume at inspiration versus expiration.

    Rationale: Deoxyhemoglobin more readily accepts the H^+ produced by the dissociation of carbonic acid. This permits more CO_2 to be carried in the form of bicarbonate ions.

    Ref: Nagelhout, J.J., & Plaus, K.L. (2014). Ch 26 *Nurse Anesthesia* (5th ed.). St. Louis, MO: Elsevier.

176. A 22-year-old male emerges from a laparoscopic appendectomy under general endotracheal anesthesia still intubated. The patient is without an oral airway. During emergence, the patient sits up bucking with teeth clamped down occluding the endotracheal tube. He forcefully attempts to breathe. Which respiratory phenomenon could occur based on this scenario?

    (A) Pulmonary embolism
    (B) Pulmonary edema
    (C) Aspiration pneumonia
    (D) Acute asthma attack

Rationale: During obstruction, forceful inspiratory effects are ineffective because of the airway obstruction. Ineffective expiration produces an increase in intrathoracic and alveolar pressure. The end result of these events is the rapid immense transudation of fluid from the pulmonary interstitium into the alveoli, which consequences pulmonary edema.
Ref: Nagelhout, J.J., & Plaus, K.L. (2014). Ch 26 *Nurse Anesthesia* (5th ed.). St. Louis, MO: Elsevier.

177. In which lung region are the alveoli most compliant in an upright healthy person?

    (A) Apex
    (B) Middle
    (C) Base
    (D) Pleura

Rationale: The smaller alveoli in dependent areas have a lower transpulmonary pressure thus are more compliant and undergo greater expansion during inspiration.
Ref: Butterworth, J.F., Mackey, D.C., & Wasnick, J.D. (2013). Ch 23 *Morgan & Mikhail's Clinical Anesthesiology* (5th ed.). New York, NY: McGraw-Hill.
Nagelhout, J.J., & Plaus, K.L. (2014). Ch 26 *Nurse Anesthesia* (5th ed.). St. Louis, MO: Elsevier.

178. A ventilation:perfusion (V:Q) ratio of zero (0) may be seen in which disorder?

    (A) Pulmonary embolism
    (B) Low cardiac output
    (C) Emphysema
    (D) Mucous plug

Rationale: Alveoli that are perfused but not ventilated have a V:Q of 0 which constitutes a intrapulmonary shunt.
Ref: Butterworth, J.F., Mackey, D.C., & Wasnick, J.D. (2013). Ch 23 *Morgan & Mikhail's Clinical Anesthesiology* (5th ed.). New York, NY: McGraw-Hill.
Nagelhout, J.J., & Plaus, K.L. (2014). Ch 26 *Nurse Anesthesia* (5th ed.). St. Louis, MO: Elsevier.

179. In what form is the majority of CO_2 transported in the blood?

    (A) Carbonic acid
    (B) Bicarbonate
    (C) Dissolved
    (D) Attached to hemoglobin

Rationale: Carbon dioxide is transported in the blood in three forms: As bicarbonate, dissolved in solution and with proteins. Bicarbonate represents the largest fraction of carbon dioxide in the blood.
Ref: Butterworth, J.F., Mackey, D.C., & Wasnick, J.D. (2013). Ch 23 *Morgan & Mikhail's Clinical Anesthesiology* (5th ed.). New York, NY: McGraw-Hill.
Nagelhout, J.J., & Plaus, K.L. (2014). Ch 26 *Nurse Anesthesia* (5th ed.). St. Louis, MO: Elsevier.

180. What would be the expected P_{50} of a patient with increased levels of 2,3-diphosphoglycerate?

    (A) P_{50} of 22 mmHg
    (B) P_{50} of 26 mmHg
    (C) P_{50} of 30 mmHg
    (D) P_{50} of 38 mmHg

Rationale: The effect of hemoglobin-O_2 interaction is expressed by the P_{50}, the O_2 tension at which hemoglobin is 50% saturated. 2,3-diphosphoglycerate will shift the hemoglobin dissociation curve to the right thus decreasing P_{50}.
Ref: Butterworth, J.F., Mackey, D.C., & Wasnick, J.D. (2013). Ch 23 *Morgan & Mikhail's Clinical Anesthesiology* (5th ed.). New York, NY: McGraw-Hill.
Nagelhout, J.J., & Plaus, K.L. (2014). Ch 26 *Nurse Anesthesia* (5th ed.). St. Louis, MO: Elsevier.

181. Which anticholinergic possesses the least antisialogogue effect?

    (A) Atropine
    (B) Glycopyrrolate
    (C) Scopolamine
    (D) Neostigmine

Rationale: Antisialogue effects are similar for glycopyrrolate and scopolamine. They are less than atropine. Neostigmine is a cholinesterase inhibitor.

TABLE 1-11. Pharmacological characteristics of anticholinergic drugs.[1]

	Atropine	Scopolamine	Glycopyrrolate
Tachycardia	+++	+	++
Bronchodilatation	++	+	++
Sedation	+	+++	0
Antisialagogue effect	++	+++	+++

[1]0, no effect; +, minimal effect; ++, moderate effect; +++, marked effect.

Ref: Butterworth, J.F., Mackey, D.C., & Wasnick, J.D. (2013). Ch 13 *Morgan & Mikhail's Clinical Anesthesiology* (5th ed.). New York, NY: McGraw-Hill.

182. The patient presents for outpatient surgery with a history of asthma. When using glycopyrrolate, what do you expect?

(A) Constriction of bronchial smooth muscle

(B) Increased gastric acid secretion

(C) Decreased body temperature

(D) Relaxation of bronchial smooth muscle

Rationale: Anticholinergics relax bronchial smooth muscle which is significant for asthma patients or those with chronic obstructive pulmonary disease. Decreased gastric acid sections and increased body temperature result from use of anticholinergics.

Ref: Butterworth, J.F., Mackey, D.C., & Wasnick, J.D. (2013). Ch 13 *Morgan & Mikhail's Clinical Anesthesiology* (5th ed.). New York, NY: McGraw-Hill.

183. What would be the expected P_{50} of a patient with a body temperature of 35.2° Celsius?

(A) P_{50} of 30 mmHg

(B) P_{50} of 26 mmHg

(C) P_{50} of 20 mmHg

(D) P_{50} of 18 mmHg

Rationale: The effect of hemoglobin-O_2 interaction is expressed by the P_{50}, the O_2 tension at which hemoglobin is 50% saturated. Hypothermia will shift the hemoglobin dissociation curve to the left thus increasing P_{50}.

Ref: Butterworth, J.F., Mackey, D.C., & Wasnick, J.D. (2013). Ch 23 *Morgan & Mikhail's Clinical Anesthesiology* (5th ed.). New York, NY: McGraw-Hill.

Nagelhout, J.J., & Plaus, K.L. (2014). Ch 26 *Nurse Anesthesia* (5th ed.). St. Louis, MO: Elsevier.

184. Which type of pneumocytes in the pulmonary epithelium contains surfactant?

(A) Type I pneumocytes

(B) Pulmonary alveolar macrophages

(C) Type II pneumocytes

(D) Mast cells

Rationale: Type II pneumocytes comprise cytoplasmic inclusions which hold surfactant, a substance that reduces surface tension in the alveoli.

Ref: Butterworth, J.F., Mackey, D.C., & Wasnick, J.D. (2013). Ch 23 *Morgan & Mikhail's Clinical Anesthesiology* (5th ed.). New York, NY: McGraw-Hill.

Nagelhout, J.J., & Plaus, K.L. (2014). Ch 26 *Nurse Anesthesia* (5th ed.). St. Louis, MO: Elsevier Saunders.

185. Which is the origin of the phrenic nerves?

(A) T10

(B) C2

(C) C3-C5

(D) T4-T6

Rationale: The diaphragm is innervated by the phrenic nerves which arise from C3-C5.

Ref: Butterworth, J.F., Mackey, D.C., & Wasnick, J.D. (2013). Ch 23 *Morgan & Mikhail's Clinical Anesthesiology* (5th ed.). New York, NY: McGraw-Hill.

Nagelhout, J.J., & Plaus, K.L. (2014). Ch 26 *Nurse Anesthesia* (5th ed.). St. Louis, MO: Elsevier.

186. What are the two lung volumes that comprise the functional residual capacity?

(A) Residual volume and tidal volume

(B) Tidal volume and expiratory reserve volume

(C) Residual volume and inspiratory reserve volume

(D) Residual volume and expiratory reserve volume

Rationale: The lung volume at the end of a normal exhalation is called functional residual capacity (FRC). The FRC is a combination of maximal volume that can be expired below tidal volume and the volume remaining after maximal exhalation.

Ref: Butterworth, J.F., Mackey, D.C., & Wasnick, J.D. (2013). Ch 23 *Morgan & Mikhail's Clinical Anesthesiology* (5th ed.). New York, NY: McGraw-Hill.

Nagelhout, J.J., & Plaus, K.L. (2014). Ch 26 *Nurse Anesthesia* (5th ed.). St. Louis, MO: Elsevier.

187. What is vital capacity?

(A) Volume remaining after maximal exhalation

(B) Maximal additional volume that can be inspired above tidal volume

(C) Maximal volume that can be expired below tidal volume

(D) Maximum volume of gas that can be expired following maximal inspiration

Rationale: Vital capacity is the maximum volume of gas that can be exhaled following maximal inspiration.

Ref: Butterworth, J.F., Mackey, D.C., & Wasnick, J.D. (2013). Ch 23 *Morgan & Mikhail's Clinical Anesthesiology* (5th ed.). New York, NY: McGraw-Hill.

Nagelhout, J.J., & Plaus, K.L. (2014). Ch 26 *Nurse Anesthesia* (5th ed.). St. Louis, MO: Elsevier.

188. Prior to rapid sequence induction of general anesthesia you plan to administer ranitidine. When is the best time to administer the medication?

(A) 0.5-1 hour preoperatively
(B) 1.0-1.5 hours preoperatively
(C) 1-2 hours preoperatively
(D) 1.5-2.5 hours preoperatively

Rationale: The onset of action of ranitidine is 1 to 2 hours following IV administration. Decreasing gastric fluid volume and increasing gastric acid pH decreases the risk of aspiration.
Ref: Butterworth, J.F., Mackey, D.C., & Wasnick, J.D. (2013). Ch 17 *Morgan & Mikhail's Clinical Anesthesiology* (5th ed.). New York, NY: McGraw-Hill.

189. Which H_2 receptor antagonist affects the metabolism of warfarin?

(A) Cimetidine
(B) Ranitidine
(C) Diphenhydramine
(D) Hydroxyzine

Rationale: Ranitidine metabolism via CP-450 pathways is less than cimetidine. Diphenhydramine and hydroxyzine are H_1 receptor antagonists.
Ref: Butterworth, J.F., Mackey, D.C., & Wasnick, J.D. (2013). Ch 17 *Morgan & Mikhail's Clinical Anesthesiology* (5th ed.). New York, NY: McGraw-Hill.

190. Which drug affects the absorption of digoxin?

(A) Cimetidine
(C) Bicitra
(C) Metoclopramide
(D) Omeprazole

Rationale: Urinary and gastric pH are altered by antacids. Absorption of digoxin, cimetidine, and ranitidine are slowed.
Ref: Butterworth, J.F., Mackey, D.C., & Wasnick, J.D. (2013). Ch 17 *Morgan & Mikhail's Clinical Anesthesiology* (5th ed.). New York, NY: McGraw-Hill.

191. What is the normal ratio of the forced expiratory volume in the first second of exhalation to the total forced vital capacity?

(A) Less than 60%
(B) Greater than 50%
(C) Greater than or equal to 80%
(D) Greater than or equal to 20%

Rationale: The normal ratio of the forced expiratory volume in the first second of exhalation to the total forced vital capacity is greater than or equal to 80%.
Ref: Butterworth, J.F., Mackey, D.C., & Wasnick, J.D. (2013). Ch 23 *Morgan & Mikhail's Clinical Anesthesiology* (5th ed.). New York, NY: McGraw-Hill.
Nagelhout, J.J., & Plaus, K.L. (2014). Ch 26 *Nurse Anesthesia* (5th ed.). St. Louis, MO: Elsevier.

192. What is the functional residual capacity in the supine position?

(A) 2,300 mL
(B) 1,300 mL
(C) 1,200 mL
(D) 500 mL

Rationale: Normal functional residual capacity is 2,300 mL. The supine position reduces the functional residual capacity by 800 to 1,000 mL.
Ref: Butterworth, J.F., Mackey, D.C., & Wasnick, J.D. (2013). Ch 23 *Morgan & Mikhail's Clinical Anesthesiology* (5th ed.). New York, NY: McGraw-Hill.
Nagelhout, J.J., & Plaus, K.L. (2014). Ch 26 *Nurse Anesthesia* (5th ed.). St. Louis, MO: Elsevier.

193. Which structure classifies local anesthetics?

(A) Lipophilic group
(B) Benzene ring
(C) Hydrophilic group
(D) Intermediate chain

Rationale: An intermediate chain separates the lipophilic and hydrophilic groups. A benzene ring is noted in the lipophilic group.

TABLE 1-12. Physicochemical properties of local anesthetics.

Generic (Proprietary)	Structure	Relative Lipid Solubility of Unchanged Local Anesthetic	pKa	Protein Binding (%)
Amides Bupivacaine (Marcaine, Sensorcaine)		8	8.2	96
Etidocaine (Duranest)		16	8.1	94
Lidocaine (Xylocaine)		1	8.2	64
Mepivacaine (Carbocaine)		0.3	7.9	78
Prilocaine (Citanest)		0.4	8.0	53
Ropivacaine (Naropin)		2.5	8.2	94

(continued)

TABLE 1-12. Physicochemical properties of local anesthetics. (continued)

Generic (Proprietary)	Structure	Relative Lipid Solubility of Unchanged Local Anesthetic	pKa	Protein Binding (%)
Esters				
Chloroprocaine (Nesacaine)		2.3	9.1	NA[1]
Cocaine		NA	8.7	91
Procaine (Novocaine)		0.3	9.1	NA
Tetracaine (Pontocaine)		12	8.6	76

*carbon atom responsible for optical isomerism.
[1]NA, not available.

Ref: Butterworth, J.F., Mackey, D.C., & Wasnick, J.D. (2013). Ch 16 *Morgan & Mikhail's Clinical Anesthesiology* (5th ed.). New York, NY: McGraw-Hill.

194. Lipid solubility is greatest with which local anesthetic?

(A) Tetracaine

(B) Procaine

(C) Cocaine

(D) Chloroprocaine

Rationale: Lipid solubility is one factor that affects the onset of local anesthetics. Tetracaine possesses the greatest lipid solubility as compared to procaine and chloroprocaine. Cocaine possesses no lipid solubility.

Ref: Butterworth, J.F., Mackey, D.C., & Wasnick, J.D. (2013). Ch 16 *Morgan & Mikhail's Clinical Anesthesiology* (5th ed.). New York, NY: McGraw-Hill.

195. Which factor most influences the duration of action for local anesthetics?

(A) pKa

(B) Ionization

(C) Lipid solubility

(D) Minimum concentration

Rationale: A longer duration of action correlates with highly lipid soluble local anesthetics. Chemical structure modifications influence potency. Onset of action is affected by ionization as well as lipid solubility. Factors influencing duration of action include lipid solubility and potency. Nerve fiber characteristics, nerve stimulation and electrolyte concentration are factors affecting the minimum concentration of local anesthetic needed to block nerve fibers.

Ref: Butterworth, J.F., Mackey, D.C., & Wasnick, J.D. (2013). Ch 16 *Morgan & Mikhail's Clinical Anesthesiology* (5th ed.). New York, NY: McGraw-Hill.

196. What two factors can shift the hemoglobin dissociation curve to the right?

Select (2) two

(A) Acidosis

(B) Hypoventilation

(C) Hyperthermia

(D) Decrease in 2,3,-DPG

Rationale: Acidosis, hyperthermia, and increased 2,3,-DPG shift the oxyhemoglobin dissociation curve to the right. Alkalosis, hypothermia, and decreased 2,3,-DPG shift the oxyhemoglobin dissociation curve to the left.

Ref: Butterworth, J.F., Mackey, D.C., & Wasnick, J.D. (2013). Ch 23 *Morgan & Mikhail's Clinical Anesthesiology* (5th ed.). New York, NY: McGraw-Hill.

Nagelhout, J.J., & Plaus, K.L. (2014). Ch 26 *Nurse Anesthesia* (5th ed.). St. Louis, MO: Elsevier.

197. What is the anatomic dead space in a 75 kg healthy adult patient?

(A) 75 mL

(B) 100 mL

(C) 150 mL

(D) 200 mL

Rationale: Anatomic dead space is 2 mL/kg

Ref: Butterworth, J.F., Mackey, D.C., & Wasnick, J.D. (2013). Ch 23 *Morgan & Mikhail's Clinical Anesthesiology* (5th ed.). New York, NY: McGraw-Hill.

Nagelhout, J.J., & Plaus, K.L. (2014). Ch 26 *Nurse Anesthesia* (5th ed.). St. Louis, MO: Elsevier.

198. What law applies when determining blood flow through an intravenous catheter?

(A) Poiseuille's Law

(B) Bernoulli's Principle

(C) LaPlace's Law

(D) Van der Wall's

Rationale: The radius of the intravenous catheter will affect flow as described by Poiseuille. Poiseuille

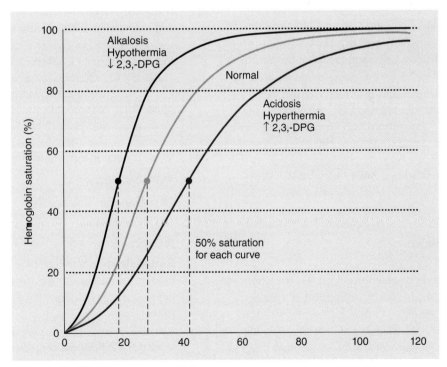

FIG. 1-6. The effects of changes in acid–base status, body temperature, and 2,3–DPG concentration on the hemoglobin–oxygen dissociation curve.

explains the relationship of fluid flow in a tube. In addition, viscosity of the fluid directly influences flow. For example, increased viscosity will decrease blood flow. Bernoulli's Principle addresses fluid and gas flow speed through a narrow orifice. The principle shares that with increased flow speed, pressure decreases. The Law of LaPlace examines the relationship of radius, pressure and wall tension. Van der Wall's principle addresses the sum of forces amongst molecules.

Ref: Nagelhout, J.J., & Plaus, K.L. (2014). Ch 14 *Nurse Anesthesia* (5th ed.). St. Louis, MO: Elsevier.

Butterworth, J.F., Mackey, D.C., & Wasnick J.D. (2013). Ch 4 & 5 *Morgan & Mikhail's Clinical Anesthesiology* (5th ed.). New York, NY: McGraw-Hill.

199. During a general anesthetic fentanyl and versed are administered. The interaction of the drugs produces a greater effect than the sum of the two medications. What is the interaction called?

    (A) Addition
    (B) Synergism
    (C) Tolerance
    (D) Tachyphylaxis

    Rationale: Synergism results when two drugs react to create a greater effect rather than an additive effect. Addition means that an equal effect results when two drugs are given after one another. Tolerance results from chronic drug exposure. Acute tolerance after a few doses of a drug results is termed tachyphylaxis.

    Ref: Butterworth, J.F., Mackey, D.C., & Wasnick, J.D. (2013). Ch 9 *Morgan & Mikhail's Clinical Anesthesiology* (5th ed.). New York, NY: McGraw-Hill.

200. Which of the following is not a Phase I reaction?

    (A) Oxidation
    (B) Reduction
    (C) Conjugation
    (D) Hydrolysis

    Rationale: Phase I reactions include oxidation, reduction, and hydrolysis. Conjugation is classified as a Phase II reaction.

    Ref: Butterworth, J.F., Mackey, D.C., & Wasnick, J.D. (2013). Ch 7 *Morgan & Mikhail's Clinical Anesthesiology* (5th ed.). New York, NY: McGraw-Hill.

    Stoelting, R.K., & Hillier, S.C. (2006). Ch 5 *Pharmacology and Physiology in Anesthetic Practice* (4th ed.). Philadelphia, PA: Elsevier.

201. Which inhalational agent's metabolism produces compound A?

    (A) Sevoflurane with low flow
    (B) Desflurane with low flow
    (C) Sevoflurane with high flow
    (D) Desflurane with high flow

    Rationale: Sevoflurane's metabolites include compound A. In long anesthetics using low flows (1L/m) production of compound A is more likely than in longer cases using high gas flows.

    Ref: Butterworth, J.F., Mackey, D.C., & Wasnick, J.D. (2013). Ch 5 *Morgan & Mikhail's Clinical Anesthesiology* (5th ed.). New York, NY: McGraw-Hill.

    Miller, R.D., & Pardo, M.C. (2011). Chapter 8 *Basics of Anesthesia* (6th ed.). Philadelphia, PA: Elsevier.

202. How is propofol classified?

    (A) Alkylphenol
    (B) Barbituric acid
    (C) Phencyclidine
    (D) Carboxylated imidazole

    Rationale: Propofol is an alkylphenol. Barbituric acid is the base chemical structure for sodium pentothal and methohexital. Ketamine is a phencyclidine derivative. Etomidate is a carboxylated imidazole.

    Ref: Butterworth, J.F., Mackey, D.C., & Wasnick, J.D. (2013). Ch 9 *Morgan & Mikhail's Clinical Anesthesiology* (5th ed.). New York, NY: McGraw-Hill.

    Miller, R.D., & Pardo, M.C. (2011). Ch 9 *Basics of Anesthesia* (6th ed.). Philadelphia, PA: Elsevier.

203. What induction agent is least protein-bound?

    (A) Ketamine
    (B) Propofol
    (C) Methohexital
    (D) Etomidate

    Rationale: Ketamine is 12% protein bound. The highest protein binding exists with propofol (97%), next with etomidate (77%), and methohexital (73%).

    Ref: Butterworth, J.F., Mackey, D.C., & Wasnick, J.D. (2013). Ch 9 *Morgan & Mikhail's Clinical Anesthesiology* (5th ed.). New York, NY: McGraw-Hill.

    Miller, R.D., & Pardo, M.C. (2011). Ch 9 *Basics of Anesthesia* (6th ed.). Philadelphia, PA: Elsevier.

204. Clearance of which benzodiazepine is greatest?

(A) Diazepam

(B) Lorazepam

(C) Midazolam

(D) Zaleplon

Rationale: Clearance for midazolam is 6.4 to 11 mL/kg/min. Clearance for lorazepam and diazepam is 0.8 to 01.2 mL/kg/min and 0.2 to 0.5 mL/kg/min respectively. Zaleplon is a nonbenzodiazepine hypnotic.

Ref: Butterworth, J.F., Mackey, D.C., & Wasnick, J.D. (2013). Ch 9 *Morgan & Mikhail's Clinical Anesthesiology* (5th ed.). New York, NY: McGraw-Hill.

Miller, R.D., & Pardo, M.C. (2011). Ch 9 *Basics of Anesthesia* (6th ed.). Philadelphia, PA: Elsevier.

Ouellette, R.G., & Joyce, J.A. (2011). Ch 5 *Pharmacology for Nurse Anesthesiology*. Sudbury, MA: Jones and Bartlett Learning.

205. Following administration of a beta-lactam antibiotic, the patient exhibits urticaria, hypotension, and arrhythmias. What is the most likely cause?

(A) Tachyphylaxis reaction

(B) Anaphylaxis reaction

(C) Atopic reaction

(D) Anaphylactoid reaction

Rationale: Anaphylaxis is commonly associated with antibiotic administration. Beta-lactam drugs including penicillin are primarily responsible for the reaction involving IgE antibodies. The signs and symptoms include: pruritus, urticaria, hypotension, wheezing, bronchospasm, abdominal pain, arrhythmias, and possibly angioedema. Individuals who exhibit greater tendencies for allergic reactions are atopic. Acute tolerance after a few doses of a drug results is termed tachyphylaxis. Tachyphylaxis results in acute tolerance following a few drug doses, but does not result in signs and symptoms associated with anaphylaxis. Anaphylactoid reactions involve non-IgE antibodies.

Ref: Ouellette, R.G., & Joyce, J.A. (2011). Ch 13 *Pharmacology for Nurse Anesthesiology*. Sudbury, MA: Jones and Bartlett Learning.

Nagelhout, J.J., & Plaus, K.L. (2014). Ch 41 *Nurse Anesthesia* (5th ed.). Philadelphia, PA: Elsevier.

Stoelting, R.K. and Hillier, SC. (2006). Ch 5 *Pharmacology and Physiology in Anesthetic Practice* (4th ed.). Philadelphia, PA: Elsevier.

206. Which would be best in the care of a patient in myxedema coma needing emergent surgery?

(A) Propylthiouracil

(B) Liothyronine

(C) Thyroxine

(D) Thyroid stimulating hormone

Rationale: Liothyronine (T_3) can be used for rapid emergent treatment of myxedema coma.

Ref: Butterworth, J.F., Mackey, D.C., & Wasnick, J.D. (2013). Ch 52 *Morgan & Mikhail's Clinical Anesthesiology* (5th ed.). New York, NY: McGraw-Hill.

Miller, R,D. Eriksson, L.I., Fleisher, L.A., Wiener-Kronish, J.P., & Young, W.L. (Eds.). (2010). Ch 35 *Miller's Anesthesia* (7th ed.). Philadelphia, PA: Elsevier.

207. Which indicates primary hypothyroidism?

(A) Decreased thyroid stimulating hormone with decreased triiodothyronine and thyroxine

(B) Increased thyroid stimulating hormone with decreased triiodothyronine and thyroxine

(C) Decreased thyroid stimulating hormone with increased triiodothyronine and thyroxine

(D) Increased thyroid stimulating hormone with increased triiodothyronine and thyroxine

Rationale: Increased thyroid stimulating hormone levels with decreased thyroid hormone levels indicate primary hypothyroidism.

Ref: Butterworth, J.F., Mackey, D.C., & Wasnick, J.D. (2013). Ch 52 *Morgan & Mikhail's Clinical Anesthesiology* (5th ed.). New York, NY: McGraw-Hill.

Hines, R.L., & Marschall, K.E. (Eds.) (2012). Ch 19 *Stoelting's anesthesia and co-existing disease* (6th ed.). Philadelphia, PA: Elsevier.

208. Which statement is true regarding phenytoin?

(A) Chronic treatment with phenytoin leads to prolonged neuromuscular blockade.

(B) Lower doses of neuromuscular blockers are required.

(C) Elimination of neuromuscular blockers is decreased.

(D) Higher doses of neuromuscular blockers are required.

Rationale: Higher doses of neuromuscular blockers are needed due to increased elimination in patients taking phenytoin.

Ref: Stoelting, R.K., & Hillier, S.C. (2006). Ch 30 *Pharmacology and Physiology in Anesthetic Practice* (4th ed.). Philadelphia, PA: Elsevier.

209. Which antiemetic will you avoid for patients with Parkinson's disease?

(A) Dolasetron

(B) Metoclopramide

(C) Odansetron

(D) Diphenhydramine

Rationale: Metoclopramide may precipitate or worsen Parkinson's disease. Dolasetron, odansetron, and diphenhydramine may be given safely to patients with Parkinson's disease.

Ref: Hines, R.L., & Marschall, K.E. (2012). Ch 28 *Stoelting's Anesthesia and Co-Exiting Disease* (6th ed.). Philadelphia, PA: Elsevier.

210. During surgery for breast cancer, the patient receives isosulfan blue dye. What will you expect?

(A) Increased SaO_2

(B) Tachycardia

(C) Decreased SaO_2

(D) Cardiac arrhythmias

Rationale: A transient decreased oxygenation is common following injection of isosulfan blue dye.

Ref: Hines, R.L., & Marschall, K.E. (2012). Ch 23 *Stoelting's Anesthesia and Co-Exiting Disease* (6th ed.). Philadelphia, PA: Elsevier Saunders.

211. Which analgesic for labor is not associated with significant respiratory depression affecting the mother or fetus?

(A) Morphine

(B) Nalbuphine

(C) Fentanyl

(D) Demerol

Rationale: Nalbuphine is a mixed agonist-antagonist. A respiratory ceiling effect negates unwanted respiratory depression in the mother and fetus. In contrast, morphine, fentanyl, and demerol are associated with significant respiratory depression for the mother and the neonate.

Ref: Butterworth, J.F., Mackey, D.C., & Wasnick, J.D. (2013). Ch 41 *Morgan & Mikhail's Clinical Anesthesiology* (5th ed.). New York, NY: McGraw-Hill.

212. Why are benzodiazepines avoided during labor and delivery?

(A) Pain on injection

(B) Prolonged neonatal respiratory depression

(C) High Apgar scores

(D) Nausea and vomiting

Rationale: Benzodiazepines should be avoided during labor due to prolonged neonatal respiratory depression following delivery. Also, mothers are affected by the amnestic properties of benzodiazepines that may affect memory of childbirth. Low Apgar scores may reflect respiratory depression.

Ref: Butterworth, J.F., Mackey, D.C., & Wasnick, J.D. (2013). Ch 41 *Morgan & Mikhail's Clinical Anesthesiology* (5th ed.). New York, NY: McGraw-Hill.

213. Which inhalational agent affects the blood pressure the least?

(A) Sevoflurane

(B) Halothane

(C) Isoflurane

(D) Desflurane

Rationale: A dose dependent decrease in blood pressures occurs with halothane. There is minimal cardiac depression with isoflurane and desflurane. Sevoflurane decreases the arterial blood pressure, but less than isoflurane or desflurane.

Ref: Butterworth, J.F., Mackey, D.C., & Wasnick, J.D. (2013). Ch 41 *Morgan & Mikhail's Clinical Anesthesiology* (5th ed.). New York, NY: McGraw-Hill.

214. Which analgesic given to renal failure patients results in prolonged respiratory depression?

(A) Remifentanil

(B) Demerol

(C) Sufentanil

(D) Morphine

Rationale: Morphine 3-glucoronide and morphine 6-glucoronide metabolites prolong respiratory depression and narcosis. Remifentanil is metabolized by plasma esterases. Demerol undergoes demethylation producing normeperidine. Seizures are linked to norpeperidine. Fentanyl metabolites are inactive.

Ref: Butterworth, J.F., Mackey, D.C., & Wasnick, J.D. (2013). Ch 10 *Morgan & Mikhail's Clinical Anesthesiology* (5th ed.). New York, NY: McGraw-Hill.

215. Which COX-2 selective agent is linked to hepatic failure?

(A) Acetaminophen

(B) Aspirin

(C) Ketorolac

(D) Celecoxib

Rationale: Acetaminophen results in production of *N*-acetyl-p-benzoquinone imine. Toxic levels cause hepatic failure. Ketorolac is metabolized in the liver with end product excreted unchanged. Inactive metabolites occur following hepatic metabolism of celecoxib. Aspirin is a COX-1 inhibitor.
Ref: Butterworth, J.F., Mackey, D.C., & Wasnick, J.D. (2013). Ch 10 *Morgan & Mikhail's Clinical Anesthesiology* (5th ed.). New York, NY: McGraw-Hill.

216. Your patient suffers from chronic renal failure. Which nondepolarizer will you avoid?

(A) Vecuronium
(B) Rocuronium
(C) Mivacron
(D) Anectine

Rationale: Prolonged neuromuscular blockade occurs due to partial renal excretion of vecuronium, pancuronium, doxacurium, and pipecuronium for patients in renal failure. Pseudocholinesterase is responsible for mivacron metabolism. The liver is the primary route of elimination for rocuronium. Anectine (Succinylcholine) is a depolarizing neuromuscular blocking drug.
Ref: Butterworth, J.F., Mackey, D.C., & Wasnick, J.D. (2013). Ch 11 *Morgan & Mikhail's Clinical Anesthesiology* (5th ed.). New York, NY: McGraw-Hill.

217. What is the mechanism of action for reversal of succinylcholine?

(A) Metabolism by acetylcholinesterase
(B) Hydrolyzed pseudocholinesterase
(C) Complex formation with steroidal nondepolarizers
(D) Chemical degradation by L-cysteine

Rationale: Succinylcholine is hydrolyzed in the plasma and liver by the enzyme pseudocholinesterase following release from the ACh receptors. Sugammadex forms complexes with steroidal nondepolarizers resulting in reversal. Investigative nondepolarizers undergo chemical degradation.
Ref: Butterworth, J.F., Mackey, D.C., & Wasnick, J.D. (2013). Ch 11 *Morgan & Mikhail's Clinical Anesthesiology* (5th ed.). New York, NY: McGraw-Hill.

218. The patient undergoing cataract extraction takes echothiophate for glaucoma. If given succinylcholine, what will you expect?

(A) Duration <5 minutes
(B) Duration <10 minutes
(C) Duration >10 minutes
(D) No effect on duration of action

Rationale: Echothiophate eye drops, an organophosphate, decrease pseudocholinesterase activity. This may increase the duration of neuromuscular blockade following administration of succinylcholine. The normal duration of action of succinylcholine is approximately 10 minutes.
Ref: Butterworth, J.F., Mackey, D.C., & Wasnick, J.D. (2013). Ch 11 *Morgan & Mikhail's Clinical Anesthesiology* (5th ed.). New York, NY: McGraw-Hill.

219. You administered propofol 2 mg/kg, succinylcholine 1.5 mg/kg, and fentanyl 2 ug/kg to a 70-kg patient undergoing emergent appendectomy. Following the 45-minute case you observe no respiratory effort. What is the best choice for this patient?

(A) Administer naloxone
(B) Maintain ventilatory support with sedation
(C) Administer neostigmine
(D) Check the ventilator settings

Rationale: Maintaining ventilator support is the best choice given this patient's lack of respiratory effort. Consider variables affecting prolonged neuromuscular blockade with succinylcholine. Depolarizing neuromuscular blockade is not reversed with neostigmine. The dose of fentanyl is not likely to produce prolonged depressed ventilation.
Ref: Butterworth, J.F., Mackey, D.C., & Wasnick, J.D. (2013). Ch 11 *Morgan & Mikhail's Clinical Anesthesiology* (5th ed.). New York, NY: McGraw-Hill.

220. Considering hyperkalemia, rhabdomyolysis, and cardiac arrest which neuromuscular blocking agent will you avoid in children?

(A) Rocuronium
(B) Succinylcholine
(C) Atracurium
(D) Cisatracurium

Rationale: Succinylcholine is strongly linked to hyperkalemia, rhabdomyolysis, and cardiac arrest particularly in children with undiagnosed myopathies. A relative contraindication exists for the routine use of succinylcholine in pediatric anesthesia. Nondepolarizing muscular blockers do not possess the same concerns.
Ref: Butterworth, J.F., Mackey, D.C., & Wasnick, J.D. (2013). Ch 11 *Morgan & Mikhail's Clinical Anesthesiology* (5th ed.). New York, NY: McGraw-Hill.

221. Which medication blocks muscarinic receptors?

(A) Atropine

(B) Rocuronium

(C) Pyridostigmine

(D) Neostigmine

Rationale: Atropine, an anticholinergic, blocks muscarinic receptors. Nondepolarizing neuromuscular blockers, also cholinergic antagonists such as rocurnoium, work at the nicotinic receptors of skeletal muscle. The cholinesterase inhibitors pyridostigmine and neostigmine act at both cholinergic and nicotinic receptors.

Ref: Butterworth, J.F., Mackey, D.C., & Wasnick, J.D. (2013). Ch 13 *Morgan & Mikhail's Clinical Anesthesiology* (5th ed.). New York, NY: McGraw-Hill.

222. What part of the structure of glycopyrrolate is responsible for binding to acetylcholine receptors?

(A) Organic base

(B) Ester linkage

(C) Aromatic base

(D) Benzene ring

Rationale: While each of the structure of anticholinergic drugs is present, the ester linkage is significant for binding thereby exerting a competitive blockade.

Ref: Butterworth, J.F., Mackey, D.C., & Wasnick, J.D. (2013). Ch 13 *Morgan & Mikhail's Clinical Anesthesiology* (5th ed.). New York, NY: McGraw-Hill.

223. What manifestation occurs as a result of anticholinergic overdose?

(A) Tachycardia

(B) Oral secretions

(C) Bradycardia

(D) Cutaneous vasoconstriction

Rationale: Central anticholinergic syndrome results in tachycardia, excessive dry mouth, and cutaneous vasodilation (also known as atropine flush).

Ref: Butterworth, J.F., Mackey, D.C., & Wasnick, J.D. (2013). Ch 13 *Morgan & Mikhail's Clinical Anesthesiology* (5th ed.). New York, NY: McGraw-Hill.

224. How is eutectic mixture of local anesthetics (EMLA) cream formulated?

(A) 1:1 mixture of 0.5% lidocaine and 0.5% prilocaine

(B) 2:1 mixture of 1.5% lidocaine and 2.5% prilocaine

(C) 1:1 mixture of 0.75% benzocaine and 0.5% lidocaine

(D) 2:1 mixture of 0.75% benzocaine and 1.5% lidocaine

Rationale: EMLA's formulation is a 1:1 mixture of prilocaine and lidocaine. The concentration of benzocaine is 20%.

Ref: Butterworth, J.F., Mackey, D.C., & Wasnick, J.D. (2013). Ch 16 *Morgan & Mikhail's Clinical Anesthesiology* (5th ed.). New York, NY: McGraw-Hill.

225. During an inguinal hernia repair, the surgeon asks how much bupivacaine is allowed for local infiltration. What is the correct maximum dose?

(A) 12 mg/kg

(B) 8 mg/kg

(C) 4.5 mg/kg

(D) 3 mg/kg

Rationale: The maximum dose for chloroprocaine is 12 mg/kg; 8 mg/kg for prilocaine; and 4.5 mg/kg for lidocaine and mepivacaine without epinephrine.

Ref: Butterworth, J.F., Mackey, D.C., & Wasnick, J.D. (2013). Ch 16 *Morgan & Mikhail's Clinical Anesthesiology* (5th ed.). New York, NY: McGraw-Hill.

226. How does the duration of epidural ropivacaine differ from lidocaine?

(A) The duration of lidocaine is shorter than ropivacaine.

(B) The duration of lidocaine and ropivacaine is similar.

(C) The duration of lidocaine is longer than ropivacaine.

(D) Ropivacaine is similar to all amides.

Rationale: The duration of action of lidocaine is shorter than ropivacaine. Ropivacaine is longer acting than other amides including lidocaine, mepivacaine, and prilocaine. The duration is similar to bupivacaine.

Ref: Butterworth, J.F., Mackey, D.C., & Wasnick, J.D. (2013). Ch 16 *Morgan & Mikhail's Clinical Anesthesiology* (5th ed.). New York, NY: Lange Medical Books

227. Which local anesthetic is metabolized by pseudocholinesterase?

(A) Lidocaine

(B) Bupivacaine

(C) Ropivacaine

(D) Tetracaine

Rationale: Lidocaine, bupivacaine, and ropivacaine are amide local anesthetics. Amide local anesthetics are metabolized in the liver by P-450 microsomal enzymes.

Ref: Butterworth, J.F., Mackey, D.C., & Wasnick, J.D. (2013). Ch 16 *Morgan & Mikhail's Clinical Anesthesiology* (5th ed.). New York, NY: McGraw-Hill.

228. Prolonged neurological deficits have been associated with which local anesthetic?

(A) Epidural chloroprocaine

(B) EMLA

(C) Topical chloroprocaine

(D) Intrathecal lidocaine

Rationale: Inadvertent dural puncture with chloroprocaine has caused total spinal anesthesia, severe hypotension, severe back pain, and neurological deficits. Sodium bisulfate preservative in chloroprocaine has been implicated as the causative agent. Topical local anesthetics are not linked to neurological deficits. Chloroprocaine is administered via epidural, infiltration, peripheral nerve block, and spinal routes.

Ref: Butterworth, J.F., Mackey, D.C., & Wasnick, J.D. (2013). Ch 16 *Morgan & Mikhail's Clinical Anesthesiology* (5th ed.). New York, NY: McGraw-Hill.

229. What part of the body houses the greatest concentration of histamine?

(A) Parietal cells

(B) Circulating basophils and mast cells

(C) Gastric mucosa

(D) Peripheral tissues

Rationale: Histamine facilitates the release of hydrochloric acid by parietal cells in the gastric mucosa. While histamine can be found in the central nervous system, peripheral tissues and the gastric mucosa, the greatest concentration is found in circulating basophils and mast cells.

Ref: Butterworth, J.F., Mackey, D.C., & Wasnick, J.D. (2013). Ch 17 *Morgan & Mikhail's Clinical Anesthesiology* (5th ed.). New York, NY: McGraw-Hill.

230. Which cardiovascular effect occurs when administering diphenhydramine?

(A) Hypertension

(B) Peripheral arteriolar constriction

(C) Coronary vasoconstriction

(D) Hypotension

Rationale: H_1 receptor antagonist diphenhydramine dilates coronary arteries and peripheral arterioles. Heart rate is increased, but blood pressure falls.

Ref: Butterworth, J.F., Mackey, D.C., & Wasnick, J.D. (2013). Ch 17 *Morgan & Mikhail's Clinical Anesthesiology* (5th ed.). New York, NY: McGraw-Hill.

231. When administering promethazine, how long will sedative effects last?

(A) 3-6 hours

(B) 4-12 hours

(C) 8-24 hours

(D) 24 hours

Rationale: Diphenhydramine and dimenhydrinate's effect last 3 to 6 hours. The duration of action of meclizine is 8 to 24 hours. Loratadine acts for 24 hours.

Ref: Butterworth, J.F., Mackey, D.C., & Wasnick, J.D. (2013). Ch 17 *Morgan & Mikhail's Clinical Anesthesiology* (5th ed.). New York, NY: McGraw-Hill.

232. Which of the following medications is potentiated by hydroxyzine?

(A) Midazolam

(B) Claritin

(C) Fexofenadine

(D) Metoclopramide

Rationale: H_1 receptor antagonists potentiate central nervous system depressants. No sedative effects are linked to Claritin or fexofenadine. Rare sedative effects occur with metoclopramide.

Ref: Butterworth, J.F., Mackey, D.C., & Wasnick, J.D. (2013). Ch 17 *Morgan & Mikhail's Clinical Anesthesiology* (5th ed.). New York, NY: McGraw-Hill.

233. You include dexmedetomidine as an adjunct to general anesthesia. Which drug requirements will most likely decrease?

(A) Vecuronium

(B) Propofol

(C) Ephedrine

(D) Methoxamine

Rationale: Decreasing the dose of central nervous system depressants and anesthetic agents is needed to avoid profound hypotension. Ephedrine and methoxamine, sympathomimetic amines, are used to increase blood pressure. No interaction exists between neuromuscular blockers (vecuronium) and dexmedetomidine.

Ref: Butterworth, J.F., Mackey, D.C., & Wasnick, J.D. (2013). Ch 17 *Morgan & Mikhail's Clinical Anesthesiology* (5th ed.). New York, NY: McGraw-Hill.

234. What is the primary receptor for phenylephrine?

    (A) B_1

    (B) A_1

    (C) B_2

    (D) A_2

Rationale: Receptor selectivity for adrenergic agonist phenylephrine is primarily A_1. There is some A_2, but no beta receptor selectivity.

Ref: Butterworth, J.F., Mackey, D.C., & Wasnick, J.D. (2013). Ch 14 *Morgan & Mikhail's Clinical Anesthesiology* (5th ed.). New York, NY: McGraw-Hill.

235. How do direct and indirect adrenergic agonists differ?

    (A) Indirect agonists bind to the receptor.

    (B) Ephedrine binds to the receptor.

    (C) Direct agonists bind to the receptor.

    (D) Phenylephrine increases neurotransmitter activity.

Rationale: Direct acting adrenergic agonists bind to receptors (neosynephrine). Indirect acting adrenergic agonists (ephedrine) increase the release or decrease the reuptake of norepinephrine.

Ref: Butterworth, J.F., Mackey, D.C., & Wasnick, J.D. (2013). Ch 14 *Morgan & Mikhail's Clinical Anesthesiology* (5th ed.). New York, NY: McGraw-Hill.

236. What is the primary effect of phenylephrine?

    (A) Peripheral vasoconstriction

    (B) Decreased vascular resistance

    (C) Increased heart rate

    (D) Increased cardiac output

Rationale: The cardiac effects of phenylephrine are primarily peripheral vasoconstriction, increased vascular resistance, and arterial blood pressure due to A_1 selectivity. Reflex bradycardia may result decreasing cardiac output.

TABLE 1-13. Receptor selectivity of adrenergic agonists.[1]

Drug	α_1	α_2	β_1	β_2	DA_1	DA_2
Phenylephrine	+++	+	0	0	0	0
Methyldopa	+	+	0	0	0	0
Clonidine	+	++	0	0	0	0
Dexmedetomidine	+	+++	0	0	0	0
Epinephrine[2]	++	++	+++	++	0	0
Ephedrine[3]	++	?	++	+	0	0
Fenoldopam	0	0	0	0	+++	0
Norepinephrine[2]	++	++	++	0	0	0
Dopamine[2]	++	++	++	+	+++	+++
Dopexamine	0	0	+	+++	++	+++
Dobutamine	0/+	0	+++	+	0	0
Terbutaline	0	0	+	+++	0	0

[1]0, no effect; +, agonist effect (mild, moderate, marked); ?, unknown effect; DA_1 and DA_2, dopaminergic receptors.
[2]The α_1-effects of epinephrine, norepinephrine, and dopamine become more prominent at high doses.
[3]The primary mode of action of ephedrine is indirect stimulation.

TABLE 1-14. Effects of adrenergic agonists on organ systems.[1]

Drug	Heart Rate	Mean Arterial Pressure	Cardiac Output	Peripheral Vascular Resistance	Bronchodilation	Renal Blood Flow
Phenylephrine	↓	↑↑↑	↓	↑↑↑	0	↓↓↓
Epinephrine	↑↑	↑	↑↑	↑/↓	↑↑	↓↓
Ephedrine	↑↑	↑↑	↑↑	↑	↑↑	↓↓
Fenoldopam	↑↑	↓↓↓	↓/↑	↓↓	0	↑↑↑
Norepinephrine	↓	↑↑↑	↓/↑	↑↑↑	0	↓↓↓
Dopamine	↑/↑↑	↑	↑↑↑	↑	0	↑↑↑
Dopexamine	↑/↑↑	↓/↑	↑↑	↑	0	↑
Isoproterenol	↑↑↑	↓	↑↑↑	↓↓	↑↑↑	↓/↑
Dobutamine	↑	↑	↑↑↑	↓	0	↑

[1]0, no effect; ↑, increase (mild, moderate, marked); ↓, decrease (mild, moderate, marked); ↓/↑, variable effect; ↑/↑↑, mild-to-moderate increase.

Ref: Butterworth, J.F., Mackey, D.C., & Wasnick, J.D. (2013). Ch 14 *Morgan & Mikhail's Clinical Anesthesiology* (5th ed.). New York, NY: McGraw-Hill.

237. Which of the following halogenated agents potentiates the effects of epinephrine the most?

   (A) Desflurane

   (B) Sevoflurane

   (C) Isoflurane

   (D) Halothane

   Rationale: Halothane sensitizes the myocardium to catecholamines. Myocardial sensitization to catecholamines is minimal with other halogenated agents.
   Ref: Butterworth, J.F., Mackey, D.C., & Wasnick, J.D. (2013). Ch 14 *Morgan & Mikhail's Clinical Anesthesiology* (5th ed.). New York, NY: McGraw-Hill.

238. You plan to administer ephedrine for hypotension following spinal anesthesia. What do you expect?

   (A) Decreased heart rate

   (B) Decreased cardiac output

   (C) Increased heart rate

   (D) Short duration of action

   Rationale: Administration of ephedrine results in increased heart rate, blood pressure, cardiac output, and cardiac contractility. Duration of action is longer compared to other sympathomimetics (neosynephrine).
   Ref: Butterworth, J.F., Mackey, D.C., & Wasnick, J.D. (2013). Ch 14 *Morgan & Mikhail's Clinical Anesthesiology* (5th ed.). New York, NY: McGraw-Hill.

239. How is ephedrine classified?

   (A) Indirect $Beta_1$, $Beta_2$ agonist

   (B) Direct Beta agonist

   (C) Direct Alpha agonist

   (D) Indirect $Alpha_1$, $Beta_1$, $Beta_2$ agonist

   Rationale: Ephedrine is classified as an indirect-acting adrenergic agonist. Receptivity includes moderate $Alpha_1$, $Beta_1$, and mild $Beta_2$.
   Ref: Butterworth, J.F., Mackey, D.C., & Wasnick, J.D. (2013). Ch 14 *Morgan & Mikhail's Clinical Anesthesiology* (5th ed.). New York, NY: McGraw-Hill.

240. What cardiac effect do you expect following administration of norepinephrine?

   (A) Decreased heart rate

   (B) Decreased mean arterial pressure

   (C) Increased heart rate

   (D) Decreased peripheral vascular resistance

   Rationale: Norepinephrine results in a decreased heart rate, increased mean arterial pressure and increased peripheral vascular resistance.
   Ref: Butterworth, J.F., Mackey, D.C., & Wasnick, J.D. (2013). Ch 14 *Morgan & Mikhail's Clinical Anesthesiology* (5th ed.). New York, NY: McGraw-Hill.

241. You are planning to use clonidine during a general anesthetic. Primary receptor selectivity for clonidine includes with of the following?

   (A) $Alpha_2$

   (B) $Beta_1$

   (C) $Beta_2$

   (D) $Alpha_1$

   Rationale: Receptor selectivity for clonidine is primarily $Alpha_2$. Mild $Alpha_1$ receptor selectivity exists. There is no beta receptor selectivity for clonidine.
   Ref: Butterworth, J.F., Mackey, D.C., & Wasnick, J.D. (2013). Ch 14 *Morgan & Mikhail's Clinical Anesthesiology* (5th ed.). New York, NY: McGraw-Hill.

242. Your patient is taking phenelzine. What is your primary concern when administering epinephrine to this patient?

   (A) Profound increase in heart rate

   (B) Lowered heart rate

   (C) Increased heart rate

   (D) Profound decrease in heart rate

   Rationale: When administering a catecholamine (epinephrine) to patients taking phenelzine (monoamine oxidase inhibitor) expect a profound cardiac response. Epinephrine is metabolized by monoamine oxidase and catechol-o-transferase.
   Ref: Butterworth, J.F., Mackey, D.C., & Wasnick, J.D. (2013). Ch 14 *Morgan & Mikhail's Clinical Anesthesiology* (5th ed.). New York, NY: McGraw-Hill.

243. You are administering an infusion of dopamine (0.5-3 μg/kg/min). What do you anticipate?

   (A) B_1 stimulation

   (B) DA_1 stimulation

   (C) $Alpha_1$ stimulation

   (D) B_2 stimulation

   Rationale: Lower doses of dopamine result in primarily dopaminergic receptor (DA_1) stimulation resulting renal vessel dilation. Higher doses (3-10 ug/kg/min) result in B$_1$ stimulation effects. Increases in peripheral vascular resistance with a decreased renal blood flow result due to Alpha$_1$ effects include dopamine administered in doses 10–20 ug/kg/min.

Ref: Butterworth, J.F., Mackey, D.C., & Wasnick, J.D. (2013). Ch 14 *Morgan & Mikhail's Clinical Anesthesiology* (5th ed.). New York, NY: McGraw-Hill.

244. A patient scheduled for an open bowel resection presents with congestive heart failure and well-documented coronary artery disease. You note the patient's heart rate is 98. Which of the following adrenergic agonists would be the best choice for this patient?

(A) Dobutamine
(B) Esmolol
(C) Phentolamine
(D) Norepinephrine

Rationale: Dobutamine improves cardiac output and assists in balancing myocardial oxygen consumption particularly in tachycardic patients or those with increased peripheral vascular resistance. While peripheral vasoconstriction and an increased blood pressure occur when using norepinephrine, an increased afterload and reflex bradycardia result. Cardiac output is not improved. Phentolamine is an alpha blocker. Esmolol is a short-acting beta blocker.

Ref: Butterworth, J.F., Mackey, D.C., & Wasnick, J.D. (2013). Ch 14 *Morgan & Mikhail's Clinical Anesthesiology* (5th ed.). New York, NY: McGraw-Hill.

245. A patient presents for removal of a pheochromocytoma. Preoperatively, which medication is most useful?

(A) Phenoxybenzamine
(B) Labetalol
(C) Esmolol
(D) Norepinephrine

Rationale: Lowering the blood pressure prior to surgery is a goal for patients presenting with a pheochromocytoma. Preoperatively, the most frequently used alpha$_1$-antagonist for patients with a pheochromocytoma is phenoxybenzamine. Phenoxybenzamine is effective in lowering blood pressure due to reversal of vasoconstriction associated with tumor secreting epinephrine and norepinephrine. Esmolol's ultra-short duration as well as minimal effect on blood pressure makes it a poor choice for blood pressure control. If the patient presents with tachycardia or ventricular

arrhythmias, a Beta$_1$ blocker (labetalol) may be useful. Norepinephrine exerts the opposite effect (increased blood pressure).

Ref: Butterworth, J.F., Mackey, D.C., & Wasnick, J.D. (2013). Ch 14 *Morgan & Mikhail's Clinical Anesthesiology* (5th ed.). New York, NY: McGraw-Hill.

246. During metabolism of nitrates (nitroglycerin and sodium nitroprusside) what substance is released?

(A) Guanylyl cyclase
(B) cGMP
(C) Nitric oxide
(D) Nitrate

Rationale: Metabolism of nitrates result in release of nitric oxide. Nitric oxide activates guanylyl cyclase which synthesizes cyclic guanosine. Nitric oxide is responsible for the vasodilatory effects of nitrates. Production of nitrate may lead to conversion of hemoglobin to methemoglobin.

Ref: Butterworth, J.F., Mackey, D.C., & Wasnick, J.D. (2013). Ch 15 *Morgan & Mikhail's Clinical Anesthesiology* (5th ed.). New York, NY: McGraw-Hill.

247. You are infusing sodium nitroprusside at 3 ug/kg/min. What condition is likely to result?

(A) Cyanide toxicity
(B) Adsorption of polyvinylchloride
(C) Increased afterload
(D) Cerebral vessel constriction

Rationale: Nitroprusside in doses greater than 500 ug/kg or infusions faster than 2 ug/kg/min are associated with cyanide toxicity. Tubing and glass containers specific for the administration of nitroglycerin are used to avoid adsorption of nitroglycerin to polyvinylchloride. Administration of sodium nitroprusside results in reduced preload and afterload as well as cerebral vessel dilation.

Ref: Butterworth, J.F., Mackey, D.C., & Wasnick, J.D. (2013). Ch 15 *Morgan & Mikhail's Clinical Anesthesiology* (5th ed.). New York, NY: McGraw-Hill.

248. During esophageal surgery, the endotracheal tube catches fire. What will you do first?

(A) Call for help.
(B) Remove the endotracheal tube.
(C) Stop the gas flow and remove the endotracheal tube.
(D) Remove the surgical drapes.

Rationale: Rapidly stopping the gas flow (oxidizers) and removing the endotracheal tube is essential when an airway fire occurs. Removing surgical drapes after turning off gases is needed when a fire involves the patient's body.

Ref: Butterworth, J.F., Mackey, D.C., & Wasnick, J.D. (2013). Ch 3 *Morgan & Mikhail's Clinical Anesthesiology* (5th ed.). New York, NY: McGraw-Hill.

249. The patient with rheumatoid arthritis complains of long-term throbbing joint pain. Which fibers are activated?

    (A) Efferent A and C fibers
    (B) Alpha and Beta efferent fibers
    (C) Afferent A and C fibers
    (D) Alpha and Beta afferent fibers

    Rationale: As compared to peripheral nerve injury that results in shooting or burning pain, tissue injury or inflammation results in throbbing or aching pain. A and C afferent fibers are activated with tissue injury and inflammation. With nerve injuries, alpha and beta afferent fibers are activated.

    Ref: Butterworth, J.F., Mackey, D.C., & Wasnick, J.D. (2013). Ch 47 *Morgan & Mikhail's Clinical Anesthesiology* (5th ed.). New York, NY: McGraw-Hill.

    Brunton, L.L., Chabner, B.A., & Knollmann, B.C. (Eds) (2010). Ch 18 *Goodman & Gilman's The Pharmacological Basis of Therapeutics* (12th ed.). New York, NY: McGraw-Hill.

250. Why is the primary metabolite of tramadol significant?

    (A) Greater potency than the parent drug
    (B) Shorter elimination half-life than the parent drug
    (C) Respiratory depression is not reversible with naloxone
    (D) Safety profile when using MAO inhibitors

    Rationale: Tramadol's O-demethylated metabolite possesses greater potency than the parent drug. The elimination half-life is 7.5 hours as compared to the parent drug (6 hours). Naloxone is used effectively to reverse respiratory depression but my not entirely reverse analgesia. Tramadol should be avoided for patients taking MAO inhibitors or SSRIs due to the propensity for seizures.

    Ref: Hemmings, H.C., & Egan, T.D. (2013). *Pharmacology and Physiology for Anesthesia: Foundations and Clinical Application*. Philadelphia, PA: Elsevier.

Brunton, L.L., Chabner, B.A., & Knollmann, B.C. (Eds) (2010). Ch 18 *Goodman & Gilman's The Pharmacological Basis of Therapeutics* (12th ed.). New York, NY: McGraw-Hill.

251. Following general anesthesia for right should arthroscopy, the patient complains of pain. The patient's history includes congestive heart failure. Which analgesic will you avoid?

    (A) Butorphanol
    (B) Morphine
    (C) Demerol
    (D) Nalbuphine

    Rationale: Cardiac effects following administration of butorphanol include increased pulmonary artery pressure and decreased systemic arterial pressure. It is generally avoided in patients with a history of myocardial infarction or congestive heart failure. Comparatively, morphine, demerol, and nalbuphine administration results in fewer cardiac effects.

    Ref: Brunton, L.L., Chabner, B.A., & Knollmann, B.C. (Eds) (2010). Ch 18 *Goodman & Gilman's The Pharmacological Basis of Therapeutics* (12th ed.). New York, NY: McGraw-Hill.

252. Which two drugs would you avoid in an asthmatic patient?

    Select (2) two
    (A) Volatile anesthetics
    (B) Labetalol
    (C) Morphine
    (D) Lidocaine

    Rationale: Morphine can release histamine which could cause bronchoconstriction and labetalol can produce bronchoconstriction related to the B_2 blocking effects.

    Ref: Nagelhout, J.J., & Plaus, K. L., (2014). Ch 26 *Nurse Anesthesia* (5th ed.). St. Louis, MO: Elsevier.

253. You decide to give butorphanol 2 mg to the patient postoperatively. What is the equipotent dose of morphine?

    (A) 100 mg
    (B) 8 mg
    (C) 10 mg
    (D) 80 mg

Rationale: The equipotent dose of morphine is 10 mg or demerol 80 to 100 mg.
Ref: Brunton, L.L., Chabner, B.A., & Knollmann, B.C. (Eds) (2010). Ch 18 *Goodman & Gilman's The Pharmacological Basis of Therapeutics* (12th ed.). New York, NY: McGraw-Hill.

254. Your patient has a history of asthma. Which opioid will you avoid?

   (A) Fentanyl
   (B) Morphine
   (C) Remifentanil
   (D) Tramadol

Rationale: Morphine releases histamine and is contraindicated for patients with asthma. Tramadol and fentanyl and derivatives do not release histamine.
Ref: Butterworth, J.F., Mackey D.C., & Wasnick, J.D. (2013). Ch 10 *Morgan & Mikhail's Clinical Anesthesiology* (5th ed.). New York, NY: McGraw-Hill.
Brunton, L.L., Chabner, B.A., & Knollmann, B.C. (Eds) (2010). Ch 18 *Goodman & Gilman's The Pharmacological Basis of Therapeutics* (12th ed.). New York, NY: McGraw-Hill.

255. How is remifentanil metabolized?

   (A) Hepatic cytochrome P
   (B) Hydrolysis by esterase enzymes
   (C) Hepatic conjugation
   (D) Conjugation with glucuronic acid

Rationale: The majority of opioids are metabolized in the liver. Metabolic processes include conjugation, Cytochrome P, or a combination. Remifentanil is the exception, whereby metabolism undergoes hydrolysis in the blood and tissue.
Ref: Butterworth, J.F., Mackey, D.C., & Wasnick, J.D. (2013). Ch 10 *Morgan & Mikhail's Clinical Anesthesiology* (5th ed.). New York, NY: McGraw-Hill.
Nagelhout, J.J., & K.L., Plaus.(2014) Ch 11 *Nurse Anesthesia* (5th ed.). St. Louis, MO: Elsevier.

256. How does digoxin control atrial arrhythmias?

   (A) Enhancing vagal tone
   (B) Addition of calcium
   (C) Decreased intracellular sodium
   (D) Decreasing vagal tone

Rationale: Vagal effects result in decreased heart rate, prolonged AV conduction, slowed impulse through the AV node, and a prolonged effective refractory period. Because of the vagal effects it is used to control atrial arrhythmias.
Ref: Nagelhout, J.J., & Plaus, K.L. (2014) Ch 13 *Nurse Anesthesia* (5th ed.). St. Louis, MO: Elsevier.

257. Your patient is undergoing a cholecystectomy with general endotracheal anesthesia. The patient takes digoxin for chronic congestive heart failure. What is the first sign of digitalis toxicity under anesthesia?

   (A) Bradycardia
   (B) Hypotension
   (C) Arrhythmias
   (D) Hypertension

Rationale: Signs and symptoms associated with digitalis toxicity include headache, CNS dysfunction, diarrhea, nausea and vomiting, fatigue, and arrhythmias. Specifically, when a patient is anesthetized premature ventricular contractions may be the first sign of digitalis toxicity.
Ref: Nagelhout, J.J., & Plaus, K.L. (2014) Ch 13 *Nurse Anesthesia* (5th ed.). St. Louis, MO: Elsevier Saunders.
Brunton, L.L., Chabner, B.A., & Knollmann, B.C. (Eds) (2010). Ch 18 *Goodman & Gilman's The Pharmacological Basis of Therapeutics* (12th ed.). New York, NY: McGraw-Hill.

258. What medication is indicated for treatment of ventricular fibrillation?

   (A) Vasopressin
   (B) Verapamil
   (C) Ibutilide
   (D) Adenosine

Rationale: Vasopressin may be used in place of epinephrine for treatment of ventricular fibrillation. Verapamil is indicated for rate control in atrial flutter, atrial fibrillation and for stopping paroxysmal supraventricular tachycardia. For cardioversion of atrial fibrillation or atrial flutter, ibutilide is used. Adenosine is used to treat stable supraventricular tachycardia, narrow and wide-complex tachycardias.
Ref: Butterworth, J.F., Mackey, D.C., & Wasnick, J.D. (2013). Ch 55 *Morgan & Mikhail's Clinical Anesthesiology* (5th ed.). New York, NY: McGraw-Hill.

259. Why is terbutaline preferred for the treatment of asthma over isoetharine?

(A) Isoetharine B_1 adrenergic activity is less than terbutaline.

(B) Either bronchodilator is acceptable.

(C) Terbutaline's B_1 adrenergic activity is less than isoetharine.

(D) Isoetharine B_2 activity is greater than terbutaline.

Rationale: The preference for using terbutaline is due to more selective beta$_2$ activity. Bronkosol's increased B_1 activity makes it less useful than terbutaline.

Ref: Butterworth, J.F., Mackey, D.C., & Wasnick, J.D. (2013). Ch 24 *Morgan & Mikhail's Clinical Anesthesiology* (5th ed.). New York, NY: McGraw-Hill.

260. During the preoperative interview you learn the patient takes daily lithium. How will lithium affect drugs used for general anesthesia?

(A) Shorten the duration of action of vecuronium.

(B) Increase the MAC of isoflurane.

(C) Increase the duration of action of vecuronium.

(D) No interaction with lithium exists for drugs used during general anesthesia.

Rationale: Lithium decreases MAC and increases the duration of action of neuromuscular blockers. Neuromuscular monitoring is essential.

Ref: Butterworth, J.F., Mackey, D.C., & Wasnick, J.D. (2013). Ch 24 *Morgan & Mikhail's Clinical Anesthesiology* (5th ed.). New York, NY: Lange Medical Books McGraw-Hill.

Brunton, L.L., Chabner, B.A., & Knollmann, B.C. (Eds) (2010). Ch 18 *Goodman & Gilman's The Pharmacological Basis of Therapeutics* (12th ed.). New York, NY: McGraw-Hill.

261. In reviewing the patient's record, you note daily use of lithium and hydrochlorothiazide. What do you expect?

(A) Hypernatremia

(B) Therapeutic lithium levels

(C) Decrease lithium levels

(D) Hyponatremia

Rationale: Patient concomitantly taking lithium and a loop or thiazide diuretic may experience lithium toxicity. Lithium toxicity results from hyponatremia that decreases renal excretion of lithium. Due to the lithium's narrow therapeutic range (0.8-1.0 mEq/L), preoperative lithium levels should be checked.

Ref: Butterworth, J.F., Mackey, D.C., & Wasnick, J.D. (2013). Ch 28 *Morgan & Mikhail's Clinical Anesthesiology* (5th ed.). New York, NY: Lange Medical Books McGraw-Hill.

Brunton, L.L., Chabner, B.A., & Knollmann, B.C. (Eds) (2010). Ch 18 *Goodman & Gilman's The Pharmacological Basis of Therapeutics* (12th ed.). New York, NY: McGraw-Hill.

262. You are called for an emergency exploratory laparoscopy. The patient was involved in a motor vehicle accident and appears intoxicated. What do you expect?

(A) Increased requirements for fentanyl

(B) Decreased requirements for midazolam

(C) Increased requirements for sodium pentothal

(D) Decreased requirements for amphetamines

Rationale: The patient is acutely intoxicated. Acute intoxication results in decreased requirements for opioids, barbiturates, benzodiazepines, and phencyclidine derivatives. By comparison patients with chronic alcoholism require higher requirements for opioids, barbiturates, and benzodiazepines.

TABLE 1-15. Effect of acute and chronic substance abuse on anesthetic requirements.[1]

Substance	Acute	Chronic
Opioids	↓	↑
Barbiturates	↓	↑
Alcohol	↓	↑
Marijuana	↓	0
Benzodiazepines	↓	↑
Amphetamines	↑[2]	↓
Cocaine	↑[2]	0
Phencyclidine	↓	?

[1] ↓, decreases; ↑, increases; 0, no effect; ?, unknown.
[2] Associated with marked sympathetic stimulation.

Ref: Butterworth, J.F., Mackey, D.C., & Wasnick, J.D. (2013). Ch 28 *Morgan & Mikhail's Clinical Anesthesiology* (5th ed.). New York, NY: McGraw-Hill.

Brunton, L.L., Chabner, B.A., & Knollmann, B.C. (Eds) (2010). Ch 16 *Goodman & Gilman's The Pharmacological Basis of Therapeutics* (12th ed.). New York, NY: McGraw-Hill.

263. Why do patients who take tranylcypromine need to avoid eating cheese?

(A) Hypotensive crisis due to tyramine

(B) Decreased agitation

(C) Hypertensive crisis due to tyramine

(D) Jaundice

Rationale: Tyramine containing foods such as cheese and red wine, may result in a hypertensive crisis secondary to generation of norepinephrine for patients taking MAO inhibitors (tranylcypromine). Side effects of MAO inhibitors may include orthostatic hypotension, increased agitation, jaundice, urinary retention, muscle spasms, tremors, and seizures.
Ref: Butterworth, J.F., Mackey, D.C., & Wasnick, J.D. (2013). Ch 28 *Morgan & Mikhail's Clinical Anesthesiology* (5th ed.). New York, NY: McGraw-Hill.
Brunton, L.L., Chabner, B.A., & Knollmann, B.C. (Eds) (2010). Ch 16 *Goodman & Gilman's The Pharmacological Basis of Therapeutics* (12th ed.). New York, NY: McGraw-Hill.

264. Which narcotic will you avoid in patients taking MAO inhibitors?

(A) Demerol
(B) Fentanyl
(C) Morphine
(D) Sufentanil

Rationale: Administration of demerol to patients taking MAO inhibitors may result in hyperthermia, seizures, coma and death. All narcotics should be used with caution for patients taking MAO inhibitors.
Ref: Butterworth, J.F., Mackey, D.C., & Wasnick, J.D. (2013). Ch 28 *Morgan & Mikhail's Clinical Anesthesiology* (5th ed.). New York, NY: McGraw-Hill.
Brunton, L.L., Chabner, B.A., & Knollmann, B.C. (Eds) (2010). Ch 16 *Goodman & Gilman's The Pharmacological Basis of Therapeutics* (12th ed.). New York, NY: McGraw-Hill.
Nagelhout, J.J., & Plaus, K.L. (2014). Ch 11 *Nurse Anesthesia* (5th ed.). St. Louis, MO: Elsevier.

265. Which of the follow medications does not prolong the QT interval?

(A) Fluoxetine
(B) Sertraline
(C) Azithromycin
(D) Gentamicin

Rationale: Classifications of psychiatric drugs known to prolong the QT interval include butyrophenones, phenothiazines, antipsychotics, and SSRIs (fluoxetine, sertraline). Antibiotic classifications associated with prolonging the QT interval include macrolides (azithromycin). Gentamicin, an aminoglycoside, may cause auditory dysfunction.

Ref: Butterworth, J.F., Mackey, D.C., & Wasnick, J.D. (2013). Ch 28 *Morgan & Mikhail's Clinical Anesthesiology* (5th ed.). New York, NY: McGraw-Hill.
Nagelhout, J.J., & Plaus, K.L. (2014). Ch 54 *Nurse Anesthesia* (5th ed.). St. Louis, MO: Elsevier.

266. When treating hypotension for a patient taking doxepin what will you use?

(A) Neosynephrine 10 ug IV
(B) Ephedrine 5 mg IV
(C) Neosynephrine 100 ug IV
(D) Ephedrine 10 mg IV

Rationale: Doxepin, a tricyclic antidepressant, results in an exaggerated response when given indirect-acting vasopressors or sympathetic stimulants. Small doses of direct acting vasopressors (neosynephrine) are the appropriate treatment for hypotension.
Ref: Butterworth, J.F., Mackey, D.C., & Wasnick, J.D. (2013). Ch 28 *Morgan & Mikhail's Clinical Anesthesiology* (5th ed.). New York, NY: McGraw-Hill.

267. Your patient is taking Amitriptyline. What will you tell your patient about taking this drug?

(A) Continue taking Amitriptyline preoperatively.
(B) Stop taking Amitryptyline 24 hours before surgery.
(C) Stop taking Amitriptyline 1 week before surgery.
(D) Stop taking Amitryptiline 2 weeks before surgery.

Rationale: Amitriptyline (Elavil) is a tricyclic antidepressant. Informing the patient to take continue taking the medication will avoid possible cholinergic symptoms, cardiac arrhythmias, and extrapyramidal side effects.
Ref: Butterworth, J.F., Mackey, D.C., & Wasnick, J.D. (2013). Ch 28 *Morgan & Mikhail's Clinical Anesthesiology* (5th ed.). New York, NY: McGraw-Hill.
Nagelhout, J.J., & Plaus, K.L. (2014). Ch 19 & 51 *Nurse Anesthesia* (5th ed.). St. Louis, MO: Elsevier.
Brunton, L.L., Chabner, B.A., & Knollmann, B.C. (Eds) (2010). Ch 16 *Goodman & Gilman's The Pharmacological Basis of Therapeutics* (12th ed.). New York, NY: McGraw-Hill.

268. Contractions weaken despite use of oxytocin. Prostaglandin is administered. What do you expect?

(A) Constipation
(B) Hypotension
(C) Headache
(D) Bronchodilation

Rationale: Side effects of prostaglandin (Hemabate or Carboprost) may result in diarrhea, nausea, and vomiting and bronchoconstriction. Hypotension results due to vascular relaxation of smooth muscle.

Ref: Butterworth, J.F., Mackey, D.C., & Wasnick, J.D. (2013). Ch 40 *Morgan & Mikhail's Clinical Anesthesiology* (5th ed.). New York, NY: McGraw-Hill.

Nagelhout, J.J., & Plaus, K.L. (2014). Ch 46 *Nurse Anesthesia* (5th ed.). St. Louis, MO: Elsevier.

269. The patient is scheduled for a cesarean section. You plan to use sevoflurane. How will this choice affect the uterus?

   (A) Increase uterine constriction
   (B) Decrease uterine bleeding
   (C) Increase uterine relaxation
   (D) Inhalational agents have no effect on the uterus.

Rationale: Volatile anesthetics relax the uterus. For this reason, decrease the concentration to 0.5 MAC.

Ref: Butterworth, J.F., Mackey, D.C., & Wasnick, J.D. (2013). Ch 40 *Morgan & Mikhail's Clinical Anesthesiology* (5th ed.). New York, NY: McGraw-Hill.

270. Dantrolene was administered for malignant hyperthermia. What is the most serious complication?

   (A) Respiratory insufficiency
   (B) Aspiration pneumonia
   (C) Hepatic dysfunction
   (D) Generalized muscle weakness

Rationale: Generalized muscle weakness may result in respiratory insufficiency and aspiration pneumonia. It is also associated with hepatic dysfunction.

Ref: Butterworth, J.F., Mackey, D.C., & Wasnick, J.D. (2013). Ch 52 *Morgan & Mikhail's Clinical Anesthesiology* (5th ed.). New York, NY: McGraw-Hill.

Nagelhout, J.J., & Plaus, K.L. (2014). Ch 32 *Nurse Anesthesia* (5th ed.). St. Louis, MO: Elsevier Saunders.

271. What is the result of an excess of glucocorticoids?

   (A) Cushing's syndrome
   (B) Addison's disease
   (C) Conn syndrome
   (D) Pheochromocytoma

Rationale: Excess production or administration of glucocorticoids results in Cushing's syndrome. A deficiency of glucocorticoids results in Addison's disease. Conn syndrome is caused by increased aldosterone (mineralocorticoid) whereas an excess in catecholamines results in a pheochromocytoma.

Ref: Butterworth, J.F., Mackey, D.C., & Wasnick, J.D. (2013). Ch 34 *Morgan & Mikhail's Clinical Anesthesiology* (5th ed.). New York, NY: McGraw-Hill.

Nagelhout, J.J., & Plaus, K.L. (2014). Ch 33 *Nurse Anesthesia* (5th ed.). St. Louis, MO: Elsevier.

272. What is the most effective treatment for moderate to severe Parkinson's disease?

   (A) Levodopa
   (B) Non-ergot derivatives
   (C) Levodopa with a decarboxylase inhibitor
   (D) Dopamine receptor agonists

Rationale: Levodopa given with a decarboxylase inhibitor increases the central delivery and allows for decreased doses of Levodopa. Dopamine receptor agonists including ergot and nonergot derivatives are useful. Nonergot derivatives are used in early Parkinson's disease treatment.

Ref: Butterworth, J.F., Mackey, D.C., & Wasnick, J.D. (2013). Ch 28 *Morgan & Mikhail's Clinical Anesthesiology* (5th ed.). New York, NY: McGraw-Hill.

273. The patient is scheduled for a thoracotomy. Upon review of the patient's medical history you note lovastatin as part of the medical management. What will you tell the patient preoperatively?

   (A) Take the statin as directed prior to surgery.
   (B) Stop the statin immediately.
   (C) Stop the statin 1 week prior to surgery.
   (D) Stop the statin 2 weeks prior to surgery.

Rationale: Anti-lipid lowering medications offer benefits for patients undergoing surgery that include decreasing the length of hospital stay, stroke, MI, renal dysfunction, and death. The anti-inflammatory effects, stabilizing atherosclerotic plaquing and improved endothelial function offer benefit to high-risk surgical patients. Stopping statins prior to surgery may result in a rebound effect.

Ref: Nagelhout, J.J., & Plaus, K.L. (2014). Ch 19 *Nurse Anesthesia* (5th ed.). St. Louis, MO: Elsevier.

Miller, R.D., & Pardo, M.C. (2011). Ch 13 *Basics of Anesthesia* (6th ed.). Philadelphia, PA: Elsevier.

Hines, R.L., & Marschall K.E. (2012). Ch 1 *Stoelting's Anesthesia and Co-Existing Disease* (6th ed.). Philadelphia, PA: Elsevier.

274. What is the percent of total body water in the intracellular compartment?

(A) 25%

(B) 8%

(C) 100%

(D) 67%

Rationale: The total body water in the extracellular compartment is comprised of 25% interstitial and 8% intravascular. The total body water of the intracellular compartment is 67%.

TABLE 1-16. Body fluid compartments (based on average 70-kg male).

Compartment	Fluid as Percent Body Weight (%)	Total Body Water (%)	Fluid Volume (L)
Intracellular	40	67	28
Extracellular			
Interstitial	15	25	10.5
Intravascular	5	8	3.5
Total	60	100	42

Ref: Butterworth, J.F., Mackey, D.C., & Wasnick, J.D. (2013). Ch 49 *Morgan & Mikhail's Clinical Anesthesiology* (5th ed.). New York, NY: McGraw-Hill.
Nagelhout, J.J., & Plaus, K.L. (2014). Ch 20 *Nurse Anesthesia* (5th ed.). St. Louis, MO: Elsevier.

275. What is the major extracellular cation?

(A) Sodium

(B) Potassium

(C) Magnesium

(D) Chloride

Rationale: The major intracellular cation is potassium whereas sodium is the major extracellular cation. Magnesium comprises about 50% of the intracellular compartment as compared to potassium. The

anion chloride comprises approximately 60% of the extracellular compartment.

Ref: Butterworth, J.F., Mackey, D.C., & Wasnick, J.D. (2013). Ch 49 *Morgan & Mikhail's Clinical Anesthesiology* (5th ed.). New York, NY: McGraw-Hill.
Nagelhout, J.J., & Plaus, K.L. (2014). Ch 20 *Nurse Anesthesia* (5th ed.). St. Louis, MO: Elsevier.

276. What substance poorly penetrates through the capillary endothelium?

(A) Oxygen

(B) Water

(C) Lipid-soluble substances

(D) Plasma proteins

Rationale: Oxygen, water, lipid-soluble freely as well as low molecular weight substances (sodium, chloride, potassium, and glucose) penetrate the capillary endothelium. High molecular weight substances (plasma proteins) poorly penetrate the endothelial clefts.

Ref: Butterworth, J.F., Mackey, D.C., & Wasnick, J.D. (2013). Ch 49 *Morgan & Mikhail's Clinical Anesthesiology* (5th ed.). New York, NY: McGraw-Hill.
Nagelhout, J.J., & Plaus, K.L. (2014). Ch 20 *Nurse Anesthesia* (5th ed.). St. Louis, MO: Elsevier.

277. At what value do serious complications of hyponatremia manifest?

(A) 150 mEq/L

(B) 145 mEq/L

(C) 130 mEq/L

(D) 120 mEq/L

Rationale: Hypernatremia is sodium >145 mEq/L where as hyponatremia is sodium <135 mEq/L. Severe hyponatremia (<120 mEq/L) manifests neurologically with cerebral edema, confusion, seizures, coma, and death.

TABLE 1-17. The composition of fluid compartments.

	Gram-Molecular Weight	Intracellular (mEq/L)	Extracellular	
			Intravascular (mEq/L)	Interstitial (mEq/L)
Sodium	23.0	10	145	142
Potassium	39.1	140	4	4
Calcium	40.1	<1	3	3
Magnesium	24.3	50	2	2
Chloride	35.5	4	105	110
Bicarbonate	61.0	10	24	28
Phosphorus	31.0[1]	75	2	2
Protein (g/dL)		16	7	2

[1]PO_4^{3-} is 95 g.

Ref: Butterworth, J.F., Mackey, D.C., & Wasnick, J.D. (2013). Ch 49 *Morgan & Mikhail's Clinical Anesthesiology* (5th ed.). New York, NY: McGraw-Hill.

Nagelhout, J.J., & Plaus, K.L. (2014). Ch 20 *Nurse Anesthesia* (5th ed.). St. Louis, MO: Elsevier.

278. The patient presents for surgery and you note a potassium level of 6 mEq/L. You choose to administer calcium gluconate. Which drug interaction is most concerning for this patient when administering potassium?

    (A) Digoxin
    (B) Furosemide
    (C) Kayexalate
    (D) Sodium polystyrene sulfonate

    Rationale: Digoxin toxicity is potentiated by calcium. Furosemide, kayexalate, and sodium bicarbonate assist with decreasing potassium.

    Ref: Butterworth, J.F., Mackey, D.C., & Wasnick, J.D. (2013). Ch 49 *Morgan & Mikhail's Clinical Anesthesiology* (5th ed.). New York, NY: McGraw-Hill.

279. The patient presents with hypercalcemia secondary to a malignancy. What is the most effective means for lower serum calcium?

    (A) A loop diuretic followed by rehydration
    (B) Bisphosphonate
    (C) Rehydration followed by a loop diuretic
    (D) Etidronate

    Rationale: Rehydrate the patient first. Giving the loop diuretic first will worsen hypovolemia and the hypercalcemia. Bisphosphonate and etidronate may be used to lower calcium levels.

    Ref: Butterworth, J.F., Mackey, D.C., & Wasnick, J.D. (2013). Ch 49 *Morgan & Mikhail's Clinical Anesthesiology* (5th ed.). New York, NY: McGraw-Hill.

    Nagelhout, J.J., & Plaus, K.L. (2014). Ch 20 *Nurse Anesthesia* (5th ed.). St. Louis, MO: Elsevier.

280. What target range is required for therapeutic effects of heparin?

    (A) ACT 200 to 400 seconds
    (B) aPTT 1.5-2.5 times the control value
    (C) ACT 100-200 seconds
    (D) aPTT 2.5-3.5 times the control value

    Rationale: The aPTT is typically used to determine a therapeutic range for heparin. Activated Coagulation Time (ACT) is also available with values above 400 to 800 seconds.

    Ref: Hemmings, H, & Egan, T. (2013). Ch 37 *Pharmacology and Physiology for Anesthesia: Foundations and Clinical Application*. Philadelphia, PA: Elsevier.

281. Which statement is false regarding low molecular weight heparins (LMWHs)?

    (A) LMWHs prevent formation of prothrombinase.
    (B) Thrombolytic doses do not significantly cross the placenta.
    (C) Bioavailability is greater with LMWHs as compared to heparin.
    (D) Protamine is the antidote of choice for LMWHs.

    Rationale: Protamine reverses the effects of heparin. There is no antidote for LMWHs.

    Ref: Butterworth, J.F., Mackey, D.C., & Wasnick, J.D. (2013). Ch 24 *Morgan & Mikhail's Clinical Anesthesiology* (5th ed.). New York, NY: McGraw-Hill.

    Hemmings, H, & Egan, T. (2013). Ch 37 *Pharmacology and Physiology for Anesthesia: Foundations and Clinical Application*. Philadelphia, PA: Elsevier.

282. The patient is taking subcutaneous unfractionated heparin. When is the best time to administer a spinal anesthetic?

    (A) 4-6 hours after heparin administration
    (B) 2-4 hours after heparin administration
    (C) 12-24 hours after heparin administration
    (D) 6 to 8 hours after heparin administration

    Rationale: For patients taking unfractionated heparin, it is advisable to wait 6 to 8 hours before proceeding with a regional anesthetic technique. For patients taking low molecular weight heparin, wait 12 to 24 hours.

    Ref: Butterworth, J.F., Mackey, D.C., & Wasnick, J.D. (2013). Ch 24 *Morgan & Mikhail's Clinical Anesthesiology* (5th ed.). New York, NY: McGraw-Hill.

    Hemmings, H, & Egan, T. (2013). Ch 37 *Pharmacology and Physiology for Anesthesia: Foundations and Clinical Application*. Philadelphia, PA: Elsevier.

283. What test is used to measure the effect of warfarin on blood coagulation?

    (A) aPTT
    (B) ACT
    (C) AT
    (D) INR

Rationale: The aPTT and ACT determine the therapeutic range of heparin. The INR or PT measure the effect of warfarin on blood coagulation. Antithrombin (AT) is the plasma co-factor needed to exert anticoagulation action by heparin.

Ref: Hemmings, H. & Egan, T. (2013). Ch 37 *Pharmacology and Physiology for Anesthesia: Foundations and Clinical Application.* Philadelphia, PA: Elsevier.

284. How does renal impairment affect insulin requirements?

    (A) Insulin requirements decrease.

    (B) No relationship exists between insulin requirements and renal impairment.

    (C) Insulin requirements increase.

    (D) The kidneys break down insulin to a greater extent.

    Rationale: Insulin is broken down in the liver, kidneys, and muscle. For patients with renal disease, the insulin requirements decrease.

    Ref: Butterworth, J.F., Mackey, D.C., & Wasnick, J.D. (2013). Ch 34 *Morgan & Mikhail's Clinical Anesthesiology* (5th ed.). New York, NY: McGraw-Hill.

    Hemmings, H, & Egan, T. (2013). Ch 31 *Pharmacology and Physiology for Anesthesia: Foundations and Clinical Application.* Philadelphia, PA: Elsevier.

285. What oral hypoglycemic is relatively contraindicated for patients with renal impairment?

    (A) Glyburide

    (B) Glipizide

    (C) Tolbutamide

    (D) Metformin

Rationale: First generation sulfonylureas (Tolbutamide) are used cautiously for patient with renal disease. Second generation sulfonylureas are better suited for patients with renal disease. Metformin, a biguanide, is relatively contraindicated for patients with renal disease due to unchanged urinary excretion.

Ref: Butterworth, J.F., Mackey, D.C., & Wasnick, J.D. (2013). Ch 34 *Morgan & Mikhail's Clinical Anesthesiology* (5th ed.). New York, NY: McGraw-Hill.

Hemmings, H, & Egan, T. (2013). Ch 31 *Pharmacology and Physiology for Anesthesia: Foundations and Clinical Application.* Philadelphia, PA: Elsevier.

286. A patient with preexisting hypertension is undergoing an exploratory laparotomy. The blood pressure increases intraoperatively. What will you do first?

    (A) Give esmolol

    (B) Increase the concentration of isoflurane

    (C) Give labetalol

    (D) Decrease the concentration of isoflurane

    Rationale: Deepening the anesthetic typically precedes pharmacological intervention.

    Ref: Butterworth, J.F., Mackey, D.C., & Wasnick, J.D. (2013). Ch 21 *Morgan & Mikhail's Clinical Anesthesiology* (5th ed.). New York, NY: McGraw-Hill.

287. A patient states they take nitroglycerin for angina. What statement is true regarding nitroglycerin's effect on the heart?

    (A) Decreases preload

    (B) Increases afterload

    (C) Increases preload

    (D) Decreases coronary vasodilatation

    Rationale: Patients taking nitrates for angina benefit due to decreasing preload and afterload as well as dilating the coronary and systemic circulation.

TABLE 1-18. Comparison of antianginal agents.[1]

Cardiac Parameter	Nitrates	Verapamil	Nifedipine Nicardipine Nimodipine	Diltiazem	β-Blockers
			Calcium Channel Blockers		
Preload	↓↓	—	—	—	—/↑
Afterload	↓	↓	↓↓	↓	—/↓
Contractility	—	↓↓	—	↓	↓↓↓
SA node automaticity	↑/—	↓↓	↑/—	↓↓	↓↓↓
AV conduction	—	↓↓↓	—	↓↓	↓↓↓
Vasodilatation					
Coronary	↑	↑↑	↑↑↑	↑↑	—/↓
Systemic	↑↑	↑	↑↑	↑	—/↓

[1]SA, sinoatrial; AV, atrioventricular; ↑, increases; —, no change; ↓, decreases.

Ref: Butterworth, J.F., Mackey, D.C., & Wasnick, J.D. (2013). Ch 21 *Morgan & Mikhail's Clinical Anesthesiology* (5th ed.). New York, NY: McGraw-Hill.

288. What patient history represents the greatest risk for cardiac complications?

(A) Recent angina

(B) Coronary artery disease involving two vessels

(C) History of MI 1 year ago

(D) Coronary artery disease involving three vessels

Rationale: Patients whose history includes extensive coronary artery disease involving three or more vessels or left main, recent history of myocardial infarction, or ventricular dysfunction pose the greatest risk for cardiac complications.

Ref: Butterworth, J.F., Mackey, D.C., & Wasnick, J.D. (2013). Ch 21 *Morgan & Mikhail's Clinical Anesthesiology* (5th ed.). New York, NY: McGraw-Hill.

289. What characterizes a second-degree burn?

Select (3) three

(A) Penetrate epidermis

(B) Blisters form

(C) Replace fluids for burns >20% of the total body surface area

(D) Full thickness

(E) Requires debridement

Rationale: First-degree burns do not penetrate the epidermis. In comparison, second-degree burns penetrate the epidermis with blister formation. Fluids are replaced for second-degree burns involving more than 20% of the total body surface area. Third-degree burns involve full thickness of the dermis requiring debridement and skin grafting.

Ref: Butterworth, J.F., Mackey, D.C., & Wasnick, J.D. (2013). Ch 39 *Morgan & Mikhail's Clinical Anesthesiology* (5th ed.). New York, NY: McGraw-Hill.

290. An adult male who weighs 100 kg is burned over 50% of his body. Using the Parkland formula, calculate the fluid requirements for the first 24 hours.
Answer: 20,000 mL

Rationale: The Parkland Formula is used to calculate the fluids needed for resuscitation of burn patients. The calculation includes 4 mL/kg × body weight × percent burned 4 × 100 × 50 = 20,000 mL

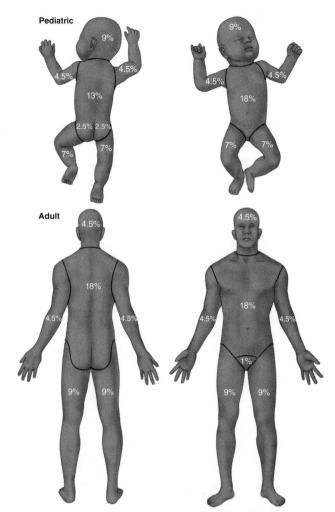

FIG. 1-7. The rule of nines, utilized to estimate burned surface area as a percentage of total body surface area (TBSA). (Reproduced, with permission, from American College of Surgeons: *ATLS: Advanced Trauma Life Support for Doctors (Student Course Manual)*, 9th ed. ACS, 2012.)

Ref: Butterworth, J.F., Mackey, D.C., & Wasnick, J.D. (2013). Ch 39 *Morgan & Mikhail's Clinical Anesthesiology* (5th ed.). New York, NY: McGraw-Hill.

291. Which of the following medications decrease the production of aqueous humor in glaucoma patients?

Select (2) two

(A) Pilocarpine

(B) Timolol

(C) Acetazolamide

(D) Echothiophate

Rationale: Beta blockers (Timolol, betaxolol) and carbonic anhydrase inhibitors (acetazolamide, dorzolamide) aid glaucoma patients by decreasing the production of aqueous humor. Pilocarpine is a cholinergic agonist biotic used for pupillary constriction.

Echothiophate, a cholinesterase inhibitor, is useful for patients with glaucoma. The drug causes miosis that improves the outflow of aqueous humor.

Ref: Nagelhout, J.J., & Plaus, K.L. (2014). Ch 39 *Nurse Anesthesia* (5th ed.). St. Louis, MO: Elsevier.

292. What signs and symptoms are associated with acute opioid intoxication?

    Select (2) two

    (A) Tachypnea
    (B) Hypotension
    (C) Dilated pupils
    (D) Pinpoint pupils

    Rationale: Acute opioid use is associated with respiratory depression, hypotension, euphoria, bradycardia, pinpoint pupils, and marked decreased consciousness.

    Ref: Butterworth, J.F., Mackey, D.C., & Wasnick, J.D. (2013). Ch 28 *Morgan & Mikhail's Clinical Anesthesiology* (5th ed.). New York, NY: McGraw-Hill.
    Nagelhout, J.J., & Plaus, K.L. (2014). Ch 19 *Nurse Anesthesia* (5th ed.). St. Louis, MO: Elsevier.

293. How does chronic alcohol ingestion affect anesthetic requirements including central nervous system hypnotics?

    (A) Decreases requirements
    (B) Increases requirements
    (C) No effect on anesthetic requirements
    (D) No affect with central nervous system hypnotics

    Rationale: Acute ingestion of alcohol decreases anesthetic requirements whereas chronic ingestion increases the requirements due to tolerance.

TABLE 1-19. Effect of acute and chronic substance abuse on anesthetic requirements.[1]

Substance	Acute	Chronic
Opioids	↓	↑
Barbiturates	↓	↑
Alcohol	↓	↑
Marijuana	↓	0
Benzodiazepines	↓	↑
Amphetamines	↑[2]	↓
Cocaine	↑[2]	0
Phencyclidine	↓	?

[1] ↓, decreases; ↑, increases; 0, no effect; ?, unknown.
[2] Associated with marked sympathetic stimulation.

Ref: Butterworth, J.F., Mackey, D.C., & Wasnick, J.D. (2013). Ch 28 *Morgan & Mikhail's Clinical Anesthesiology* (5th ed.). New York, NY: McGraw-Hill.
Nagelhout, J.J., & Plaus, K.L. (2014). Ch 19 *Nurse Anesthesia* (5th ed.). St. Louis, MO: Elsevier.

294. Which of the following statements regarding cigarette smoking is true?

    Select (3) three

    (A) Carbon monoxide's affinity for hemoglobin is 300 times greater than oxygen.
    (B) Carboxyhemoglobin returns to normal following one night without smoking.
    (C) Smoking cessation within 12 to 48 hours of surgery decreases circulating catecholamines.
    (D) Nicotine causes hypotension and tachycardia.
    (E) Oxygen transport to tissues is increased.

    Rationale: Nicotine's effects on the cardiovascular system include tachycardia, hypertension, myocardial oxygen consumption, and decreased delivery of oxygen to the tissue.

    Ref: Nagelhout, J.J., & Plaus, K.L. (2014). Ch 19 *Nurse Anesthesia* (5th ed.). St. Louis, MO: Elsevier.

295. During the preoperative interview the patient admits to the use of anabolic steroids. What implications for anesthesia are most concerning?

    Select (2) two

    (A) Impaired liver function
    (B) Myocardial infarction
    (C) Behavioral disturbances
    (D) Atherosclerosis

    Rationale: Use of anabolic steroids predisposes patients to liver disorders that directly affect selection of medications that require liver metabolism. Risk factors are numerous including psychiatric conditions, cardiac dysfunction including myocardial infarction, stroke, liver cancer, and hypercoagulopathy.

    Ref: Nagelhout, J.J., & Plaus, K.L. (2014). Ch 19 *Nurse Anesthesia* (5th ed.). St. Louis, MO: Elsevier.

296. The patient has a history of porphyria. What drugs will you avoid?

    Select (2) two

    (A) Methohexital
    (B) Propofol
    (C) Thiopental
    (D) Nitrous oxide

Rationale: Metabolism of thiobarbiturates results in production of aminolevulinic acid synthetase. Porphyrin is formed by aminolevulinic acid synthetase. Porphyrin may precipitate an acute porphyric crisis.

Ref: Butterworth, J.F., Mackey, D.C., & Wasnick, J.D. (2013). Ch 28 *Morgan & Mikhail's Clinical Anesthesiology* (5th ed.). New York, NY: McGraw-Hill.

Hines, R.L., & Marschall, K.E. (2012). Chapter 15 *Stoelting's Anesthesia and Co-Exiting Disease*, (6th ed.). Philadelphia, PA: Elsevier.

297. Which risk factors exist for latex allergy?

Select (3) three

(A) Allergy to passion fruit
(B) Greater than 5 surgical procedures
(C) Spina bifida
(D) Greater than 9 surgical procedures
(E) Acute exposure to latex

Rationale: Chronic, rather than acute, exposure to latex products represents a significant risk factor for latex allergy. Factors including spina bifida and urologic reconstructive surgery as well as food allergies (mainly fruits) may predispose an individual to latex allergy.

Ref: Nagelhout, J.J., & Plaus, K.L. (2014). Ch 19 *Nurse Anesthesia* (5th ed.). St. Louis, MO: Elsevier.

298. What statements are true regarding trauma-induced coagulopathy?

Select (2) two

(A) Tissue hyperperfusion results in coagulopathy.
(B) Thrombomodulin and activated protein C are released from the endothelium.
(C) Tissue hypoperfusion results in coagulopathy.
(D) Thrombomodulin binds to protein C.

Rationale: Tissue hypoperfusion results in trauma-induced coagulopathy. Thrombomodulin and activated protein C are released from the endothelium. Thombomodulin binds to thrombin resulting in impaired clot formation. However, several mechanisms exist.

Ref: Butterworth, J.F., Mackey, D.C., & Wasnick, J.D. (2013). Ch 39 *Morgan & Mikhail's Clinical Anesthesiology* (5th ed.). New York, NY: McGraw-Hill.

Nagelhout, J.J., & Plaus, K.L. (2014). Ch 36 *Nurse Anesthesia* (5th ed.). St. Louis, MO: Elsevier.

299. Which statement is false regarding epidural hematomas?

(A) Typically associated with skull fractures
(B) Patient may present conscious and then lapse into an unconscious state.
(C) When supratentorial hematomas exceed 30 mL volume, surgical decompression is used.
(D) Typically associated with blunt force injury

Rationale: Acute subdural hematomas are associated with deceleration or blunt force injury. Mortality is highest with subdural hematomas. Surgical evacuation is employed regardless of the volume.

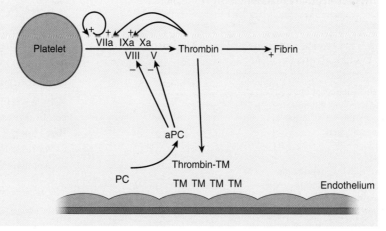

FIG. 1-8. Mechanism of trauma-induced coagulopathy. During periods of tissue hypoperfusion, thrombomodulin (TM) released by the endothelium complexes with thrombin. The thrombin-TM complexes prevent cleavage of fibrinogen to fibrin and also activate protein C (PC), reducing further thrombin generation through COfactors V and VIII. (Reproduced, with permission, from Brohi K, Cohen MJ, Davenport RA: Acute coagulopathy of trauma: mechanism, identification and effect. Curr Opln Crlt Care2007;13:680.)

Ref: Butterworth, J.F., Mackey, D.C., & Wasnick, J.D. (2013). Ch 39 *Morgan & Mikhail's Clinical Anesthesiology* (5th ed.). New York, NY: McGraw-Hill.

300. What condition results from a deficiency of complement 1 esterase inhibitor?

(A) Angioedema

(B) Neutropenia

(C) Chronic granulomatous disease

(D) Chediak-Higashi syndrome

Rationale: Angioedema is an autosomal dominant disorder. Complement 1 esterase inhibitor deficiency or dysfunction causes increased vascular permeability, facial and/or laryngeal edema.
Ref: Hines, R.L., & Marschall, K.E. (2012). Ch 24 *Stoelting's Anesthesia and Co-Exiting Disease*, (6th ed.). Philadelphia, PA: Elsevier.

301. What statements are true regarding allergic reactions?

Select (3) three

(A) Anaphylaxis is a Type I hypersensitivity reaction.

(B) Type II hypersensitivity include transfusion reactions.

(C) Anaphylactic reactions result due to an interaction with IgE.

(D) Angioedema is a Type II hypersensitivity reaction.

(E) Anaphylactoid reactions result due to an interaction with IgE.

Rationale: Angioedema is classified as a Type I hypersensitivity reaction. Anaphylactoid reactions are not due to an interaction with IgE.

TABLE 1-20. Hypersensitivity reactions.

Type I (immediate)
  Atopy
  Urticaria—angioedema
  Anaphylaxis
Type II (cytotoxic)
  Hemolytic transfusion reactions
  Autoimmune hemolytic anemia
  Heparin-induced thrombocytopenia
Type III (immune complex)
  Arthus reaction
  Serum sickness
  Acute hypersensitivity pneumonitis
Type IV (delayed, cell-mediated)
  Contact dermatitis
  Tuberculin-type hypersensitivity
  Chronic hypersensitivity pneumonitis

Ref: Butterworth, J.F., Mackey, D.C., & Wasnick, J.D. (2013). Ch 54 *Morgan & Mikhail's Clinical Anesthesiology* (5th ed.). New York, NY: McGraw-Hill.

Hines, R.L., & Marschall, K.E. (2012). Ch 24 *Stoelting's Anesthesia and Co-Exiting Disease* (6th ed.). Philadelphia, PA: Elsevier.

302. Which classification of anesthetic agents is most commonly linked to anaphylactic reactions?

(A) Thiobarbiturates

(B) Narcotics

(C) Benzodiazepines

(D) Muscle relaxants

Rationale: All anesthetic agents may cause anaphylactic reactions, muscle relaxants (rocuronium, atracurium, succinylcholine) remain the most common. This is primarily due to repeated use of this drug group.
Ref: Butterworth, J.F., Mackey, D.C., & Wasnick, J.D. (2013). Ch 54 *Morgan & Mikhail's Clinical Anesthesiology* (5th ed.). New York, NY: McGraw-Hill.

Hines, R.L., & Marschall, K.E. (2012). Ch 24 *Stoelting's Anesthesia and Co-Exiting Disease*, (6th ed.). Philadelphia, PA: Elsevier.

303. What statements about HIV and AIDS are true?

Select (3) three

(A) AIDS is caused by a retrovirus

(B) Seroconversion occurs 2-3 months following transmission of the HIV virus

(C) Highly active antiretroviral therapy (HAART) stops HIV replication

(D) Seroconversion occurs 2-3 weeks following transmission of the HIV virus

(E) There is no contraindication for the use of spinal anesthesia

Rationale: Neuraxial anesthesia may be contraindicated for patients with HIV/AIDS when neurologic lesions are present. Neurologic lesions increase intercerebral pressure (ICP).
Ref: Hines, R.L., & Marschall, K.E. (2012). Ch 24 *Stoelting's Anesthesia and Co-Exiting Disease*, (6th ed.). Philadelphia, PA: Elsevier.

304. What signs and symptoms are linked to the pathophysiology of septic shock?

Select (3) three

(A) Hypervolemia

(B) Bounding pulse

(C) Wide pulse pressure

(D) Bradycardia

(E) Hypotension

Rationale: Systemic venodilation and fluid shift to the tissues exists in septic shock resulting in hypovolemia and hypotension. Hemodynamic instability is prominent.

Ref: Butterworth, J.F., Mackey, D.C., & Wasnick, J.D. (2013). Ch 57 *Morgan & Mikhail's Clinical Anesthesiology* (5th ed.). New York, NY: McGraw-Hill.

Hines, R.L., & Marschall, K.E. (2012). Ch 22 *Stoelting's Anesthesia and Co-Exiting Disease* (6th ed.). Philadelphia, PA: Elsevier Saunders.

305. What is the recommended minimum liter flow to avoid renal injury when using sevoflurane?

(A) 1 L/min

(B) 2 L/min

(C) 3 L/min

(D) 4 L/min

Rationale: To avoid renal injury use a minimum flow of 2 L/min of sevoflurane.

Ref: Butterworth, J.F., Mackey, D.C., & Wasnick, J.D. (2013). Ch 29 *Morgan & Mikhail's Clinical Anesthesiology* (5th ed.). New York, NY: McGraw-Hill.

Hines, R.L., & Marschall, K.E. (2012). Ch 17 *Stoelting's Anesthesia and Co-Exiting Disease* (6th ed.). Philadelphia, PA: Elsevier.

306. What percent of the total cardiac output flows through the kidneys?

(A) 10-15%

(B) 20-25%

(C) 30-35%

(D) 40-45%

Rationale: Twenty to 25% of the cardiac output flows through the kidneys.

Ref: Butterworth, J.F., Mackey, D.C., & Wasnick, J.D. (2013). Ch 29 *Morgan & Mikhail's Clinical Anesthesiology* (5th ed.). New York, NY: Lange Medical Books McGraw-Hill.

Hines, R.L., & Marschall, K.E. (2012). Ch 17 *Stoelting's Anesthesia and Co-Exiting Disease* (6th ed.). Philadelphia, PA: Elsevier.

307. What is the normal glomerular filtration rate (GFR)?

(A) 440 mL/min

(B) 660 mL/min

(C) 1,200 mL/min

(D) 120 mL/min

Rationale: Renal plasma flow is 660 mL/min; renal blood flow is 1,200 mL/min; and the glomerular filtration rate in men is 120 +/− 25 mL/min. In women, the GFR is 95 +/−20 mL/min.

Ref: Butterworth, J.F., Mackey, D.C., & Wasnick, J.D. (2013). Ch 29 *Morgan & Mikhail's Clinical Anesthesiology* (5th ed.). New York, NY: McGraw-Hill.

Hines, R.L., & Marschall, K.E. (2012). Ch 17 *Stoelting's Anesthesia and Co-Exiting Disease* (6th ed.). Philadelphia, PA: Elsevier Saunders.

308. What drugs are associated with acute kidney injury?

Select (2) two

(A) Halothane

(B) Demerol

(C) Radiocontrast agents

(D) NSAIDs

Rationale: Inhalational agents decrease renal vascular resistance but are not linked to acute kidney injury. The exception is sevoflurane's breakdown product compound A. The effects of opioids on the kidney are minimal. Radiocontrast agents decrease renal perfusion and cause direct tubular injury and intratubular obstruction. NSAIDs inhibit prostaglandin synthesis and decrease renal perfusion.

TABLE 1-21. Drugs and toxins associated with acute kidney injury.[1]

Type of Injury	Drug or Toxin
Decreased renal perfusion	Nonsteroidal antiinflammatory drugs (NSAIDs), angiotensin-converting enzyme inhibitors, radiocontrast agents, amphotericin B, cyclosporine, tacrolimus
Direct tubular injury	Aminoglycosides, radiocontrast agents, amphotericin B, methotrexate, cisplatin, foscarnet, pentamidine, heavy metals, myoglobin, hemoglobin, intravenous immunoglobulin, HIV protease inhibitors
Intratubular obstruction	Radiocontrast agents, methotrexate, acyclovir, sulfonamides, ethylene glycol, uric acid, cocaine, lovastatin
Immunological-Inflammatory	Penicillin, cephalosporins, allopurinol, NSAIDs, sulfonamides, diuretics, rifampin, ciprofloxacin, cimetidine, proton pump inhibitors, tetracycline, phenytoin

[1]Reproduced, with permission, from Anderson RJ, Barry DW: Clinical and laboratory diagnosis of acute renal failure. Best Pract Res Clin Anaesthesiol 2004;18:1.

Ref: Butterworth, J.F., Mackey, D.C., & Wasnick, J.D. (2013). Ch 30 *Morgan & Mikhail's Clinical Anesthesiology* (5th ed.). New York, NY: McGraw-Hill.

Hines, R.L., & Marschall, K.E. (2012). Ch 17 *Stoelting's Anesthesia and Co-Exiting Disease* (6th ed.). Philadelphia, PA: Elsevier.

309. What narcotic metabolites are most likely to accumulate in patients with renal dysfunction?

    (A) Fentanyl
    (B) Demerol
    (C) Remifentanil
    (D) Morphine

    Rationale: The majority of narcotic metabolites are inactivated in the liver. Demerol and Morphine metabolites accumulate in patients with renal disease and increase the likelihood of respiratory depression and/or seizures.
    Ref: Butterworth, J.F., Mackey, D.C., & Wasnick, J.D. (2013). Ch 29 *Morgan & Mikhail's Clinical Anesthesiology* (5th ed.). New York, NY: McGraw-Hill.

    Hines, R.L., & Marschall, K.E. (2012). Ch 17 *Stoelting's Anesthesia and Co-Exiting Disease* (6th ed.). Philadelphia, PA: Elsevier.

310. What condition is most likely to cause complications during extracorporeal shock wave lithotripsy (ESWL)?

    (A) Renal calculi <4 mm
    (B) Cardiac arrhythmias
    (C) Ecchymosis
    (D) Skin blistering

    Rationale: ESWL is effect for renal calculi 4 mm to 2 cm. Ecchymosis and skin blistering may occur during or following the procedure. While shock waves are timed with the electrocardiogram, cardiac arrthymias may result during ESWL.
    Ref: Butterworth, J.F., Mackey, D.C., & Wasnick, J.D. (2013). Ch 31 *Morgan & Mikhail's Clinical Anesthesiology* (5th ed.). New York, NY: McGraw-Hill.

    Hines, R.L., & Marschall, K.E. (2012). Ch 17 *Stoelting's Anesthesia and Co-Exiting Disease* (6th ed.). Philadelphia, PA: Elsevier.

311. What is the normal hepatic blood flow?

    (A) 15-20%
    (B) 25-30%
    (C) 20-25%
    (D) 30-35%

Rationale: Twenty-five to 30% of the cardiac output is provided to the liver.
Ref: Butterworth, J.F., Mackey, D.C., & Wasnick, J.D. (2013). Ch 32 *Morgan & Mikhail's Clinical Anesthesiology* (5th ed.). New York, NY: McGraw-Hill.

Hines, R.L., & Marschall, K.E. (2012). Ch 13 *Stoelting's Anesthesia and Co-Exiting Disease* (6th ed.). Philadelphia, PA: Elsevier.

312. Which coagulation factor is not produced in the liver?

    (A) Factor V
    (B) Factor I
    (C) Factor VIII
    (D) Factor II

    Rationale: Factor VIII and von Willebrand Factor are the only coagulation factors not produced in the liver.
    Ref: Butterworth, J.F., Mackey, D.C., & Wasnick, J.D. (2013). Ch 32 *Morgan & Mikhail's Clinical Anesthesiology* (5th ed.). New York, NY: McGraw-Hill.

313. What factors cause a Vitamin K deficiency?

    (A) VI, IX, X
    (B) VII, IX, X
    (C) VIII, IX, X
    (D) VII, IX, VI

    Rationale: Factors causing a vitamin K deficiency include flawed prothrombin and factors VII, IX, X.
    Ref: Butterworth, J.F., Mackey, D.C., & Wasnick, J.D. (2013). Ch 32 *Morgan & Mikhail's Clinical Anesthesiology* (5th ed.). New York, NY: McGraw-Hill.

314. What albumin level is associated with chronic liver disease?

    (A) 3.5 g/dL
    (B) 4.0 g/dL
    (C) 4.5 g/dL
    (D) 2.5 g/dL

    Rationale: Normal albumin levels range from 3.5 to 5.5 g/dL. Values less than 2.5 g/dL indicate chronic liver disease.
    Ref: Butterworth, J.F., Mackey, D.C., & Wasnick, J.D. (2013). Ch 32 *Morgan & Mikhail's Clinical Anesthesiology* (5th ed.). New York, NY: McGraw-Hill.

315. Which of the following is false regarding prothrombin time (PT)?

    (A) The normal PT range is 11-14 seconds.
    (B) Measures factors V, VII, X, finbrinogen, and prothrombin

(C) Assists in the evaluation of chronic and acute liver disease

(D) PT is decreased in vitamin K deficiency

Rationale: The PT is increased in vitamin K deficiency, advanced liver disease, DIC, warfarin and heparin therapy, and factor VII deficiency.

TABLE 1-22. Coagulation test abnormalities.[1]

	PT	PTT	TT	Fibrinogen
Advanced liver disease	↑	↑	N or ↑	N or ↓
DIC	↑	↑	↑	↓
Vitamin K deficiency	↑↑	↑	N	N
Warfarin therapy	↑↑	↑	N	N
Heparin therapy	↑	↑↑	↑	N
Hemophilia				
Factor VIII deficiency	N	↑	N	N
Factor IX deficiency	N	↑	N	N
Factor VII deficiency	↑	N	N	N
Factor XIII deficiency	N	N	N	N

[1]PT, prothrombin time; PTT, partial thromboplastin time; TT, thrombin time; N, normal; DIC, disseminated intravascular coagulation.

Ref: Butterworth, J.F., Mackey, D.C., & Wasnick, J.D. (2013). Ch 32 *Morgan & Mikhail's Clinical Anesthesiology* (5th ed.). New York, NY: McGraw-Hill.

316. What are the characteristics of hepatitis B?

Select (3) three

(A) Incubation period 20-37 days

(B) Fecal-oral transmission

(C) Incubation period 60-110 days

(D) Percutaneous or body fluids

(E) Development of chronic liver disease in 80-90% of children

(F) No progression to chronic liver disease

Rationale: Characteristics of hepatitis A include fecal-oral transmission with an incubation period of 20 to 37 days. There is no progression to chronic liver disease as compared to hepatitis B.

Ref: Butterworth, J.F., Mackey, D.C., & Wasnick, J.D. (2013). Ch 32 *Morgan & Mikhail's Clinical Anesthesiology* (5th ed.). New York, NY: McGraw-Hill.

Hines, R.L., & Marschall, K.E. (2012). Ch 13 *Stoelting's Anesthesia and Co-Exiting Disease* (6th ed.). Philadelphia, PA: Elsevier.

317. What are the risk factors for halothane hepatitis?

Select (3) three

(A) >40 years

(B) Male gender

(C) Female gender

(D) Obesity

(E) Smoking

Rationale: Females, >40 years, obesity, exposure to multiple anesthetics, and familial predisposition represent risk factors linked to halothane hepatitis.

Ref: Butterworth, J.F., Mackey, D.C., & Wasnick, J.D. (2013). Ch 8 *Morgan & Mikhail's Clinical Anesthesiology* (5th ed.). New York, NY: McGraw-Hill.

Nagelhout, J.J., & Plaus K.L. (2014). Ch 30 *Nurse Anesthesia* (5th ed.). St. Louis, MO: Elsevier.

318. When evaluating a patient with cirrhosis, what laboratory findings are expected?

Select (3) three

(A) Increased bilirubin

(B) Increased albumin

TABLE 1-23. Manifestations of cirrhosis.

Gastrointestinal
Portal hypertension
  Ascites
  Esophageal varices
  Hemorrhoids
  Gastrointestinal bleeding
Circulatory
  Hyperdynamic state (high cardiac output)
  Systemic arteriovenous shunts
  Low systemic vascular resistance
  Cirrhotic cardiomyopathy; pulmonary hypertension
Pulmonary
  Increased intrapulmonary shunting; hepatopulmonary syndrome
  Decreased functional residual capacity
  Pleural effusions
  Restrictive ventilatory defect
  Respiratory alkalosis
Renal
  Increased proximal reabsorption of sodium
  Increased distal reabsorption of sodium
  Impaired free water clearance
  Decreased renal perfusion
  Hepatorenal syndrome
Hematological
  Anemia
  Coagulopathy
  Hypersplenism
  Thrombocytopenia
  Leukopenia
Infectious
  Spontaneous bacterial peritonitis
Metabolic
  Hyponatremia and hypernatremia
  Hypokalemia and hypocalcemia
  Hypomagnesemia
  Hypoalbuminemia
  Hypoglycemia
Neurological
  Encephalopathy

(C) Increased prothrombin time

(D) Decreased albumin

(E) Hyponatremia

Rationale: Laboratory findings consistent with cirrhosis include increased bilirubin, normal or increased AST/ALT, decreased albumin and PT, hyponatremia, thrombocytopenia, and decreased hemoglobin, and hematocrit.
Ref: Butterworth, J.F., Mackey, D.C., & Wasnick, J.D. (2013). Ch 32 *Morgan & Mikhail's Clinical Anesthesiology* (5th ed.). New York, NY: McGraw-Hill.
Nagelhout, J.J., & Plaus K.L. (2014). Ch 30 *Nurse Anesthesia* (5th ed.). St. Louis, MO: Elsevier.

319. The intoxicated patient arrives for an emergent exploratory laparotomy following a motor vehicle accident. What statement is true regarding this scenario?

(A) Anesthetic requirements are increased.

(B) Alcohol increases MAC.

(C) Alcohol decreases GABA receptor activity.

(D) Alcohol inhibits NMDA receptors.

Rationale: Acute alcohol intoxication decreases MAC thereby decreasing anesthetic requirements. GABA receptor activity is increased resulting in marked effects of central nervous system depressants.
Ref: Butterworth, J.F., Mackey, D.C., & Wasnick, J.D. (2013). Ch 32 *Morgan & Mikhail's Clinical Anesthesiology* (5th ed.). New York, NY: McGraw-Hill.
Nagelhout, J.J., & Plaus K.L. (2014). Ch 30 *Nurse Anesthesia* (5th ed.). St. Louis, MO: Elsevier.

320. Which statements are true regarding the pneumatic tourniquet?

Select (3) three

(A) Hypertension occurs when the tourniquet is released.

(B) Tissue hypoxia occurs within 2 minutes of application.

(C) Hypotension occurs when the tourniquet is released.

(D) Metabolic acidosis occurs after tourniquet release.

(E) Core body temperature increases upon tourniquet release.

Rationale: The pneumatic tourniquet causes hypertension and pain approximately 60 minutes after inflation. Tissue hypoxia occurs shortly after inflating the tourniquet. Once the tourniquet is released products of tissue metabolism cause a brief period of metabolic acidosis and fall in blood pressure and temperature.
Ref: Butterworth, J.F., Mackey, D.C., & Wasnick, J.D. (2013). Ch 38 *Morgan & Mikhail's Clinical Anesthesiology* (5th ed.). New York, NY: McGraw-Hill.

321. A 65-year-old patient presents for an open reduction and internal fixation following a hip fracture. The patient is short of breath, confused, and you notice petechiae on the chest. What is the most likely cause?

(A) Fat embolism syndrome

(B) Mentation changes due to aging

(C) Deep vein thrombosis

(D) Thromboembolism

Rationale: Classic signs of fat embolism include dyspnea, confusion and petechiae. The signs occur 1 to 3 days following a long-bone or pelvic fracture.
Ref: Butterworth, J.F., Mackey, D.C., & Wasnick, J.D. (2013). Ch 38 *Morgan & Mikhail's Clinical Anesthesiology* (5th ed.). New York, NY: McGraw-Hill.

322. Which congenital cardiac malformations may benefit from a modified Blalock-Taussig shunt procedure?

Select (2) two

(A) Tetralogy of Fallot

(B) Truncus arteriosus

(C) Tricuspid atresia

(D) Transposition of the great vessels

Rationale: A modified Blalock-Taussig procedure is a shunt between systemic, often subclavian, and pulmonary circulation. This procedure can be useful in tricuspid atresia or palliative in Tetralogy of Fallot.
Ref: Butterworth, J.F., Mackey, D.C., & Wasnick, J.D. (2013). Ch 21 *Morgan & Mikhail's Clinical Anesthesiology* (5th ed.). New York, NY: McGraw-Hill.
Jaffe, R.A., Samuels, S.I., Schmiesing C.A., & Golianu, B. (Eds.) (2009). Ch 12.4 *Anesthesiologist's manual of surgical procedures* (4th ed.). Philadelphia, PA: Lippincott Williams & Wilkins.

323. What is the National Asthma Education and Prevention Program Expert Panel Report 3 definition of asthma?

(A) A chronic inflammatory disorder of the airways

(B) Preventable and treatable disease state characterized by airflow limitation that is not fully reversible

(C) Mechanical obstruction to breathing that occurs during sleep

(D) Right heart failure secondary to pulmonary pathology

Rationale: The National Asthma Education and Prevention Program Expert Panel Report 3 define asthma as a chronic inflammatory disorder of the airways in which many cells and cellular elements play a role.

Ref: Butterworth, J.F., Mackey, D.C., & Wasnick, J.D. (2013). Ch 23 *Morgan & Mikhail's Clinical Anesthesiology* (5th ed.). New York, NY: McGraw-Hill.

Nagelhout, J.J., & Plaus, K.L. (2014). Ch 26 *Nurse Anesthesia* (5th ed.). St. Louis, MO: Elsevier.

324. How is the clinical diagnosis of chronic bronchitis made?

(A) Presence of a productive cough on most days of three consecutive months for at least two consecutive years

(B) Presence of an occasional productive cough for two consecutive months for at least 1 year

(C) Presence of a productive cough on most days of three consecutive weeks for a least two consecutive months

(D) Presence of a productive cough on three consecutive days for a least two consecutive weeks

Rationale: Presence of a productive cough on most days of three consecutive months for a least two consecutive years is diagnostic of chronic bronchitis.

Ref: Butterworth, J.F., Mackey, D.C., & Wasnick, J.D. (2013). Ch 23 *Morgan & Mikhail's Clinical Anesthesiology* (5th ed.). New York, NY: McGraw-Hill.

Nagelhout, J.J., & Plaus, K.L. (2014). Ch 26 *Nurse Anesthesia* (5th ed.). St. Louis, MO: Elsevier.

325. Which congenital cardiac malformation includes a right-to-left intracardiac shunt?

(A) Tetralogy of Fallot

(B) Atrial septal defect

(C) Ventricular septal defect

(D) Patent ductus arteriosus

Rationale: Tetralogy of Fallot includes a right-to-left shunt. The others result in left-to-right shunting.

Ref: Butterworth, J.F., Mackey, D.C., & Wasnick, J.D. (2013). Ch 21 *Morgan & Mikhail's Clinical Anesthesiology* (5th ed.). New York, NY: McGraw-Hill.

Hines, R.L., & Marschall, K.E. (Eds.) (2012). Ch 3 *Stoelting's anesthesia and co-existing disease* (6th ed.). Philadelphia, PA: Elsevier.

326. Which diseases place the patient at increased risk for developing Cor Pulmonale?

Select (3) three

(A) Adenotonsillar hypertrophy

(B) Chronic obstructive pulmonary disease

(C) Obesity

(D) Eaton-Lambert syndrome

Rationale: Cor Pulmonale is right-heart disease of pulmonary origin. A and C predispose to the development of obstructive sleep apnea which can eventually manifest as right-sided disease and failure. Cor Pulmonale is frequently associated with chronic obstructive pulmonary disease.

Ref: Butterworth, J.F., Mackey, D.C., & Wasnick, J.D. (2013). Ch 34 *Morgan & Mikhail's Clinical Anesthesiology* (5th ed.). New York, NY: McGraw-Hill.

Hines, R.L., & Marschall, K.E. (Eds.) (2012). Ch 6 *Stoelting's Anesthesia and Co-existing Disease* (6th ed.). Philadelphia, PA: Elsevier.

Barash, P.G., Cullen, B.F., Stoelting, R.K., Cahalan, M.K. & Stock, M.C. (Eds.). (2009) Ch 50 *Clinical anesthesia*, (6th ed.). Philadelphia, PA: Lippincott Williams & Wilkins.

327. What is indicated by an apnea/hypopnea index of 42 occurrences per hour?

(A) Normal result

(B) Mild obstructive sleep apnea

(C) Moderate sleep apnea

(D) Severe sleep apnea

Rationale: More than 30 to 40 apnea/hypopnea events per hour indicates severe obstructive disease.

Ref: Butterworth, J.F., Mackey, D.C., & Wasnick, J.D. (2013). Ch 44 *Morgan & Mikhail's Clinical Anesthesiology* (5th ed.). New York, NY: McGraw-Hill.

Miller, R.D., Eriksson, L.I., Fleisher, L.A., Weiner-Kronish, J.P., & Young, W.L. (Eds.). (2010). Ch 64 *Miller's Anesthesia* (7th ed.). Philadelphia, PA: Elsevier.

328. What is the most common cause of obstructive sleep apnea?

(A) Ondine's curse

(B) Obesity

(C) Muscular dystrophy

(D) Central apnea

Rationale: Obesity is the most common contributor to development of obstructive sleep apnea.

Ref: Butterworth, J.F., Mackey, D.C., & Wasnick, J.D. (2013). Ch 44 *Morgan & Mikhail's Clinical Anesthesiology* (5th ed.). New York, NY: McGraw-Hill.

Nagelhout, J.J., & Plaus K.L. (2014). Ch 26 *Nurse Anesthesia* (5th ed.). St. Louis, MO: Elsevier.

329. Which structure is most commonly occluded in obstructive hydrocephalus?

(A) Choroid plexus

(B) Foramen of Monro

(C) Aqueduct of Sylvius

(D) Foramen of Magendie

Rationale: Cerebrospinal fluid commonly flows through the aqueduct of Sylvius to the fourth ventricle. Narrowing or obstruction of this path can result in obstructive, or noncommunicating, hydrocephalus.

Ref: Butterworth, J.F., Mackey, D.C., & Wasnick, J.D. (2013). Ch 26 *Morgan & Mikhail's Clinical Anesthesiology* (5th ed.). New York, NY: McGraw-Hill.

Hall, J.E. (2011). Ch 61 *Guyton and Hall Textbook of Medical Physiology.* Philadelphia, PA: Elsevier.

330. Which state should be avoided during the anesthetic care of a patient with multiple sclerosis?

(A) Hyperthermia

(B) Hyperoxia

(C) Hypercapnia

(D) Hypertension

Rationale: Hyperthermia should be avoided because increases in temperature may precipitate exacerbations of this condition.

Ref: Butterworth, J.F., Mackey, D.C., & Wasnick, J.D. (2013). Ch 28 *Morgan & Mikhail's Clinical Anesthesiology* (5th ed.). New York, NY: McGraw-Hill.

331. What causes weakness in myasthenia gravis?

(A) Autoimmune damage to nerve axons

(B) Damage to presynaptic calcium channels

(C) Damage to postsynaptic cholinergic receptors

(D) Autoimmune damage to type I muscle fibers

Rationale: Weakness results from loss of postsynaptic acetylcholine receptors.

Ref: Butterworth, J.F., Mackey, D.C., & Wasnick, J.D. (2013). Ch 35 *Morgan & Mikhail's Clinical Anesthesiology* (5th ed.). New York, NY: McGraw-Hill.

Hall, J.E. (2011). Ch 7 *Guyton and Hall Textbook of Medical Physiology.* Philadelphia, PA: Elsevier.

332. What would be the effect on muscle strength if a patient with myasthenia gravis were treated with an anticholinesterase?

(A) No change

(B) Decreased strength

(C) Increased strength

Rationale: Pyridostigmine, an anticholinesterase, is used to improve weakness in patients with this disease.

Ref: Butterworth, J.F., Mackey, D.C., & Wasnick, J.D. (2013). Ch 35 *Morgan & Mikhail's Clinical Anesthesiology* (5th ed.). New York, NY: McGraw-Hill.

Longnecker, D. Brown, D. Newman, M., & Zapol, W. (Eds.) (2012). Ch 54 *Anesthesiology* (2nd ed.). New York, NY: McGraw-Hill.

333. Is an aneurysm in the brain more likely to occur in a larger vessel or a smaller vessel? Why?

(A) Equally likely in either a large or small vessel because blood pressure is constant

(B) More likely in a larger vessel due to increased diameter

(C) More likely in a smaller vessel due to increased resistance

(D) More likely in a smaller vessel due to decreased flow

Rationale: Brain aneurysms are more common in larger arteries. Application of the law of LaPlace illustrates increasing vessel wall pressure with increasing diameter.

Ref: Butterworth, J.F., Mackey, D.C., & Wasnick, J.D. (2013). Ch 27 *Morgan & Mikhail's Clinical Anesthesiology* (5th ed.). New York, NY: McGraw-Hill.

Shubert, D., & Leyba, J. (Eds.) (2013). Ch 7 *Chemistry and Physics for Nurse Anesthesia* (2nd ed.). New York, NY: Springer Publishing.

334. Which level of spinal cord injury is most associated with autonomic hyperreflexia?

(A) T5-T8

(B) T10-L1

(C) L1-L4

(D) L4-S1

Rationale: Autonomic hyperreflexia is most associated with spinal cord injuries at or above the midthoracic spine.

Ref: Butterworth, J.F., Mackey, D.C., & Wasnick, J.D. (2013). Ch 28 *Morgan & Mikhail's Clinical Anesthesiology* (5th ed.). New York, NY: McGraw-Hill.

Nagelhout, J.J., & Plaus K.L. (2014). Ch 36 *Nurse Anesthesia* (5th ed.). St. Louis, MO: Elsevier.

335. What is the most important cervical radiographic finding in a patient with rheumatoid arthritis?

(A) Cervical stenosis

(B) Cervical spondylosis

(C) Atlantoaxial subluxation

(D) Lordosis

Rationale: Atlantoaxial subluxation indicates increased risk of spinal cord impingement during airway management.

Ref: Butterworth, J.F., Mackey, D.C., & Wasnick, J.D. (2013). Ch 38 *Morgan & Mikhail's Clinical Anesthesiology* (5th ed.). New York, NY: McGraw-Hill.

Hines, R.L., & Marschall, K.E. (Eds.) (2012). Ch 21 *Stoelting's Anesthesia and Co-existing Disease* (6th ed.). Philadelphia, PA: Elsevier.

336. What is the most common form of muscular dystrophy?

(A) Becker

(B) Limb-girdle

(C) Myotonic

(D) Duchenne

Rationale: Duchenne occurs most frequently.

Ref: Butterworth, J.F., Mackey, D.C., & Wasnick J.D. (2013). Ch 35 *Morgan & Mikhail's Clinical Anesthesiology* (5th ed.). New York, NY: Lange Medical Books McGraw-Hill.

Nagelhout, J.J., & Plaus K.L. (2014). Ch 32 *Nurse Anesthesia* (5th ed). St. Louis, MO: Elsevier.

337. Which statement is true regarding Duchenne muscular dystrophy?

(A) The disease is X-linked and occurs more frequently in girls.

(B) The disease occurs equally in boys and girls and is diagnosed in early childhood.

(C) The disease is X-linked and symptoms occur only in boys.

(D) The disease primarily manifests as contractures of the large joints.

Rationale: Duchenne muscular dystrophy is an X-linked disease manifesting clinically in young boys while girls can be carriers who are asymptomatic.

Ref: Butterworth, J.F., Mackey, D.C., & Wasnick, J.D. (2013). Ch 35 *Morgan & Mikhail's Clinical Anesthesiology* (5th ed.). New York, NY: McGraw-Hill.

Nagelhout, J.J., & Plaus K.L. (2014). Ch 32 *Nurse Anesthesia* (5th ed). St. Louis, MO: Elsevier.

338. What is the anesthetic implication of a patient taking tricyclic antidepressants who is scheduled to receive general anesthesia?

(A) Meperidine will produce skeletal muscle rigidity and hyperpyrexia.

(B) Tricyclic antidepressants should be discontinued 2 weeks before surgery.

(C) MAC requirements may be increased for inhaled anesthetics.

(D) Ephedrine is preferred agent to treat post-induction hypotension.

Rationale: MAC requirements are increased for patients taking tricyclic antidepressants, possibly related to the enhanced catecholamine activity.

Ref: Butterworth, J.F., Mackey, D.C., & Wasnick, J.D. (2013). Ch 21 *Morgan & Mikhail's Clinical Anesthesiology* (5th ed.). New York, NY: McGraw-Hill.

Stoelting, S. & Hillier, S. (2006). Ch 19 *Pharmacology & Physiology in Anesthetic Practice* (4th ed.). Philadelphia, PA: Lippincott Williams & Wilkins.

339. Which characteristic is not shared by malignant hyperthermia and neuroleptic malignant syndrome?

(A) Generalized muscular rigidity

(B) Flaccid paralysis after vecuronium administration

(C) Effectively treated with dantrolene

(D) Hyperthermia

Rationale: The ability of NDMRs to produce flaccid paralysis distinguishes neuroleptic malignant syndrome (NMS) from malignant hyperthermia (MH). MH and NMS share the features such as generalized muscular rigidity and hyperthermia. Further, like MH, supportive measures including dantrolene administration are effective.

Ref: Butterworth, J.F., Mackey, D.C., & Wasnick, J.D. (2013). Ch 52 *Morgan & Mikhail's Clinical Anesthesiology* (5th ed.). New York, NY: McGraw-Hill.

Stoelting, S & Hillier, S. (2006). Ch 19 *Pharmacology & Physiology in Anesthetic Practice* (4th ed). Philadelphia, PA: Lippincott Williams & Wilkins.

340. A patient is taking a MAO inhibitor. What anesthetic agent can be safely used in this patient?

(A) Phenylephrine

(B) Ketamine

(C) Bupivacaine with epinephrine

(D) Pancuronium

Rationale: Any drug than enhances sympathetic activity, such as ketamine, pancuronium, and epinephrine (including epinephrine in local anesthetics) should be avoided. Phenylephrine, if necessary, can be used in small doses and is preferable to using an indirect-acting agent for treating anesthetic-induced hypotension.
Ref: Butterworth, J.F., Mackey, D.C., & Wasnick J.D. (2013). Ch 28 *Morgan & Mikhail's Clinical Anesthesiology* (5th ed.). New York, NY: McGraw-Hill.
Stoelting, S., & Hillier, S. (2006). Ch 19 *Pharmacology & Physiology in Anesthetic Practice* (4th ed). Philadelphia, PA: Lippincott Williams & Wilkins.

341. A 25-year-old, 50-kg, otherwise healthy patient complains of nausea and demonstrates vomiting, refractory to ondansetron, and dexamethasone therapy. Which dose of droperidol will achieve a safe therapeutic response?

    (A) 1.25 mg IV
    (B) 0.625 mg/kg IV
    (C) 0.5 mg IV
    (D) 12.5 mg IV

    Rationale: 1.25 mg IV is associated with greater effectiveness and is the upper limit of therapeutic dosing. 0.625 mg *per* kg (i.e., 31.25 mg is an overdose). A flat dose of 0.625 mg total would be acceptable. 0.5 mg is a sub therapeutic dose.
    Ref: Butterworth, J.F., Mackey, D.C., & Wasnick, J.D. (2013). Ch 19 *Morgan & Mikhail's Clinical Anesthesiology* (5th ed.). New York, NY: McGraw-Hill.
    Stoelting, S & Hillier, S., (2006). Ch 37 *Pharmacology & Physiology in Anesthetic Practice* (4th ed.). Philadelphia, PA: Lippincott Williams & Wilkins.

342. Which statement about phenytoin is correct?

    (A) Chronic phenytoin therapy requires higher dose requirements of vecuronium.
    (B) Chronic phenytoin therapy requires lower dose requirements of vecuronium.
    (C) Chronic phenytoin therapy requires higher dose requirements of succinylcholine.
    (D) Chronic phenytoin therapy requires lower dose requirements of succinylcholine.

    Rationale: Patients taking anticonvulsants regularly demonstrate resistance to non depolarizing agents and possess higher dosing requirements.

Ref: Butterworth, J.F., Mackey, D.C., & Wasnick, J.D. (2013). Ch 11 *Morgan & Mikhail's Clinical Anesthesiology* (5th ed.). New York, NY: McGraw-Hill.
Stoelting, S., & Hillier, S. (2006). Ch 30 *Pharmacology & Physiology in Anesthetic Practice* (4th ed). Philadelphia, PA: Lippincott Williams & Wilkins.

343. Which statement about gabapentin is false?

    (A) Gabapentin is not bound to plasma proteins.
    (B) Gabapentin is an effective monotherapy for partial seizures.
    (C) Gabapentin is unable to cross blood-brain barrier.
    (D) Gabapentin undergoes no metabolism.

    Rationale: Gabapentin is a lipid soluble anticonvulsant that can cross the blood-brain barrier (BBB), is not bound to plasma proteins, and is an effective monotherapy for partial seizures.
    Ref: Stoelting, S & Hillier, S., (2006). Ch 30 *Pharmacology & Physiology in Anesthetic Practice* (4th ed.). Philadelphia, PA: Lippincott Williams & Wilkins.
    Nagelhout, J.J., & Plaus K.L. (2014). Ch 51 *Nurse Anesthesia* (5th ed.). St. Louis, MO: Elsevier.

344. For which pathophysiologic state would gabapentin not be prescribed for management?

    (A) Postherpatic neuralgia
    (B) Diabetic neuropathy
    (C) Acute postoperative pain adjuvant
    (D) Status epilepticus

    Rationale: Gabapentin, which comes in oral form, is used for the management of postherpetic neuralgiadiabetic neuropathy, and acute postoperative pain. This agent would not be utilized in the treatment of an acute seizure, such as status epilepticus where an intravenous agent would be more appropriate.
    Ref: Butterworth, J.F., Mackey, D.C., & Wasnick, J.D. (2013). Ch 47 *Morgan & Mikhail's Clinical Anesthesiology* (5th ed.). New York, NY: McGraw-Hill.
    Nagelhout, J.J., & Plaus K.L. (2014). Ch 51 *Nurse Anesthesia* (5th ed). St. Louis, MO: Elsevier.
    Stoelting, S & Hillier, S. (2006). Ch 30 *Pharmacology & Physiology in Anesthetic Practice* (4th ed) Philadelphia, PA: Lippincott Williams & Wilkins.

345. Which neuromuscular disease is associated with increased resistance to succinylcholine?

(A) Myasthenic syndrome

(B) Myasthenia gravis

(C) Myotonic dystrophy

(D) Muscular dystrophy

Rationale: Patients with myasthenia gravis have fewer acetylcholine receptors and therefore are resistant to succinylcholine. Patients with myasthenic syndrome are sensitive to succinylcholine. In patients with myotonic syndrome, succinylcholine results in prolonged skeletal muscle contraction, indicating a lack of resistance to succinylcholine. Muscular dystrophy patient are very sensitive to succinylcholine.
Ref: Butterworth, J.F., Mackey, D.C., & Wasnick, J.D. (2013). Ch 11 *Morgan & Mikhail's Clinical Anesthesiology* (5th ed.). New York, NY: McGraw-Hill.
Hines, R.L., & Marschall, K.E. (Eds.) (2012). Ch 2 *Stoelting's Anesthesia and Co-existing Disease* (6th ed.). Philadelphia, PA: Elsevier.

346. What is the initial dose of dantrolene for a 74-kg man in acute malignant hyperthermia crisis?

(A) 150 mg

(B) 185 mg

(C) 200 mg

(D) 215 mg

Rationale: The first dose of dantrolene should be 2.5 mg/kg.
Ref: Butterworth, J.F., Mackey, D.C., & Wasnick, J.D. (2013). Ch 52 *Morgan & Mikhail's Clinical Anesthesiology* (5th ed.). New York, NY: McGraw-Hill.
Hines, R.L., & Marschall, K.E. (Eds.) (2012). Ch 27 *Stoelting's Anesthesia and Co-existing Disease* (6th ed.). Philadelphia, PA: Elsevier.

347. Which are early signs of malignant hyperthermia?

Select (3) three

(A) Increased end-tidal carbon dioxide

(B) Increased heart rate

(C) Increased temperature

(D) Masseter rigidity

Rationale: Hyperthermia is not among the early manifestations of malignant hyperthermia crisis.
Ref: Butterworth, J.F., Mackey, D.C., & Wasnick, J.D. (2013). Ch 52 *Morgan & Mikhail's Clinical Anesthesiology* (5th ed.). New York, NY: McGraw-Hill.

Hines, R.L., & Marschall, K.E. (Eds.) (2012). Ch 27 *Stoelting's Anesthesia and Co-existing Disease* (6th ed.). Philadelphia, PA: Elsevier.

348. Which disease is least likely to be associated with malignant hyperthermia?

(A) King syndrome

(B) Central-core disease

(C) Multi-minicore myopathy

(D) Duchenne muscular dystrophy

Rationale: King, or King-Denborough syndrome, central-core disease, and multi-minicore myopathy are more strongly associated with malignant hyperthermia than Duchenne's.
Ref: Butterworth, J.F., Mackey, D.C., & Wasnick, J.D. (2013). Ch 52 *Morgan & Mikhail's Clinical Anesthesiology* (5th ed.). New York, NY: McGraw-Hill.
Baum, V.C., & O'Flaherty, J.E. (2007). *Anesthesia for Genetic, Metabolic, & Dysmorphic Syndromes of Childhood.* pp. 65, 110, 199. Philadelphia, PA: Lippincott Williams & Wilkins.
Hines, R.L., & Marschall, K.E. (Eds.) (2012). Ch 21 *Stoelting's Anesthesia and Co-existing Disease* (6th ed.). Philadelphia, PA: Elsevier.

349. Which would be expected in a patient with Graves' disease?

(A) Increased thyroid stimulating hormone with decreased thyroid hormone

(B) Increased thyroid stimulating hormone with increased thyroid hormone

(C) Decreased thyroid stimulating hormone with decreased thyroid hormone

(D) Decreased thyroid stimulating hormone with increased thyroid hormone

Rationale: Graves' disease is autoimmune; antibodies stimulate the thyroid. Increased thyroid release into circulation decreases pituitary release of thyroid stimulating hormone.
Ref: Butterworth, J.F., Mackey, D.C., & Wasnick, J.D. (2013). Ch 34 *Morgan & Mikhail's Clinical Anesthesiology* (5th ed.). New York, NY: McGraw-Hill.
Hall J.E.(2011). Ch 76 *Guyton and Hall Textbook of Medical Physiology.* Philadelphia, PA: Elsevier.

350. Which diagnosis indicates adrenal insufficiency?

(A) Addison's disease

(B) Conn syndrome

(C)   Cushing's disease

(D)   Mendelsohn syndrome

Rationale: Addison's disease is glucocorticoid shortage from decreased adrenal function.

Ref: Butterworth, J.F., Mackey, D.C., & Wasnick, J.D. (2013). Ch 34 *Morgan & Mikhail's Clinical Anesthesiology* (5th ed.). New York, NY: McGraw-Hill.

Hall, J. E. (2011). Ch 77 *Guyton and Hall textbook of medical physiology.* Philadelphia, PA: Elsevier.

351.   Which is secreted from the posterior pituitary?

(A)   Antidiuretic hormone

(B)   Adrenocorticotropic hormone

(C)   Prolactin

(D)   Thyroid stimulating hormone

Rationale: Oxytocin and antidiuretic hormone are stored in the posterior pituitary.

Ref: Butterworth, J.F., Mackey, D.C., & Wasnick, J.D. (2013). Ch 27 *Morgan & Mikhail's Clinical Anesthesiology* (5th ed.). New York, NY: McGraw-Hill.

Hemmings, H.C. Jr., & Egan, T.D. (Eds.) (2013). Ch 31 *Pharmacology and Physiology for Anesthesia.* Philadelphia, PA: Elsevier.

352.   What causes acromegaly?

(A)   Hypersecretion of adrenocorticotropic hormone

(B)   Hypersecretion of thyroid stimulating hormone

(C)   Hypersecretion of growth hormone

(D)   Hypersecretion of prolactin

Rationale: Excess growth hormone in an adult results in acromegaly.

Ref: Butterworth, J.F., Mackey, D.C., & Wasnick, J.D. (2013). Ch 27 *Morgan & Mikhail's Clinical Anesthesiology* (5th ed.). New York, NY: McGraw-Hill.

Hemmings, H.C. Jr., & Egan, T.D. (Eds.) (2013). Ch 30 *Pharmacology and Physiology for Anesthesia.* Philadelphia, PA: Elsevier.

353.   What condition results from hypersecretion of growth hormone in a child?

(A)   Acromegaly

(B)   Dwarfism

(C)   Osteomalacia

(D)   Gigantism

Rationale: Pituitary hypersecretion of growth hormone in a child results in gigantism.

Ref: Butterworth, J.F., Mackey, D.C., & Wasnick, J.D. (2013). Ch 27 *Morgan & Mikhail's Clinical Anesthesiology* (5th ed.). New York, NY: McGraw-Hill.

Hall J.E.(2011). Ch 75 *Guyton and Hall Textbook of Medical Physiology.* Philadelphia, PA: Elsevier.

354.   Which common anesthetic medications should be avoided during the induction of a patient diagnosed with acute intermittent porphyria?

Select (2) two

(A)   Thiopental

(B)   Propofol

(C)   Etomidate

(D)   Fentanyl

Rationale: Barbiturates and etomidate should be avoided. Propofol and opioids are commonly regarded as safe for use with this condition.

Ref: Butterworth, J.F., Mackey, D.C., & Wasnick, J.D. (2013). Ch 9 *Morgan & Mikhail's Clinical Anesthesiology* (5th ed.). New York, NY: McGraw-Hill.

Baum, V.C., & O'Flaherty, J.E. (2007). *Anesthesia for Genetic, Metabolic, & Dysmorphic Syndromes of Childhood.* p. 305. Philadelphia, PA: Lippincott Williams & Wilkins.

Hines, R.L., & Marschall, K.E. (Eds.) (2012). Ch 15 *Stoelting's Anesthesia and Co-existing Disease* (6th ed.). Philadelphia, PA: Elsevier.

355.   Which correctly describes acute intermittent porphyria?

(A)   Accumulation of delta-aminolevulinic acid and porphobilinogen secondary to porphobilinogen deaminase deficiency.

(B)   Accumulation of protoporphyrin secondary to protoporphyrinogen oxidase deficiency.

(C)   Accumulation of delta-aminolevulinic acid and protoporphyrin secondary to ferrochelatase deficiency.

(D)   Accumulation of delta-aminolevulinic acid and coproporphyrinogen secondary to coproporphyrinogen oxidase deficiency.

Rationale: Induction of delta-aminolevulinic acid synthetase and overproduction of heme precursors called porphyrins results in various forms of porphyria. Acute intermittent porphyria is specifically related to porphobilinogen deaminase deficiency which causes accumulation of the preceding prophyrin, porphobilinogen, as well as delta-aminolevulinic acid.

Ref: Butterworth, J.F., Mackey, D.C., & Wasnick, J.D. (2013). Ch 9 *Morgan & Mikhail's Clinical Anesthesiology* (5th ed.). New York, NY: McGraw-Hill.

Hines, R.L., & Marschall, K.E. (Eds.) (2012). Ch 15 *Stoelting's Anesthesia and Co-existing Disease* (6th ed.). Philadelphia, PA: Elsevier.

Harvey, R., & Ferrier, D. (Eds.) (2011). Ch 17 *Lippincott's Illustrated Reviews: Biochemistry* (5th ed.). Philadelphia, PA: Lippincott Williams & Wilkins.

Baum, V.C., & O'Flaherty, J.E. (2007). *Anesthesia for Genetic, Metabolic, & Dysmorphic Syndromes of Childhood.* p. 304 Philadelphia, PA: Lippincott Williams& Wilkins.

356. Which are secreted by tumors in carcinoid syndrome?

Select (3) three

(A) Octreotide

(B) Serotonin

(C) Kallikrein

(D) Histamine

Rationale: Octreotide is a treatment option not a substance secreted by the tumor itself.

Ref: Butterworth, J.F., Mackey, D.C., & Wasnick J.D. (2013). Ch 34 *Morgan & Mikhail's Clinical Anesthesiology* (5th ed.). New York, NY: McGraw-Hill.

Nagelhout, J.J., & K.L. Plaus (2014). Ch 30 *Nurse Anesthesia* (5th ed.). St. Louis, MO: Elsevier.

357. What is the most likely location of a carcinoid tumor?

(A) Kidney

(B) Lung

(C) Ovary

(D) Appendix

Rationale: More than half of carcinoid tumors occur in the gastrointestinal tract with the appendix being the most common location.

Ref: Butterworth, J.F., Mackey, D.C., & Wasnick J.D. (2013). Ch 34 *Morgan & Mikhail's Clinical Anesthesiology* (5th ed.). New York, NY: McGraw-Hill.

Nagelhout, J.J., & Plaus K.L. (2014). Ch 30 *Nurse Anesthesia* (5th ed.). St. Louis, MO: Elsevier.

358. What is the typical progression of Guillain-Barré syndrome?

(A) Descending paralysis

(B) Unilateral hemiparesis

(C) Ascending paralysis

(D) Concurrent upper and lower extremity weakness

Rationale: Guillain-Barré syndrome progresses from the feet up.

Ref: Butterworth, J.F., Mackey, D.C., & Wasnick, J.D. (2013). Ch 28 *Morgan & Mikhail's Clinical Anesthesiology* (5th ed.). New York, NY: McGraw-Hill.

Hines, R.L., & Marschall, K.E. (Eds.) (2012). Ch 12 *Stoelting's Anesthesia and Co-existing Disease* (6th ed.). Philadelphia, PA: Elsevier.

359. Which neuromuscular blocking agent is most appropriate for use in severe cirrhosis?

(A) Cisatracurium

(B) Rocuronium

(C) Vecuronium

(D) Pancuronium

Rationale: Cisatracurium metabolism is not dependent upon normal liver function.

Ref: Butterworth, J.F., Mackey, D.C., & Wasnick, J.D. (2013). Ch 33 *Morgan & Mikhail's Clinical Anesthesiology* (5th ed.). New York, NY: McGraw-Hill.

Hemmings, H.C. Jr., & Egan, T.D. (Eds.). (2013). Ch 19 *Pharmacology and physiology for anesthesia.* Philadelphia, PA: Elsevier.

360. Which drugs will be prolonged in the glaucoma patient treated with echothiophate?

Select (2) two

(A) Cocaine

(B) Succinylcholine

(C) Glycopyrrolate

(D) Chloroprocaine

Rationale: Echothiophate is a cholinesterase inhibitor. Drugs dependent upon this enzyme, like succinylcholine and ester local anesthetics, will be prolonged. Cocaine is an ester but is dependent upon the liver for metabolism.

Ref: Butterworth, J.F., Mackey, D.C., & Wasnick, J.D. (2013). Ch 36 *Morgan & Mikhail's Clinical Anesthesiology* (5th ed.). New York, NY: McGraw-Hill.

Hemmings, H.C. Jr., & Egan, T.D. (Eds.). (2013). Ch 17 *Pharmacology and Physiology for Anesthesia.* Philadelphia, PA: Elsevier.

361. What causes Eaton-Lambert syndrome?

(A) Autoimmune destruction of calcium channels

(B) Atypical pseudocholinesterase

(C) Autoimmune destruction of cholinergic receptors

(D) Autoimmune destruction of thyroid tissue

Rationale: Eaton-Lambert, or Lambert-Eaton Myasthenic Syndrome, is caused by destruction of calcium channels.
Ref: Butterworth, J.F., Mackey, D.C., & Wasnick J.D. (2013). Ch 11 *Morgan & Mikhail's Clinical Anesthesiology* (5th ed.). New York, NY: McGraw-Hill.
Hemmings, H.C. Jr., & Egan, T.D. (Eds.). (2013). Ch 18 *Pharmacology and Physiology for Anesthesia.* Philadelphia, PA: Elsevier.

362. Which abnormality is associated with syringomyelia?

(A) Craniosynostosis
(B) Crouzon Syndrome
(C) Arnold-Chiari malformation
(D) Apert syndrome

Rationale: There is increased incidence of Arnold-Chiari malformation in patients with cysts within the spinal cord.
Ref: Butterworth, J.F., Mackey, D.C., & Wasnick, J.D. (2013). Ch 28 *Morgan & Mikhail's Clinical Anesthesiology* (5th ed.). New York, NY: McGraw-Hill.
Hines, R.L., & Marschall, K.E. (Eds.) (2012). Ch 11 *Stoelting's Anesthesia and Co-existing Disease* (6th ed.). Philadelphia, PA: Elsevier.

363. Which causes Zollinger-Ellison syndrome?

(A) Gastrinoma
(B) Pheochromocytoma
(C) Pituitary adenoma
(D) Osteosarcoma

Rationale: Hypersecretion of gastrin due to a gastrinoma causes increased stomach acid secretion.
Ref: Butterworth, J.F., Mackey, D.C., & Wasnick, J.D. (2013). Ch 17 *Morgan & Mikhail's Clinical Anesthesiology* (5th ed.). New York, NY: McGraw-Hill.
Hines, R.L., & Marschall, K.E. (Eds.) (2012). Ch 14 *Stoelting's Anesthesia and Co-existing Disease* (6th ed.). Philadelphia, PA: Elsevier.

364. A patient's cardiac assessment reveals a functional capacity of four metabolic equivalents. What activity can she most likely perform?

(A) Walk one to two blocks on level ground
(B) Singles tennis
(C) Cross-country skiing
(D) Swimming

Rationale: A patient with 4 metabolic equivalents has the capacity to walk on level ground for a short at 4 miles per hour or run a short distance. B, C, and D are associated with a functional capacity of 10 or more.
Ref: Butterworth, J.F., Mackey, D.C., & Wasnick, J.D. (2013). Ch 21 *Morgan & Mikhail's Clinical Anesthesiology* (5th ed.). New York, NY: McGraw-Hill.
Nagelhout, J.J., & Plaus, K.L. (2014). Ch 19 *Nurse Anesthesia* (5th ed.). St. Louis, MO: Elsevier.

CHAPTER 2

Equipment, Instrumentation, and Technology
Questions

1. What is the maximum allowable current leakage in the operating room?

   (A) 10 uA
   (B) 20 mA
   (C) <1 mA
   (D) 100 mA

2. What monitor alarms when a high current flow to the ground exists?

   (A) Isolation transformer
   (B) Line isolation monitor
   (C) Leak current
   (D) High-efficiency particulate filter

3. What humidity levels are appropriate for the operating room?

   (A) 20-25%
   (B) 30-35%
   (C) 40-45%
   (D) 50-55%

4. Which of the following is true about heat and moisture exchangers?

   (A) Dead space increases.
   (B) Heat and moisture exchangers increase heat loss.
   (C) Dead space decreases.
   (D) Heat and moisture exchangers increase water loss.

5. What is the best method to avoid perioperative heat loss?

   (A) Preoperative warming blankets
   (B) Head wrapping
   (C) Forced air warming
   (D) Heated intraoperative warming blankets

6. During infusion of multiple units of packed red blood cells, what temperature is needed to avoid hypothermia?

   (A) 37°C
   (B) 36°C
   (C) 35°C
   (D) 34°C

7. What is the capacity of nitrous oxide in an E-cylinder?

   (A) 1,590 L
   (B) 700 L
   (C) 625 L
   (D) 950 L

8. What is the color in the United States for an air cylinder?

   (A) Blue
   (B) Black
   (C) Green
   (D) Yellow

9. What is the only reliable way to determine residual volume of nitrous oxide?

   (A) Calculate the pressure constant.
   (B) Measure the amount of liquid.
   (C) Calculate the gas flow.
   (D) Weigh the cylinder.

10. Which statement is true regarding the pin index safety system?

   (A) Avoid incorrect attachment of E-cylinders to the yoke.
   (B) Pin configuration consists of three pins.
   (C) Pin configurations may be converted to accommodate cylinder gas.
   (D) H-cylinders are attached to the yoke.

11. Which statement is false regarding the fail-safe valve?

   (A) Is part of the high-pressure system.
   (B) Prevents delivery of a hypoxic gas mixture.
   (C) Shuts off when pressure in oxygen supply circuit is <25 psi.
   (D) Triggers an alarm.

12. Which principle is not included in radiation safety?

   (A) Time
   (B) Distance
   (C) Shielding
   (D) Temperature

13. What component is not included in a Mapleson circuit?

   (A) Fresh gas inlet
   (B) Adjustable pressure-limiting valve
   (C) Reservoir bag
   (D) Low-resistance vaporizer

14. What component of the circle system is not present in a Mapleson circuit?

   (A) CO_2 absorber
   (B) Reservoir
   (C) Fresh gas inlet
   (D) APL valve

15. What breathing circuit affords rebreathing?

   (A) Mapleson A
   (B) Mapleson D
   (C) Circle system
   (D) Bain circuit

16. How does soda lime differ from barium hydroxide lime?

   (A) Barium hydroxide lime contains potassium hydroxide.
   (B) Absorptive capacity of soda lime is 9-18 L of CO_2/100 g granules.
   (C) Silica is added to barium hydroxide lime.
   (D) Soda lime contains calcium hydroxide, sodium hydroxide, and potassium hydroxide.

17. The operating room lost electrical supply. Which device does not require wall-outlet electrical power?

   (A) Scavenging system
   (B) Digital flow meter displays
   (C) Mechanical ventilators
   (D) Gas/vapor blenders

18. Which of the following safety devices does not sense oxygen pressure?

   (A) Mechanically linked proportioning system
   (B) Oxygen failure protection device
   (C) Supply failure alarm
   (D) Bourdon gauge

19. How does the variable-bypass type vaporizer preoperative check procedure differ from that of the Tec 6 vaporizer?

   (A) Both check the alarm battery low indicator.
   (B) Variable-bypass vaporizer checks include the alarm battery low indicator.
   (C) Tec 6 check includes checking the alarm battery low indicator.
   (D) Neither vaporizer checks the alarm battery low indicator.

20. What type of vaporizer contains desflurane?

   (A) Vernitrol
   (B) Measured-flow
   (C) Electronic
   (D) Copper kettle

21. What results from compressing the oxygen flush valve?

    (A) Barotrauma
    (B) Ventricular fibrillation
    (C) Concentrated inhaled agent
    (D) Increased anesthetic depth

22. Which oxygen analyzer is self-calibrating?

    (A) Galvanic
    (B) Polarographic
    (C) Clark
    (D) Paramagnetic

23. Following intubation, you connect the endotracheal tube to the breathing circuit. The adjustable pressure-limiting (APL) valve is nearly closed. What is most likely to result?

    (A) Tachycardia
    (B) Hypertension
    (C) Pneumothorax
    (D) Increased cardiac output

24. What agency recommends safe levels of waste gas exposure?

    (A) U.S. Food and Drug Administration (USDA)
    (B) National Institute for Occupational Safety and Health (NIOSH) and Occupational Safety and Health Administration (OSHA)
    (C) U.S. Food and Drug Administration and Occupational Safety and Health Administration
    (D) U.S. Food and Drug Administration and National Institute for Occupational Safety and Health

25. Which anesthesia check procedure is repeated before each case?

    (A) Scavenger system check
    (B) Flow control valve check
    (C) Pipe line gas pressure check
    (D) Breathing system leak check

26. You are unable to ventilate with a mask. What should you do first?

    (A) Proceed with two-hand mask ventilation.
    (B) Awaken the patient.
    (C) Consider using a strap.
    (D) Reposition the patient's head.

27. What nerve injury may result from prolonged pressure involving bag mask ventilation?

    (A) Trigeminal and facial nerves
    (B) Greater auricular
    (C) Anterior cutaneous nerve of the neck
    (D) Lesser occipital

28. Following induction of general anesthesia, you are unable to intubate the patient. Facemask ventilation is inadequate. What should you do next?

    (A) Consider placing an LMA.
    (B) Perform cricothyrotomy.
    (C) Cancel surgery.
    (D) Re-intubate.

29. Where is the tip of the Combitube™ placed?

    (A) Trachea
    (B) Esophagus
    (C) Hypopharynx
    (D) Infraglottic

30. How do you determine the proper position of the fiberoptic bronchoscope when performing a fiberoptic intubation?

    (A) By visualizing the esophagus
    (B) By visualizing the carina
    (C) By visualizing the tracheal rings and carina
    (D) By visualizing the epiglottis

31. You plan to intubate a patient with an unstable cervical spine injury. What is the best airway management approach?

    (A) One attempt at laryngoscopy
    (B) Placement of a LMA
    (C) Lighted sylet
    (D) Flexible fiberoptic bronchoscope

32. You experience difficulty visualizing the glottic opening during endotracheal intubation. What airway device combined with direct laryngoscopy will be useful for intubation?

    (A) Classic LMA
    (B) Eschmann Stylet
    (C) Fastrach™ LMA
    (D) ProSeal™ LMA

33. When using the MacIntosh laryngoscope, where is the tip of the blade placed?

(A) Vallecula

(B) Hyoepiglottic ligament

(C) Posterior to the epiglottis

(D) Posterior pharynx

34. What statement is true about jet ventilation?

(A) Regulators allow for an increase in inspiratory pressure.

(B) Inspiratory pressure should be <50 psi.

(C) Low-pressure oxygen is delivered.

(D) Inspiratory pressure should be >50 psi.

35. In which patient condition is a nasal airway used with caution?

(A) Obesity

(B) Basilar skull fracture

(C) Hemodynamic instability

(D) Octogenarian

36. When comparing sites for placement of a central venous catheter, which site carries the greatest risk for pneumothorax?

(A) Right internal jugular vein

(B) Subclavian vein

(C) Left internal jugular vein

(D) Right external jugular vein

37. What does an "a" wave represent in a CVP tracing?

(A) Atrial contraction

(B) Tricuspid valve elevation

(C) Venous return

(D) Tricuspid valve opening

38. What is the type of ventilator bellow rises during expiration?

(A) Ascending

(B) Descending

(C) Hanging

(D) Pneumatic

39. In which patient would you avoid using an esophageal stethoscope?

(A) 50-year-old with gastroesophageal reflux disease

(B) 70-year-old with congestive heart failure

(C) 70-year-old with alcoholic liver disease

(D) 50-year-old with gastrointestinal polyps

40. Which statement is true regarding pulse oximetry?

(A) Pulse oximetry artifact is due to excessive ambient light, motion, and methylene blue dye.

(B) Pulse oximetry requires calibration.

(C) Pulse oximetry artifact is due to hyperthermia and increased cardiac output.

(D) Oxyhemoglobin and deoxyhemoglobin absorb red and infrared light equally.

41. During general anesthesia, the end-tidal CO_2 wave form stops. What is the most likely cause?

(A) Esophageal intubation

(B) Circuit disconnect

(C) Bronchial intubation

(D) Malignant hyperthermia

42. The patient is surgically anesthetized. What is the corresponding Bispectral Index (BIS)?

(A) 96

(B) 90

(C) 78

(D) 56

43. When using evoked potentials, which of the following will you avoid?

(A) Cisatracurium

(B) Nitrous oxide

(C) Sufentanil

(D) Isoflurane

44. What monitoring modality does not reflect core body temperature?

(A) Tympanic membrane

(B) Esophageal

(C) Skin adhesives

(D) Pulmonary artery

45. What results when stimulating the ulnar nerve?

    (A) Contraction of the abductor pollicis
    (B) Contraction of the orbicularis oculi
    (C) Contraction of the adductor pollicis
    (D) Contraction of the facial nerve

46. What statement about peripheral nerve stimulation is false?

    (A) The adductor pollicis recovers before the orbicularis oculi.
    (B) Clinical relaxation requires approximately 90% blockade.
    (C) The orbiculari oculi recovers before the adductor pollicis.
    (D) Abrasion and skin irritation may result from peripheral nerve stimulation.

47. What statement is true about blood pressure measurement accuracy?

    (A) The cuff's bladder should extend at least 40% around the extremity.
    (B) The width of the cuff should be 20-25% greater than the diameter of the extremity.
    (C) Blood pressure is a measure of perfusion.
    (D) The doppler probe is the preferred noninvasive blood pressure measuring technique.

48. In what range is the left ventricular end diastolic pressure?

    (A) 1-10
    (B) 10-20
    (C) 5-15
    (D) 4-12

49. When monitoring central venous pressure (CVP), what causes the loss of "a" waves?

    (A) Atrial fibrillation
    (B) Tricuspid regurgitation
    (C) PVCs
    (D) Myocardial ischemia

50. In the normal capnograph, what does Phase III indicate?

    (A) Decreased CO_2
    (B) Dead space
    (C) Dead space and alveolar gas
    (D) Alveolar gas plateau

51. What causes an increased end-tidal carbon dioxide?

    (A) CNS depression
    (B) Decreased cardiac output
    (C) Hypotension
    (D) V/Q mismatch

52. What factor results in a shift to the right in an oxyhemoglobin dissociation curve?

    (A) Decreased CO_2
    (B) Elevated temperature
    (C) Alkalosis
    (D) Decreased temperature

53. What statement about pressure-controlled ventilation is false?

    (A) Limited peak inspiratory pressure exists.
    (B) Inspiratory pressure is controlled.
    (C) Tidal volume is uncontrolled.
    (D) Tidal volume is controlled.

54. Which Mapleson circuit is the most efficient for controlled ventilation?

    (A) Mapleson D
    (B) Mapleson A
    (C) Mapleson B
    (D) Mapleson C

55. What mechanism facilitates heat loss through air currents?

    (A) Radiation
    (B) Convection
    (C) Conduction
    (D) Evaporation

56. When is cell salvage contraindicated?

    (A) Sepsis

    (B) Benign tumors

    (C) Connective tissue disorders

    (D) Orthopedic conditions

57. How much blood loss is recommended for the use of cell salvage?

    (A) 250 mL

    (B) 500 mL

    (C) 750 mL

    (D) 1,000 mL

58. Where is the best location to monitor blood pressure for patients undergoing right shoulder arthroscopy in the beach chair position?

    (A) Right lower extremity

    (B) Left lower extremity

    (C) Left upper extremity

    (D) Right upper extremity

59. Which principle is not included in radiation safety?

    (A) Time

    (B) Distance

    (C) Shielding

    (D) Temperature

60. What is a disadvantage of the Bain circuit?

    (A) Increases circuit bulk

    (B) Partial warming of inspiratory gas

    (C) Kinking of the fresh gas inlet tube

    (D) Requires low fresh gas flow

61. The E-cylinder oxygen gauge pressure reads 850 psi. How many liters are remaining presuming that the E-cylinder was full at 2,000 psi and 660 L?

    (A) 300 L

    (B) 660 L

    (C) 240 L

    (D) 280 L

62. How many liters of CO_2 per 100 g of absorbent can soda lime absorb?

    (A) 23 L

    (B) 32 L

    (C) 44 L

    (D) 18 L

63. What does the National Institute for Occupational Safety and Health (NIOSH) recommend for the room concentration of a halogenated agent when nitrous oxide is used?

    (A) 25 ppm

    (B) 2 ppm

    (C) 0.5 ppm

    (D) 2.5 ppm

64. Which selection pertains to a closed waste gas scavenging system with active scavenging?

    (A) Must have a negative-pressure relief valve

    (B) Must have both a negative and positive pressure relief valve

    (C) Must have a positive-pressure relief valve

    (D) Requires no pressure relief valves

65. What is the approximate cylinder pressure delivered to the anesthesia machine?

    (A) 45 psi

    (B) 50 psi

    (C) 1,900 psi

    (D) 745 psi

66. How many liters per minute will the oxygen flush valve provide to the common gas outlet?

    (A) 10 L/min

    (B) 80-100 L/min

    (C) 20-30 L/min

    (D) 35-75 L/min

67. What is the outer diameter of the scavenger tubing?

    (A) 22- mm

    (B) 32- mm

    (C) 19- mm

    (D) 10- mm

68. Which Mapleson circuit is most efficient for spontaneous ventilation?

(A) Mapleson D

(B) Mapleson A

(C) Mapleson B

(D) Mapleson C

69. What are the benefits of the Bain circuit?

(A) Decreases the circuit bulk and retains heat and humidity

(B) Decreases resistance

(C) Decreases fresh gas flow

(D) Scavenges waste gas

70. What is the granule size commonly used in CO_2 absorbent?

(A) 2-4 mesh

(B) 6-8 mesh

(C) 4-8 mesh

(D) 1-2 mesh

71. What does the American Society of Anesthesiologists' Closed Claims Project database identify as the most common single source of injury pertaining to the anesthesia gas machine?

(A) Failure of the anesthesia delivery equipment

(B) Faulty ventilator

(C) Inaccurate calibration of the oxygen analyzer

(D) Misconnect or disconnect of breathing circuit components

72. What are three functions of the hanger yoke?

(A) Shuts off nitrous oxide when oxygen pressure falls below 20 psi, provides a gas tight seal, and ensures unidirectional flow

(B) Monitors inspired oxygen level, reduces pressure to 45-47 psi, and ensures unidirectional flow

(C) Orients cylinders, provides a gas tight seal, and ensures unidirectional flow

(D) Ensures at least 25% oxygen is given when using nitrous oxide, provides a gas tight seal, and ensure sunidirectional flow

73. Which oxygen analyzer works by using the oxygen molecules' unique attraction into magnetic fields?

(A) Electrogalvanic cell

(B) Polarographic electrode

(C) Paramagnetic oxygen sensor

(D) Fluorescence quenching

74. Which classification of breathing circuits has complete rebreathing?

(A) Open

(B) Semi-open

(C) Semi-closed

(D) Closed

75. How many liters does an oxygen E-cylinder tank hold?

(A) 660 L

(B) 1,590 L

(C) 625 L

(D) 750 L

76. What are the appropriate measures to reduce the amount of oxygen consumed and prolong the duration of your backup oxygen supply when the oxygen supply fails?

(A) Turn off the ventilator and ventilate manually through the circle system.

(B) Increase oxygen flows to 5 L per minute.

(C) Place the patient on pressure control ventilation.

(D) Reduce tidal volume and increase respiratory rate on the ventilator.

77. When the pressure gauge drops below 745 psig on a nitrous oxide E-cylinder at room temperature, approximately how much nitrous oxide is left in the tank?

(A) 1,590 L

(B) 660 L

(C) 400 L

(D) 625 L

78. What is size of the transfer tubing in the scavenger system?

(A) 22 mm

(B) 20 mm

(C) 19 mm

(D) 9 mm

79. What is the only piece of equipment that will ensure that oxygen is present in the pipelines or cylinder?

    (A) Oxygen analyzer
    (B) Hypoxic guard
    (C) Oxygen fail-safe device
    (D) Cylinder gauge

80. What is the ideal value for the scavenging vacuum?

    (A) 10-15 L/min
    (B) 1-2 L/min
    (C) 2-5 L/min
    (D) 30-40 L/min

81. Which type of waste-gas scavenger interface requires negative and positive pressure relief valves?

    (A) Open interface
    (B) Passive closed interface
    (C) Active closed interface
    (D) Active open interface

82. Which organization published a generic checkout procedure for anesthesia gas machines and breathing circuits?

    (A) American Association of Nurse Anesthetists (AANA)
    (B) Department of Transportation (DOT)
    (C) Food and Drug Administration (FDA)
    (D) American Society for Testing and Materials (ASTM)

83. What piece of equipment provides unidirectional flow to prevent retrograde flow of gases from the anesthesia machine to the pipeline or atmosphere?

    (A) Pressure relief valve
    (B) Pressure regulator valve
    (C) Hypoxic guard
    (D) Check valve

84. After checking your oxygen E-cylinder on the back of the anesthesia machine, what is the next step?

    (A) Keep open in case of pipeline failure.
    (B) The oxygen E-cylinder is only for emergency so it does not matter if you leave it open or closed.
    (C) Leave partly open.
    (D) Close the cylinder.

85. What circuit design incorporates a fresh gas inlet tube inside the breathing tube?

    (A) Mapleson D
    (B) Bain circuit
    (C) Mapleson A
    (D) Mapleson B

86. Which of the following minimizes Phase I temperature loss?

    (A) Warm blankets
    (B) Forced air warming
    (C) Heat and moisture exchanger
    (D) Warm IV fluids

87. The formation of carbon monoxide by the degradation of volatile anesthetic by dry soda lime is greatest with which volatile anesthetic?

    (A) Desflurane
    (B) Isoflurane
    (C) Sevoflurane
    (D) Nitrous oxide

88. Compound A is one of the by-products of degradation of which volatile anesthetic?

    (A) Desflurane
    (B) Isoflurane
    (C) Sevoflurane
    (D) Nitrous oxide

89. What is the end product of the soda lime reaction?

    (A) CO_2
    (B) Carbonic acid
    (C) Calcium carbonate
    (D) Ethyl violet

90. When should the LMA be removed?

(A) When the patient moves

(B) When the patient regains airway reflexes

(C) When the surgery is completed

(D) In the Post Anesthesia Care Unit

91. Which Mapleson circuit is a modification of the Mapleson D?

(A) Jackson-Reese

(B) Mapleson A

(C) Bain

(D) Mapleson C

92. Which statement is true regarding the diameter-index safety system (DISS)?

(A) The DISS prevents accidental connection of a wrong gas cylinder.

(B) The DISS is attached to the machine via a hanger-yoke assembly nitrous oxide 2-5, air 1-5, and oxygen 3-5.

(C) The DISS prevents incorrect hose attachment nitrous oxide 3-5, air 1-5, and oxygen 2-5.

(D) The DISS fittings for the oxygen inlet and the oxygen power outlet are different and cannot be interchanged.

93. What is your greatest concern when inflating the pulmonary artery balloon?

(A) Conduction abnormalities

(B) Pulmonary artery rupture

(C) Catheter knotting

(D) Bacteremia

94. Following intubation you are unable to palpate the tracheal tube cuff in the sternal notch. The breathing bag compliance is decreased. Breath sounds are unilateral. Where is the endotracheal tube most likely positioned?

(A) Hypopharynx

(B) Esophagus

(C) Supraglottic

(D) Bronchus

Answers and Explanations: Equipment, Instrumentation, and Technology

1. What is the maximum allowable current leakage in the operating room?

   (A) 10 uA
   (B) 20 mA
   (C) <1 mA
   (D) 100 mA

   Rationale: The maximum allowable current leak in the operating room is 10 uA.
   Ref: Butterworth, J.F., Mackey, D.C., & Wasnick, J.D. (2013). Ch 2 *Morgan & Mikhail's Clinical Anesthesiology* (5th ed.). New York, NY: McGraw-Hill.

2. What monitor alarms when a high current flow to the ground exists?

   (A) Isolation transformer
   (B) Line isolation monitor
   (C) Leak current
   (D) High-efficiency particulate filter

   Rationale: The line isolation monitor affords protection from electrical shocks in the operating room. The isolation transformer affords isolation between the power supply in the operating room and the ground. High efficiency particulate (HEPA) filters are used to maintain air quality in the operating room.
   Ref: Butterworth, J.F., Mackey, D.C., & Wasnick, J.D. (2013). Ch 3 *Morgan & Mikhail's Clinical Anesthesiology* (5th ed.). New York, NY: McGraw-Hill.

3. What humidity levels are appropriate for the operating room?

   (A) 20-25%
   (B) 30-35%
   (C) 40-45%
   (D) 50-55%

   Rationale: Humidity levels between 50-55% foster infection control in the operating room. Sterile drapes may be affected by high humidity causing dampness, whereas low humidity may accelerate movement of particulate matter.
   Ref: Butterworth, J.F., Mackey, D.C., & Wasnick, J.D. (2013). Ch 3 *Morgan & Mikhail's Clinical Anesthesiology* (5th ed.). New York, NY: McGraw-Hill.

4. Which of the following is true about heat and moisture exchangers?

   (A) Dead space increases.
   (B) Heat and moisture exchangers increase heat loss.
   (C) Dead space decreases.
   (D) Heat and moisture exchangers increase water loss.

   Rationale: When using a heat and moisture exchanger, dead space increases.
   Ref: Butterworth, J.F., Mackey, D.C., & Wasnick, J.D. (2013). Ch 42 *Morgan & Mikhail's Clinical Anesthesiology* (5th ed.). New York, NY: McGraw-Hill.
   Miller, R.D., & Pardo, M.C. (2011). Ch 15 *Basics of Anesthesia* (6th ed.). Philadelphia, PA: Elsevier.

5. What is the best method to avoid perioperative heat loss?

   (A) Preoperative warming blankets
   (B) Head wrapping
   (C) Forced air warming
   (D) Heated intraoperative warming blankets

   Rationale: All methods in combination help conserve body heat. Active warming fosters greater heat conservation than passive methods.
   Ref: Butterworth, J.F., Mackey, D.C., & Wasnick, J.D. (2013). Ch 52 *Morgan & Mikhail's Clinical Anesthesiology* (5th ed.). New York, NY: McGraw-Hill.
   Nagelhout, J.J., & Plaus, K.L. (2014). Ch 50 *Nurse Anesthesia* (5th ed.). St. Louis, MO: Elsevier.

TABLE 2-1. Characteristics of medical gas cylinders.

Gas	E-Cylinder Capacity[1] (L)	H-Cylinder Capacity[1] (L)	Pressure[1] (psig at 20°C)	Color (USA)	Color (International)	Form
O_2	625-700	6,000-8,000	1,800-2,200	Green	White	Gas
Air	625-700	6,000-8,000	1,800-2,200	Yellow	White and black	Gas
N_2O	1590	15,900	745	Blue	Blue	Liquid
N_2	625-700	6,000-8,000	1,800-2,200	Black	Black	Gas

[1]Depending on the manufacturer.

6. During infusion of multiple units of packed red blood cells, what temperature is needed to avoid hypothermia?

   (A) 37°C

   (B) 36°C

   (C) 35°C

   (D) 34°C

   Rationale: Hypothermia results with multiple transfusions when the infused products are not warmed. Warming fluids (37°C) assists in minimizing body temperature loss.

   Ref: Butterworth, J.F., Mackey, D.C., & Wasnick, J.D. (2013). Ch 52 *Morgan & Mikhail's Clinical Anesthesiology* (5th ed.). New York, NY: McGraw-Hill.

7. What is the capacity of nitrous oxide in an E-cylinder?

   (A) 1,590 L

   (B) 700 L

   (C) 625 L

   (D) 950 L

   Rationale: The capacity of nitrous oxide in an E-cylinder is 1,590 L as compared to an H-cylinder (15,900 L). The capacity of oxygen, air, and nitrogen in an E-cylinder is 625-700 L.

   Ref: Butterworth, J.F., Mackey, D.C., & Wasnick, J.D. (2013). Ch 2 *Morgan & Mikhail's Clinical Anesthesiology* (5th ed.). New York, NY: McGraw-Hill.

8. What is the color (United States) for an air cylinder?

   (A) Blue

   (B) Black

   (C) Green

   (D) Yellow

   Rationale: Air cylinders are yellow; oxygen is green; nitrous oxide is blue; and nitrogen is black.

   Ref: Butterworth, J.F., Mackey, D.C., & Wasnick, J.D. (2013). Ch 2 *Morgan & Mikhail's Clinical Anesthesiology* (5th ed.). New York, NY: McGraw-Hill.

9. What is the only reliable way to determine residual volume of nitrous oxide?

   (A) Calculate the pressure constant.

   (B) Measure the amount of liquid.

   (C) Calculate the gas flow.

   (D) Weigh the cylinder.

   Rationale: Weighing the cylinder is the best means to determine the residual volume of nitrous oxide. The liquid volume of nitrous oxide is not proportional to the pressure in the cylinder.

   Ref: Butterworth, J.F., Mackey, D.C., & Wasnick, J.D. (2013). Ch 2 *Morgan & Mikhail's Clinical Anesthesiology* (5th ed.). New York, NY: McGraw-Hill.

10. Which statement is true regarding the pin index safety system?

    (A) Avoid incorrect attachment of E-cylinders to the yoke.

    (B) Pin configuration consists of three pins.

    (C) Pin configurations may be converted to accommodate cylinder gas.

    (D) H-cylinders are attached to the yoke.

    Rationale: The Pin Index Safety system is designed to ensure attachment of E-cylinders to the yoke. A two-pin

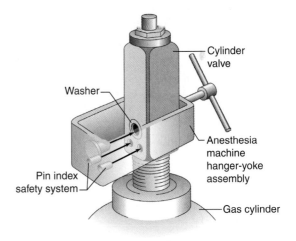

FIG. 2-1. Pin index safety system interlink between the anesthesia machine and gas cylinder.

system connects the correct E-cylinder to the correct holes on the yoke. E-cylinders are never attached or forced into reconfigured holes on the yoke.

Ref: Butterworth, J.F., Mackey, D.C., & Wasnick, J.D. (2013). Ch 2 *Morgan & Mikhail's Clinical Anesthesiology* (5th ed.). New York, NY: McGraw-Hill.

Longnecker, D.E., Brown, D.L., Newman, M.F., & Zapol, W.M. (2012). Ch 39 *Anesthesiology* (2nd ed.). New York, NY: McGraw-Hill.

11. Which statement is false regarding the fail-safe valve?

   (A) Is part of the high-pressure system.

   (B) Prevents delivery of a hypoxic gas mixture.

   (C) Shuts off when pressure in oxygen supply circuit is <25 psi.

   (D) Triggers an alarm.

   Rationale: The fail-safe valve, part of the high pressure system, does not prevent delivery of a hypoxic gas mixture. The valve shuts off or decreases gas flow when oxygen pressure decreases to less than 30 psi. The fail-safe device triggers an alarm.

   Ref: Butterworth, J.F., Mackey, D.C., & Wasnick, J.D. (2013). Ch 2 *Morgan & Mikhail's Clinical Anesthesiology* (5th ed.). New York, NY: McGraw-Hill.

   Longnecker, D.E., Brown, D.L., Newman, M.F., & Zapol, W.M. (2012). Ch 39 *Anesthesiology* (2nd ed.). New York, NY: McGraw-Hill.

12. Which principle is not included in radiation safety?

   (A) Time

   (B) Distance

   (C) Shielding

   (D) Temperature

   Rationale: Time, distance, and shielding guide the need for anesthesia providers to avoid the hazards of radiation in the operating room. No relationship exists between the operating room temperature and radiation safety.

   Ref: Butterworth, J.F., Mackey, D.C., & Wasnick, J.D. (2013). Ch 3 *Morgan & Mikhail's Clinical Anesthesiology* (5th ed.). New York, NY: McGraw-Hill.

13. What component is not included in a Mapleson circuit?

   (A) Fresh gas inlet

   (B) Adjustable pressure-limiting valve

   (C) Reservoir bag

   (D) Low-resistance vaporizer

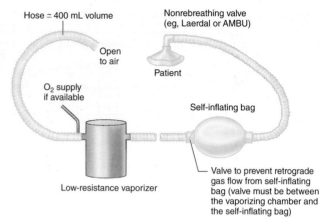

FIG. 2-2. Schematic diagram of a draw-over anesthesia device/circuit.

   Rationale: Components of Mapleson circuits include the breathing tube, fresh gas inlet, adjustable pressure-limiting valve, and reservoir bag. A low-resistance vaporizer is a component of the draw-over anesthesia device/circuit.

   Ref: Butterworth, J.F., Mackey, D.C., & Wasnick, J.D. (2013). Ch 3 *Morgan & Mikhail's Clinical Anesthesiology* (5th ed.). New York, NY: McGraw-Hill.

   Miller, R.D., & Pardo, M.C. (2011). Ch 15 *Basics of Anesthesia* (6th ed.). Philadelphia, PA: Elsevier.

14. What component of the circle system is not present in a Mapleson circuit?

   (A) CO_2 absorber

   (B) Reservoir

   (C) Fresh gas inlet

   (D) APL valve

   Rationale: CO_2 absorbers are present in the circle system but not the Mapleson circuit. Also included in the circle system but not the Mapleson system are an inspiratory unidirectional valve and breathing tube, Y-connector, and an expiratory unidirectional valve and breathing tube.

   Ref: Butterworth, J.F., Mackey, D.C., & Wasnick, J.D. (2013). Ch 3 *Morgan & Mikhail's Clinical Anesthesiology* (5th ed.). New York, NY: McGraw-Hill.

   Miller, R.D., & Pardo, M.C. (2011). Ch 15 *Basics of Anesthesia* (6th ed.). Philadelphia, PA: Elsevier.

15. What breathing circuit affords rebreathing?

   (A) Mapleson A

   (B) Mapleson D

   (C) Circle system

   (D) Bain circuit

TABLE 2-2. Classification and characteristics of Mapleson circuits.

Mapleson Class	Other Names	Configuration[1]	Required Fresh Gas Flows — Spontaneous	Required Fresh Gas Flows — Controlled	Comments
A	Magill attachment	(diagram: FGI → Breathing tube, APL valve, Breathing bag, Mask)	Equal to minute ventilation (≈80 mL/kg/min)	Very high and difficult to predict	Poor choice during cotrolled ventilaton. Enclosed Magill system is a modification that improves efficiency. Coaxial Mapleson A (Lack breathing system) provides waste gas scavenging.
B		(diagram: FGI, APL valve)	2 × minute ventilation	2-2½ × minute ventilation	
C	Waters' to-and-fro	(diagram: FGI, APL valve)	2 × minute ventilation	2-2½ × minute ventilation	
D	Bain circuit	(diagram: APL valve, FGI)	2-3 × minute ventilation	1-2 × minute ventilation	Bain coaxial modification: fresh gas tube inside breathing tube (see Figure 3-7).
E	Ayre's T-piece	(diagram: FGI)	2-3 × minute ventilation	3 × minute ventilation (I:E-1:2)	Exhalation tubing should provide a larger volume than tidal volume to prevent rebreathing. Scavenging is difficult.
F	Jackson–Rees' modification	(diagram: FGI, APL valve)	2-3 × minute ventilation	2 × minute ventilation	A Mapleson E with a breathing bag connected to the end of the breathing tube to allow controlled ventilation and scavenging.

[1]FGI, fresh gas inlet; APL, adjustable pressure-limiting (value).

Rationale: There is no rebreathing with the Mapleson circuits. Rebreathing occurs with circle systems specifically with high fresh gas flows.

Ref: Butterworth, J.F., Mackey, D.C., & Wasnick, J.D. (2013). Ch 3 *Morgan & Mikhail's Clinical Anesthesiology* (5th ed.). New York, NY: McGraw-Hill.

Miller, R.D., & Pardo, M.C. (2011). Ch 15 *Basics of Anesthesia* (6th ed.). Philadelphia, PA: Elsevier.

TABLE 2-3. Characteristics of breathing circuits.

	Insufflation and Open Drop	Mapleson	Circle
Complexity	Very simple	Simple	Complex
Control of anesthetic depth	Poor	Variable	Good
Ability to scavenge	Very poor	Variable	Good
Conservation of heat and humidity	No	No	Yes[1]
Rebreathing of exhaled gases	No	No[1]	Yes[1]

[1]These properties depend on the rate of fresh gas flow.

16. How does soda lime differ from barium hydroxide lime?

(A) Barium hydroxide lime contains potassium hydroxide.

(B) Absorptive capacity of soda lime is 9-18 L of CO_2/100 g granules.

(C) Silica is added to barium hydroxide lime.

(D) Soda lime contains calcium hydroxide, sodium hydroxide, and potassium hydroxide.

Rationale: Soda lime is hardened with silica, whereas barium hydroxide lime's hardness is due to its water of crystallization. Barium hydroxide contains barium hydroxide and calcium hydroxide, but no potassium hydroxide. The absorptive capacity of barium hydroxide is 9-18 L of CO_2/100 g granules and 14-23 L of CO_2/100 g granules for soda lime.

TABLE 2-4. Comparison of soda lime and barium hydroxide lime.

	Soda Lime	Barium Hydroxide Lime
Mesh size[1]	4-8	4-8
Method of hardness	Silica added	Water of crystallization
Content	Calcium hydroxide Sodium hydroxide Potassium hydroxide	Barium hydroxide Calcium hydroxide
Usual indicator dye	Ethyl violet	Ethyl violet
Absorptive capacity (liters of CO_2/100 g granules)	14-23	9-18

[1]The number of openings per linear inch in a wire screen used to grade particle size.

Ref: Butterworth, J.F., Mackey, D.C., & Wasnick, J.D. (2013). Ch 3 *Morgan & Mikhail's Clinical Anesthesiology* (5th ed.). New York, NY: McGraw-Hill.
Miller, R.D., & Pardo, M.C. (2011). Ch 15 *Basics of Anesthesia* (6th ed.). Philadelphia, PA: Elsevier.

17. The operating room lost electrical supply. Which device does not require wall-outlet electrical power?

(A) Scavenging system
(B) Digital flow meter displays
(C) Mechanical ventilators
(D) Gas/Vapor blenders

Rationale: Electrical wall outlet power is required for most physiologic monitors, mechanical ventilators, gas/vapor blenders in the operating room. Items not requiring electric power include the scavenging system, variable bypass vaporizers, and mechanical flow meters.
Ref: Nagelhout, J.J., & Plaus, K.L. (2014). Ch 15 *Nurse Anesthesia* (5th ed.). St. Louis, MO: Elsevier.

18. Which of the following safety devices does not sense oxygen pressure?

(A) Mechanically linked proportioning system
(B) Oxygen failure protection device
(C) Supply failure alarm
(D) Bourdon gauge

Rationale: Option A is a proportioning chain between the nitrous oxide flow control and the oxygen flow control, which limits the oxygen concentration without detecting pressures. Option B is a diaphragm device dependent upon minimum oxygen pressure to remain open. Option C operates above a minimum pressure threshold. Option D is a pressure gauge.
Ref: Butterworth, J.F., Mackey, D.C., & Wasnick, J.D. (2013). Ch 54 *Morgan & Mikhail's Clinical Anesthesiology* (5th ed.). New York, NY: Lange Medical Books McGraw-Hill.

19. How does the variable-bypass type vaporizer preoperative check procedure differ from that of the Tec 6 vaporizer?

(A) Both check the alarm battery low indicator.
(B) Variable-bypass vaporizer checks include the alarm battery low indicator.
(C) Tec 6 check includes checking the alarm battery low indicator.
(D) Neither vaporizer checks the alarm battery low indicator.

Rationale: As compared to other variable-bypass type vaporizers, the Tec 6 vaporizer contains an alarm battery low indicator light.
Ref: Nagelhout, J.J., & Plaus, K.L. (2014). Ch 15 *Nurse Anesthesia* (5th ed.). St. Louis, MO: Elsevier.

20. What type of vaporizer contains desflurane?

(A) Vernitrol
(B) Measured-flow
(C) Electronic
(D) Copper kettle

Rationale: Unlike the vapor pressures of the other inhalational agents, Desflurane's high vapor pressure requires a special electronic vaporizer. Measured-flow vaporizers include the copper kettle and vernitrol.
Ref: Butterworth, J.F., Mackey, D.C., & Wasnick, J.D. (2013). Ch 4 *Morgan & Mikhail's Clinical Anesthesiology* (5th ed.). New York, NY: McGraw-Hill.
Miller, R.D., & Pardo, M.C. (2011). Ch 15 *Basics of Anesthesia* (6th ed.). Philadelphia, PA: Elsevier.
Nagelhout, J.J., & Plaus, K.L. (2014). Ch 15 *Nurse Anesthesia* (5th ed.). St. Louis, MO: Elsevier.

21. What results from compressing the oxygen flush valve?

(A) Barotrauma
(B) Ventricular fibrillation
(C) Concentrated inhaled agent
(D) Increased anesthetic depth

Rationale: Compressing the oxygen flush valve (35-75 L/min) results in filling the breathing circuit. If the circuit is connected to the endotracheal tube during general anesthesia, barotrauma may result. The oxygen flush dilutes the inhaled agent and promotes the likelihood of decreased anesthetic depth.

Ref: Butterworth, J.F., Mackey, D.C., & Wasnick, J.D. (2013). Ch 4 *Morgan & Mikhail's Clinical Anesthesiology* (5th ed.). New York, NY: McGraw-Hill.

Nagelhout, J.J., & Plaus, K.L. (2014). Ch 15 *Nurse Anesthesia* (5th ed.). St. Louis, MO: Elsevier.

22. Which oxygen analyzer is self-calibrating?

    (A) Galvanic
    (B) Polarographic
    (C) Clark
    (D) Paramagnetic

    Rationale: Galvanic and polarographic (Clark) oxygen analyzers are electrochemical sensors requiring calibration. Components of the electrochemical sensors include anode and cathode electrodes, electrolyte gel, and an oxygen-permeable membrane. Quick oxygen analysis, no additional components, and self-calibration serve as advantages of paramagnetic oxygen analyzers

    Ref: Butterworth, J.F., Mackey, D.C., & Wasnick, J.D. (2013). Ch 4 *Morgan & Mikhail's Clinical Anesthesiology* (5th ed.). New York, NY: McGraw-Hill.

23. Following intubation, you connect the endotracheal tube to the breathing circuit. The adjustable pressure-limiting (APL) valve is nearly closed. What is most likely to result?

    (A) Tachycardia
    (B) Hypertension
    (C) Pneumothorax
    (D) Increased cardiac output

    Rationale: Hypotension and pneumothorax may result from increased pressure when the APL valve is nearly closed or closed completely.

    Ref: Butterworth, J.F., Mackey, D.C., & Wasnick, J.D. (2013). Ch 4 *Morgan & Mikhail's Clinical Anesthesiology* (5th ed.). New York, NY: McGraw-Hill.

    Miller, R.D., & Pardo, M.C. (2011). Ch 15 *Basics of Anesthesia* (6th ed.). Philadelphia, PA: Elsevier.

24. What agency recommends safe levels of waste gas exposure?

    (A) U.S. Food and Drug Administration (USDA)
    (B) National Institute for Occupational Safety and Health (NIOSH) and Occupational Safety and Health Administration (OSHA)
    (C) U.S. Food and Drug Administration and Occupational Safety and Health Administration
    (D) U.S. Food and Drug Administration and National Institute for Occupational Safety and Health

    Rationale: NIOSH and OSHA recommend that the concentration of nitrous oxide in the operating room be less than 25 ppm and 2 ppm for halogenated agents.

    Ref: Butterworth, J.F., Mackey, D.C., & Wasnick, J.D. (2013). Ch 4 *Morgan & Mikhail's Clinical Anesthesiology* (5th ed.). New York, NY: McGraw-Hill.

    Nagelhout, J.J., & Plaus, K.L. (2014). Ch 15 *Nurse Anesthesia* (5th ed.). St. Louis, MO: Elsevier.

25. Which anesthesia check procedure is repeated before each case?

    (A) Scavenger system check
    (B) Flow control valve check
    (C) Pipe line gas pressure check
    (D) Breathing system leak check

    Rationale: Although the scavenger, flow control valve, and pipeline gas pressure are checked daily, the breathing system leak check is conducted prior to each anesthetic.

    Ref: Butterworth, J.F., Mackey, D.C., & Wasnick, J.D. (2013). Ch 4 *Morgan & Mikhail's Clinical Anesthesiology* (5th ed.). New York, NY: McGraw-Hill.

    Nagelhout, J.J., & Plaus, K.L. (2014). Ch 15 *Nurse Anesthesia* (5th ed.). St. Louis, MO: Elsevier.

26. You are unable to ventilate with a mask. What should you do first?

    (A) Proceed with two-hand mask ventilation.
    (B) Awaken the patient.
    (C) Consider using a strap.
    (D) Reposition the patient's head.

    Rationale: Each of the options will assist with proper bag mask ventilation. Repositioning the patient's head will optimize the ability to ventilate. If after repositioning, it remains difficult to ventilate using a head strap, consider placing an oropharyngeal airway, using two-hand mask ventilation or using an alternative airway.

    Ref: Butterworth, J.F., Mackey, D.C., & Wasnick, J.D. (2013). Ch 19 *Morgan & Mikhail's Clinical Anesthesiology* (5th ed.). New York, NY: McGraw-Hill.

    Nagelhout, J.J., & Plaus, K.L. (2014). Ch 22 *Nurse Anesthesia* (5th ed.). St. Louis, MO: Elsevier.

TABLE 2-5. Anesthesia apparatus checkout recommendations.[1,2]

This checkout, or a reasonable equivalent, should be conducted before administration of anesthesia. These recommendations are valid only for an anesthesia system that conforms to current and relevant standards and includes an ascending bellows ventilator and at least the following monitors: capnograph, pulse oximeter, oxygen analyzer, respiratory volume monitor (spirometer), and breathing-system pressure monitor with high- and low-pressure alarms. Users are encouraged to modify this guideline to accommodate differences in equipment design and variations in local clinical practice. Such local modifications should have appropriate peer review. Users should refer to the appropriate operator manuals for specific procedures and precautions.

Emergency Ventilation Equipment
*1. Verify backup ventilation equipment is available and functioning.

High-Pressure System
*2. Check O_2 cylinder supply.
   a. Open O_2 cylinder and verify at least half full (about 1000 psig).
   b. Close cylinder.
*3. Check central pipeline supplies; check that hoses are connected and pipeline gauges read about 50 psig.

Low-Pressure System
*4. Check initial status of low-pressure system.
   a. Close flow control valves and turn vaporizers off.
   b. Check fill level and tighten vaporizers' filler caps.
*5. Perform leak check of machine low-pressure system.
   a. Verify that the machine master switch and flow control valves are off.
   b. Attach suction bulb to common (fresh) gas outlet.
   c. Squeeze bulb repeatedly until fully collapsed.
   d. Verify bulb stays *fully* collapsed for at least 10 seconds.
   e. Open one vaporizer at a time and repeat steps c and d.
   f. Remove suction bulb, and reconnect fresh gas hose.
*6. Turn on machine master switch and all other necessary electrical equipment.
*7. Test flow meters
   a. Adjust flow of all gases through their full range, checking for smooth operation of floats and undamaged flow tubes.
   b. Attempt to create a hypoxic O_2/N_2O mixture and verify correct changes in flow and/or alarm.

Scavenging System
*8. Adjust and check scavenging system.
   a. Ensure proper connections between the scavenging system and both APL (pop-off) valve and ventilator relief valve.
   b. Adjust waste-gas vacuum (if possible).
   c. Fully open APL valve and occlude Y-piece.
   d. With minimum O_2 flow, allow scavenger reservoir bag to collapse completely and verify that absorber pressure gauge reads about zero.
   e. With the O_2 flush activated, allow scavenger reservoir bag to distend fully, and then verify that absorber pressure gauge reads <10 cm H_2O.

Breathing System
*9. Calibrate O_2 monitor.
   a. Ensure monitor reads 21% in room air.
   b. Verify low-O_2 alarm is enabled and functioning.
   c. Reinstall sensor in circuit and flush breathing system with O_2.
   d. Verify that monitor now reads greater than 90%.

10. Check initial status breathing system
   a. Set selector switch to Bag mode.
   b. Check that breathing circuit is complete, undamaged, and unobstructed.
   c. Verify that CO_2 absorbent is adequate.
   d. Install breathing-circuit accessory equipment (e.g., humidifier, PEEP valve) to be used during the case.
11. Perform leak check of the breathing system
   a. Set all gas flows to zero (or minimum).
   b. Close APL (pop-off) valve and occlude Y-piece.
   c. Pressurize breathing system to about 30 cm H_2O with O_2 flush.
   d. Ensure that pressure remains fixed for at least 10 seconds.
   e. Open APL (pop-off) valve and ensure that pressure decreases.

Manual and Automatic Ventilation Systems
12. Test ventilation systems and unidirectional valves.
   a. Place a second breathing bag on Y-piece.
   b. Set appropriate ventilator parameters for next patient.
   c. Switch to automatic-ventilation (ventilator) mode.
   d. Turn ventilator on and fill bellows and breathing bag with O_2 flush.
   e. Set O_2 flow to minimum, other gas flows to zero.
   f. Verify that during inspiration bellows deliver appropriate tidal volume and that during expiration bellows fill completely.
   g. Set fresh gas flow to about 5 L/min.
   h. Verify that the ventilator bellows and simulated lungs fill and empty appropriately without sustained pressure at end expiration.
   i. Check for proper action of unidirectional valves.
   j. Exercise breathing circuit accessories to ensure proper function.
   k. Turn ventilator off and switch to manual ventilation (Bag/APL) mode.
   l. Ventilate manually and ensure inflation and deflation of artificial lungs and appropriate feel of system resistance and compliance.
   m. Remove second breathing bag from Y-piece.

Monitors
13. Check, calibrate, and/or set alarm limits of all monitors: capnograph, pulse oximeter, O_2 analyzer, respiratory-volume monitor (spirometer), pressure monitor with high and low airway-pressure alarms.

Final Position
14. Check final status of machine.
   a. Vaporizers off
   b. APL valve open
   c. Selector switch to Bag mode
   d. All flow meters to zero (or minimum)
   e. Patient suction level adequate
   f. Breathing system ready to use

[1]Data from http://www.fda.gov/cdrh/humfac/anesckot.html.
[2]APL, adjust pressure-limiting; PEEP, positive end-expiratory pressure.
*If an anesthesia provider uses the same machine in successive cases, these steps need not be repeated, or they can be abbreviated after the initial checkout.

27. What nerve injury may result from prolonged pressure involving bag mask ventilation?

(A) Trigeminal and facial nerves

(B) Greater auricular

(C) Anterior cutaneous nerve of the neck

(D) Lesser occipital

Rationale: Nerve injuries result from improper positioning. In addition, pressure may result in nerve injury from various devices including the facemask.

Ref: Butterworth, J.F., Mackey, D.C., & Wasnick, J.D. (2013). Ch 19 *Morgan & Mikhail's Clinical Anesthesiology* (5th ed.). New York, NY: McGraw-Hill.

Nagelhout, J.J., & Plaus, K.L. (2014). Ch 22 *Nurse Anesthesia* (5th ed.). St. Louis, MO: Elsevier.

28. Following induction of general anesthesia, you are unable to intubate the patient. Facemask ventilation is inadequate. What should you do next?

(A) Consider placing an LMA.

Difficult Airway Algorithm

1. Assess the likelihood and clinical impact of basic management problems.
   A. Difficult ventilation
   B. Difficult intubation
   C. Difficulty with patient cooperation or consent
   D. Difficult tracheostomy
2. Actively pursue opportunities to deliver supplemental oxygen throughout the process of difficult airway management.
3. Consider the relative merits and feasibility of basic management choices:

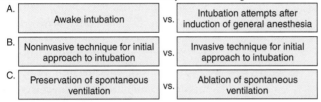

A. Awake intubation   vs.   Intubation attempts after induction of general anesthesia

B. Noninvasive technique for initial approach to intubation   vs.   Invasive technique for initial approach to intubation

C. Preservation of spontaneous ventilation   vs.   Ablation of spontaneous ventilation

4. Develop primary and alternative strategies.

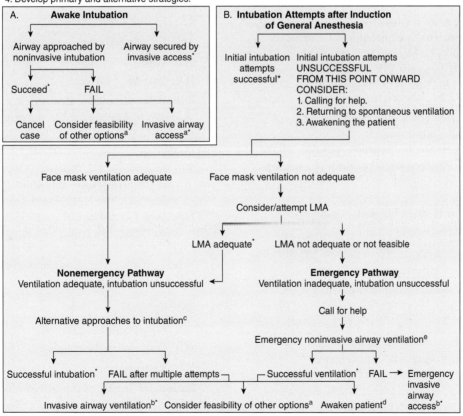

FIG. 2-3. Difficult Airway Algorithm developed by the American Society of Anesthesiologists. *Confirm tracheal intubation or LMA placement with exhaled CO_2. (Reproduced, with permission, from the American Society of Anesthesiologists Task Force on Management of the Difficult Airway. Practice guidelines for management of the difficult airway: an updated report by the American Society of Anesthesiologists Task Force on Management of the Difficult Airway. Anesthesiology 2003;98:1269.)

(B) Perform cricothyrotomy.

(C) Cancel surgery.

(D) Re-intubate.

Rationale: The American Society of Anesthesiologists Difficult Airway Algorithm informs how to manage difficult airway scenarios. For this case, calling for help, returning the patient to spontaneous ventilation, or awakening the patient is considered. If inadequate mask ventilation persists, consider or attempt LMA placement. If an LMA attempt fails, proceed to the emergency airway pathway.

Ref: Butterworth, J.F., Mackey, D.C., & Wasnick, J.D. (2013). Ch 19 *Morgan & Mikhail's Clinical Anesthesiology* (5th ed.). New York, NY: McGraw-Hill.

Nagelhout, J.J., & Plaus, K.L. (2014). Ch 22 *Nurse Anesthesia* (5th ed.). St. Louis, MO: Elsevier.

29. Where is the tip of the Combitube™ placed?

(A) Trachea

(B) Esophagus

(C) Hypopharynx

(D) Infraglottic

Rationale: The double lumen combitube is a supraglottic alternative airway device that is blindly placed in the hypopharynx. The tip is placed in the esophagus.

Ref: Butterworth, J.F., Mackey, D.C., & Wasnick, J.D. (2013). Ch 19 *Morgan & Mikhail's Clinical Anesthesiology* (5th ed.). New York, NY: McGraw-Hill.

Nagelhout, J.J., & Plaus, K.L. (2014). Ch 22 *Nurse Anesthesia* (5th ed.). St. Louis, MO: Elsevier.

30. How do you determine the proper position of the fiberoptic bronchoscope when performing a fiberoptic intubation?

(A) By visualizing the esophagus

(B) By visualizing the carina

(C) By visualizing the tracheal rings and carina

(D) By visualizing the epiglottis

Rationale: Successful fiberoptic intubation is dependent on the identification of airway structures. Once the glottis opening is identified, the fiberoptic bronchoscope is advanced. Visualization of the tracheal rings and carina inform proper placement.

Ref: Butterworth, J.F., Mackey, D.C., & Wasnick, J.D. (2013). Ch 19 *Morgan & Mikhail's Clinical Anesthesiology* (5th ed.). New York, NY: McGraw-Hill.

Nagelhout, J.J., & Plaus, K.L. (2014). Ch 22 *Nurse Anesthesia* (5th ed.). St. Louis, MO: Elsevier.

31. You plan to intubate a patient with an unstable cervical spine injury. What is the best airway management approach?

(A) One attempt at laryngoscopy

(B) Placement of a LMA

(C) Lighted sylet

(D) Flexible fiberoptic bronchoscope

Rationale: For patients where an awake intubation is indicated, a flexible fiberoptic bronchoscope facilitates intubation. Patients with conditions including cervical spine injuries, congenital abnormalities, or certain temporomandibular joint conditions benefit from this approach.

Ref: Butterworth, J.F., Mackey, D.C., & Wasnick, J.D. (2013). Ch 19 *Morgan & Mikhail's Clinical Anesthesiology* (5th ed.). New York, NY: McGraw-Hill.

Nagelhout, J.J., & Plaus, K.L. (2014). Ch 22 *Nurse Anesthesia* (5th ed.). St. Louis, MO: Elsevier.

32. You experience difficulty visualizing the glottic opening during endotracheal intubation. What airway device combined with direct laryngoscopy will be useful for intubation?

(A) Classic LMA

(B) Eschmann Stylet

(C) Fastrach™ LMA

(D) ProSeal™ LMA

Rationale: Alternative airway devices include each of the options. As compared to the variety of LMAs, the Eschmann Stylet uses direct laryngoscopy to facilitate intubation.

Ref: Butterworth, J.F., Mackey, D.C., & Wasnick, J.D. (2013). Ch 19 *Morgan & Mikhail's Clinical Anesthesiology* (5th ed.). New York, NY: McGraw-Hill.

Nagelhout, J.J., & Plaus, K.L. (2014). Ch 22 *Nurse Anesthesia* (5th ed.). St. Louis, MO: Elsevier.

33. When using the MacIntosh laryngoscope, where is the tip of the blade placed?

(A) Vallecula

(B) Hyoepiglottic ligament

(C) Posterior to the epiglottis

(D) Posterior pharynx

Rationale: The tip of the curved MacIntosh laryngoscope is place in the vallecula. The straight Miller blade is positioned posterior to the epiglottis.

Ref: Butterworth, J.F., Mackey, D.C., & Wasnick, J.D. (2013). Ch 19 *Morgan & Mikhail's Clinical Anesthesiology* (5th ed.). New York, NY: McGraw-Hill.

Nagelhout, J.J., & Plaus, K.L. (2014). Ch 22 *Nurse Anesthesia* (5th ed.). St. Louis, MO: Elsevier.

34. What statement is true about jet ventilation?

    (A) Regulators allow for an increase in inspiratory pressure.

    (B) Inspiratory pressures should be <50 psi.

    (C) Low-pressure oxygen is delivered.

    (D) Inspiratory pressure should be >50 psi.

    Rationale: Transtracheal jet ventilation is accomplished through a high-pressure oxygen source. Regulators allow for a decrease in inspiratory pressure.

    Ref: Butterworth, J.F., Mackey, D.C., & Wasnick, J.D. (2013). Ch 19 *Morgan & Mikhail's Clinical Anesthesiology* (5th ed.). New York, NY: McGraw-Hill.

    Nagelhout, J.J., & Plaus, K.L. (2014). Ch 22 *Nurse Anesthesia* (5th ed.). St. Louis, MO: Elsevier.

35. In which patient condition is a nasal airway used with caution?

    (A) Obesity

    (B) Basilar skull fracture

    (C) Hemodynamic instability

    (D) Octogenarian

    Rationale: Nasal airways are used with caution for patients receiving anticoagulation therapy or for those with thrombocytopenia, and basilar skull fracture.

    Ref: Butterworth, J.F., Mackey, D.C., & Wasnick, J.D. (2013). Ch 19 *Morgan & Mikhail's Clinical Anesthesiology* (5th ed.). New York, NY: McGraw-Hill.

36. When comparing sites for placement of a central venous catheter, which site carries the greatest risk for pneumothorax?

    (A) Right internal jugular vein

    (B) Subclavian vein

    (C) Left internal jugular vein

    (D) Right external jugular vein

    Rationale: Each of the sites may be used for central venous catheter placement. The right internal jugular vein provides easy access and safety. Increased risk of pleural effusion and chylothorax is linked to the left internal jugular vein. Because of the anatomy of the external jugular veins, placement may be challenging.

    Ref: Butterworth, J.F., Mackey, D.C., & Wasnick, J.D. (2013). Ch 5 *Morgan & Mikhail's Clinical Anesthesiology* (5th ed.). New York, NY: McGraw-Hill.

37. What does an "a" wave represent in a CVP tracing?

    (A) Atrial contraction

    (B) Tricuspid valve elevation

    (C) Venous return

    (D) Tricuspid valve opening

    Rationale: "C" waves represent tricuspid valve elevation; "v" waves represent venous return; "x" and "y" waves represent downward tricuspid valve replacement and valve opening during diastole.

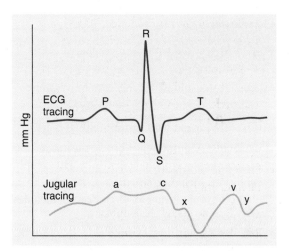

FIG. 2-4. The upward waves (*a, c, v*) and the downward descents [*x, y*] of a central venous tracing in relation to the electrocardiogram (ECG).

TABLE 2-6. Relative rating of central venous access.[1]

	Basilic	External Jugular	Internal Jugular	Subclavian	Femoral
Ease of cannulation	1	3	2	5	3
Long-term use	4	3	2	1	5
Success rate (pulmonary artery catheter placement)	4	5	1	2	3
Complications (technique-related)	1	2	4	5	3

[1]In each category, 1 = best, 5 = worst.

Ref: Butterworth, J.F., Mackey, D.C., & Wasnick, J.D. (2013). Ch 5 *Morgan & Mikhail's Clinical Anesthesiology* (5th ed.). New York, NY: McGraw-Hill.

Nagelhout, J.J., & Plaus, K.L. (2014). Ch 16 *Nurse Anesthesia* (5th ed.). St. Louis, MO: Elsevier.

38. What is the type of ventilator bellow rises during expiration?

    (A) Ascending
    (B) Descending
    (C) Hanging
    (D) Pneumatic

    Rationale: A standing (ascending) bellow rises during expiration and collapses during inspiration. A standing (ascending) bellow is preferred as it readily draws attention to a circuit disconnection by collapsing.

    Ref: Butterworth, J.F., Mackey, D.C., & Wasnick, J.D. (2013). Ch 4 *Morgan & Mikhail's Clinical Anesthesiology* (5th ed.). New York, NY: McGraw-Hill.

    Nagelhout, J.J., & Plaus, K.L., (2014). Ch 15 *Nurse Anesthesia* (5th ed.). St. Louis, MO: Elsevier.

39. In which patient would you avoid using an esophageal stethoscope?

    (A) 50-year-old with gastroesophageal reflux disease
    (B) 70-year-old with congestive heart failure
    (C) 70-year-old with alcoholic liver disease
    (D) 50-year-old with gastrointestinal polyps

    Rationale: Contraindications for using an esophageal stethoscope include patients with esophageal conditions including strictures or varices. The pathophysiology of advanced liver disease includes the presence of varices.

    Ref: Butterworth, J.F., Mackey, D.C., & Wasnick, J.D. (2013). Ch 6 *Morgan & Mikhail's Clinical Anesthesiology* (5th ed.). New York, NY: McGraw-Hill.

40. Which statement is true regarding pulse oximetry?

    (A) Pulse oximetry artifact is due to excessive ambient light, motion, and methylene blue dye.
    (B) Pulse oximetry requires calibration.
    (C) Pulse oximetry artifact is due to hyperthermia and increased cardiac output.
    (D) Oxyhemoglobin and deoxyhemoglobin absorb red and infrared light equally.

    Rationale: No calibration is required for pulse oximetry. Low-output states including any condition decreasing cardiac output will affect pulse oximetry. Oxyhemoglobin absorbs a greater amount of infrared light than deoxyhemoglobin, which absorbs a greater amount of red light.

    Ref: Butterworth, J.F., Mackey, D.C., & Wasnick, J.D. (2013). Ch 6 *Morgan & Mikhail's Clinical Anesthesiology* (5th ed.). New York, NY: McGraw-Hill.

41. During general anesthesia, the end-tidal CO_2 wave form stops. What is the most likely cause?

    (A) Esophageal intubation
    (B) Circuit disconnect
    (C) Bronchial intubation
    (D) Malignant hyperthermia

    Rationale: When the CO_2 wave form stops, a circuit disconnect is the most likely cause. During induction of anesthesia, incorrect placement of the endotracheal tube results in little to no end-tidal CO_2. An increased $ETCO_2$ is a heralding sign of malignant hyperthermia.

    Ref: Butterworth, J.F., Mackey, D.C., & Wasnick, J.D. (2013). Ch 6 *Morgan & Mikhail's Clinical Anesthesiology* (5th ed.). New York, NY: McGraw-Hill.

42. The patient is surgically anesthetized. What is the corresponding Bispectral Index (BIS)?

    (A) 96
    (B) 90
    (C) 78
    (D) 56

    Rationale: The BIS values for patients undergoing sedation are 65-85. BIS values for general anesthesia are 40-65. A BIS of 90-96 represents an awake or near awake patient.

    Ref: Butterworth, J.F., Mackey, D.C., & Wasnick, J.D. (2013). Ch 6 *Morgan & Mikhail's Clinical Anesthesiology* (5th ed.). New York, NY: McGraw-Hill.

43. When using evoked potentials, which of the following will you avoid?

    (A) Cisatracurium
    (B) Nitrous oxide
    (C) Sufentanil
    (D) Isoflurane

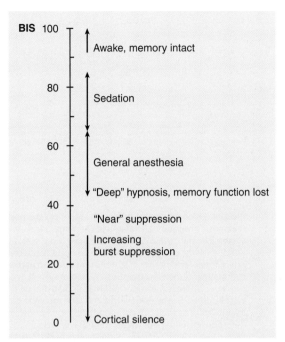

FIG. 2-5. The Bispectral Index Scale (BIS versions 3.0 and higher) is a dimensionless scale from 0 (complete cortical electroencephalographic suppression) to 100 (awake). BIS values of 65-85 have been recommended for sedation, whereas values of 40-65 have been recommended for general anesthesia. At BIS values lower than 40, cortical suppression becomes discernible in a raw electroencephalogram as a burst suppression pattern, (Reproduced, with permission from Johansen JW et al: Development and clinical application of electroencephalographic bispectrum monitoring. Anesthesiology 2000;93:1337.)

Rationale: Neuromuscular blockers, narcotics, and nitrous oxide result in small changes for evoked potentials. Although low dose volatile anesthetic agents are permissible, avoiding inhalational agents is best.

Ref: Butterworth, J.F., Mackey, D.C., & Wasnick, J.D. (2013). Ch 6 *Morgan & Mikhail's Clinical Anesthesiology* (5th ed.). New York, NY: McGraw-Hill.

44. What monitoring modality does not reflect core body temperature?

(A) Tympanic membrane

(B) Esophageal

(C) Skin adhesives

(D) Pulmonary artery

Rationale: Each of the modalities except skin temperature measurements reflects the core body temperature.

Ref: Butterworth, J.F., Mackey, D.C., & Wasnick, J.D. (2013). Ch 6 *Morgan & Mikhail's Clinical Anesthesiology* (5th ed.). New York, NY: McGraw-Hill.

45. What results when stimulating the ulnar nerve?

(A) Contraction of the abductor pollicis

(B) Contraction of the orbicularis oculi

(C) Contraction of the adductor pollicis

(D) Contraction of the facial nerve

Rationale: When using a nerve stimulator, stimulation of the facial nerve results in contraction of the orbicularis oculi. Stimulation of the ulnar nerve results in adductor pollicis muscle contraction.

Ref: Butterworth, J.F., Mackey, D.C., & Wasnick, J.D. (2013). Ch 6 *Morgan & Mikhail's Clinical Anesthesiology* (5th ed.). New York, NY: McGraw-Hill.

46. What statement about peripheral nerve stimulation is false?

(A) The adductor pollicis recovers before the orbicularis oculi.

(B) Clinical relaxation requires approximately 90% blockade.

(C) The orbicularis oculi recovers before the adductor pollicis.

(D) Abrasion and skin irritation may result from peripheral nerve stimulation.

Rationale: Recovery from neuromuscular blockade is observed in the orbicularis oculi prior to the adductor pollicis when using peripheral nerve stimulation.

Ref: Butterworth, J.F., Mackey, D.C., & Wasnick, J.D. (2013). Ch 6 *Morgan & Mikhail's Clinical Anesthesiology* (5th ed.). New York, NY: McGraw-Hill.

47. What statement is true about blood pressure measurement accuracy?

(A) The cuff's bladder should extend at least 40% around the extremity.

(B) The width of the cuff should be 20-25% greater than the diameter of the extremity.

(C) Blood pressure is a measure of perfusion.

(D) The Doppler probe is the preferred noninvasive blood pressure measuring technique.

Rationale: The bladder of the blood pressure cuff should extend at least half-way around the extremity. The blood pressure is an indicator of perfusion rather than a measure of perfusion. Oscillometric devices are the preferred noninvasive blood pressure measuring technique.

Ref: Butterworth, J.F., Mackey, D.C., & Wasnick, J.D. (2013). Ch 5 *Morgan & Mikhail's Clinical Anesthesiology* (5th ed.). New York, NY: McGraw-Hill.

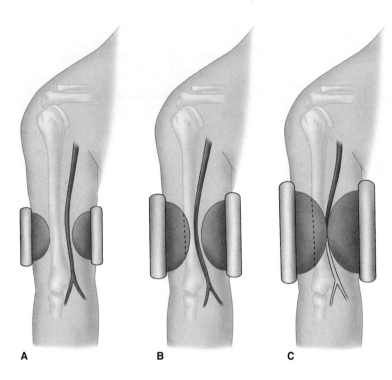

A   **B**   **C**

FIG. 2-6. Blood pressure cuff width influences the pressure readings. Three cuffs, all inflated to the same pressure, are shown. The narrowest cuff (**A**) will require more pressure, and the widest cuff (**C**) less pressure, to occlude the brachial artery for determination of systolic pressure. Too narrow a cuff may produce a large overestimation of systolic pressure. Whereas the wider cuff may underestimate the systolic pressure, the error with a cuff 20% too wide is not as significant as the error with a cuff 20% too narrow. (Reproduced, with permission, from Gravensrein J.S., &, Paulus D.A. (1987). *Clinical Monitoring Practice* (2nd ed.). Philadelphia, PA: Lippincott.)

Nagelhout, J.J., & Plaus, K.L. (2014). Ch 16 *Nurse Anesthesia* (5th ed.). St. Louis, MO: Elsevier.

48. In what range is the left ventricular end diastolic pressure?

   (A) 1-10
   (B) 10-20
   (C) 5-15
   (D) 4-12

   Rationale: Ranges are as follows: Mean right atrial pressure (1-10); Mean pulmonary artery pressure (10-20); Pulmonary artery occlusive pressure (5-15).
   Ref: Butterworth, J.F., Mackey, D.C., & Wasnick, J.D. (2013). Ch 20 *Morgan & Mikhail's Clinical Anesthesiology* (5th ed.). New York, NY: McGraw-Hill.
   Nagelhout, J.J., & Plaus, K.L. (2014). Ch 16 *Nurse Anesthesia* (5th ed.). St. Louis, MO: Elsevier.

49. When monitoring central venous pressure (CVP), what causes the loss of "a" waves?

   (A) Atrial fibrillation
   (B) Tricuspid regurgitation
   (C) PVCs
   (D) Myocardial ischemia

Rationale: The loss of "a" waves is due to atrial fibrillation or ventricular pacing during asystole. Large "v" waves may be caused by tricuspid or mitral regurgitation as well as increased intravascular volume. Cannon "a" waves result from myocardial ischemia and numerous arrhythmias.
Ref: Butterworth, J.F., Mackey, D.C., & Wasnick, J.D. (2013). Ch 5 *Morgan & Mikhail's Clinical Anesthesiology* (5th ed.). New York, NY: McGraw-Hill.
Nagelhout, J.J., & Plaus, K.L. (2014). Ch 16 *Nurse Anesthesia* (5th ed.). St. Louis, MO: Elsevier.

50. In the normal capnograph, what does Phase III indicate?

   (A) Decreased CO_2
   (B) Dead space
   (C) Dead space and alveolar gas
   (D) Alveolar gas plateau

Rationale: Phases of capnography include: Phase I—dead space; Phase II—Dead space and alveolar gas; Phase III—alveolar gas plateau; Final phase—rapid decrease in CO_2.
Ref: Butterworth, J.F., Mackey, D.C., & Wasnick, J.D. (2013). Ch 6 *Morgan & Mikhail's Clinical Anesthesiology* (5th ed.). New York, NY: McGraw-Hill.
Nagelhout, J.J., & Plaus, K.L. (2014). Ch 17 *Nurse Anesthesia* (5th ed.). St. Louis, MO: Elsevier.

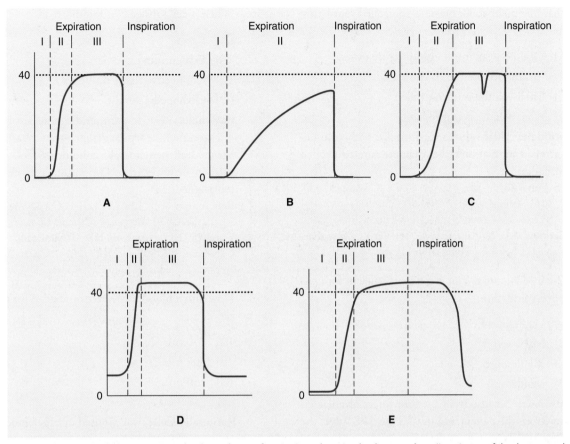

FIG. 2-7. A: A normal capnograph demonstrating the three phases of expiration: phase I—dead space; phase II—mixture of dead space and alveolar gas; phase III—alveolar gas plateau. **B:** Capnograph of a patient with severe chronic obstructive pulmonary disease. No plateau is reached before the next inspiration. The gradient between end-tidal CO_2, and arterial CO_2, is increased. **C:** Depression during phase III indicates spontaneous respiratory effort. **D:** Failure of the inspired CO_2; to return to zero may represent an incompetent expiratory valve or exhausted CO_2; absorbent. **E:** The persistence of exhaled gas during part of the inspiratory cycle signals the presence of an incompetent inspiratory valve.

51. What causes an increased end-tidal carbon dioxide?

(A) CNS depression

(B) Decreased cardiac output

(C) Hypotension

(D) VQ mismatch

Rationale: Increases in CO_2 production and conditions related to hypoventilation (CNS depression) increase CO_2. Conditions related to hyperventilation decrease CO_2 as well as production or delivery of CO_2 (tourniquet release; bicarbonate; sepsis; instillation of gas during laparoscopy; hypermetabolic conditions; seizures; fever). Technical or equipment malfunctions including airway leaks, circuit disconnect esophageal intubation, or airway equipment kinks or leaks result in deceased end-tidal CO_2.

Ref: Butterworth, J.F., Mackey, D.C., & Wasnick, J.D. (2013). Ch 6 *Morgan & Mikhail's Clinical Anesthesiology* (5th ed.). New York, NY: McGraw-Hill.

Nagelhout, J.J., & Plaus, K.L. (2014). Ch 17 *Nurse Anesthesia* (5th ed.). St. Louis, MO: Elsevier.

52. What factor results in a shift to the right in an oxyhemoglobin dissociation curve?

(A) Decreased CO_2

(B) Elevated temperature

(C) Alkalosis

(D) Decreased temperature

Rationale: Elevated temperature; 2,3 –DPG; increased CO_2 and acidosis (decreased pH) shift the oxyhemoglobin dissociation curve to the right. Alkalosis (increased pH), decreased 2,3 DPG, decreased CO_2, and decreased temperature shift the oxyhemoglobin dissociation curve to the left.

Ref: Butterworth, J.F., Mackey, D.C., & Wasnick, J.D. (2013). Ch 6 *Morgan & Mikhail's Clinical Anesthesiology* (5th ed.). New York, NY: McGraw-Hill.

Nagelhout, J.J., & Plaus, K.L. (2014). Ch 17 *Nurse Anesthesia* (5th ed.). St. Louis, MO: Elsevier.

53. What statement about pressure-controlled ventilation is false?

    (A) Limited peak inspiratory pressure exists.
    (B) Inspiratory pressure is controlled.
    (C) Tidal volume is uncontrolled.
    (D) Tidal volume is controlled.

    Rationale: Tidal volume is controlled with volume-controlled ventilation rather than pressure-controlled ventilation.

    Ref: Butterworth, J.F., Mackey, D.C., & Wasnick, J.D. (2013). Ch 6 *Morgan & Mikhail's Clinical Anesthesiology* (5th ed.). New York, NY: McGraw-Hill.

    Nagelhout, J.J., & Plaus, K.L. (2014). Ch 17 *Nurse Anesthesia* (5th ed.). St. Louis, MO: Elsevier.

54. Which Mapleson circuit is the most efficient for controlled ventilation?

    (A) Mapleson D
    (B) Mapleson A
    (C) Mapleson B
    (D) Mapleson C

    Rationale: Because fresh gas flow forces alveolar air away from the patient and toward the APL valve, the Mapleson D circuit is the most efficient for controlled ventilation.

    Ref: Butterworth, J.F., Mackey, D.C., & Wasnick, J.D. (2013). Ch 3 *Morgan & Mikhail's Clinical Anesthesiology* (5th ed.). New York, NY: McGraw-Hill.

    Nagelhout, J.J., & Plaus, K.L., (2014). Ch 15 *Nurse Anesthesia* (5th ed.). St. Louis, MO: Elsevier.

55. What mechanism facilitates heat loss through air currents?

    (A) Radiation
    (B) Convection
    (C) Conduction
    (D) Evaporation

    Rationale: Evaporative heat loss results fluid loss through the skin and respiratory system. Conductive heat loss occurs when direct contact between cold and warm objects. Radiation involves the transfer of heat from infrared rays. Convective heat loss requires currents and is dependent on thermal gradients.

    Ref: Butterworth, J.F., Mackey, D.C., & Wasnick, J.D. (2013). Ch 52 *Morgan & Mikhail's Clinical Anesthesiology* (5th ed.). New York, NY: McGraw-Hill.

    Nagelhout, J.J., & Plaus, K.L. (2014). Ch 14 *Nurse Anesthesia* (5th ed.). St. Louis, MO: Elsevier.

56. When is cell salvage contraindicated?

    (A) Sepsis
    (B) Benign tumors
    (C) Connective tissue disorders
    (D) Orthopedic conditions

    Rationale: Relative contraindications for the use of cell saver include sepsis, malignancies, pharmacologic agents, and hematologic conditions. Cell salvage is used in orthopedic conditions such as major joint replacement.

    Ref: Butterworth, J.F., Mackey, D.C., & Wasnick, J.D. (2013). Ch 51 *Morgan & Mikhail's Clinical Anesthesiology* (5th ed.). New York, NY: McGraw-Hill.

    Nagelhout, J.J., & Plaus, K.L. (2014). Ch 20 *Nurse Anesthesia* (5th ed.). St. Louis, MO: Elsevier.

57. How much blood loss is recommended for the use of cell salvage?

    (A) 250 mL
    (B) 500 mL
    (C) 750 mL
    (D) 1,000 mL

    Rationale: Cell salvage is used in large blood loss surgeries (1,000 mL or greater).

    Ref: Butterworth, J.F., Mackey, D.C., & Wasnick, J.D. (2013). Ch 51 *Morgan & Mikhail's Clinical Anesthesiology* (5th ed.). New York, NY: McGraw-Hill.

    Nagelhout, J.J., & Plaus, K.L. (2014). Ch 20 *Nurse Anesthesia* (5th ed.). St. Louis, MO: Elsevier.

58. Where is the best location to monitor blood pressure for patients undergoing right shoulder arthroscopy in the beach chair position?

    (A) Right lower extremity
    (B) Left lower extremity
    (C) Left upper extremity
    (D) Right upper extremity

    Rationale: The upper extremity is used to monitor non invasive blood pressure for this case. There is a significant difference (40 mmHg) when using the lower extremity. Hypotension although common for this procedure and position, needs to be minimized to avoid low cerebral perfusion.

    Ref: Butterworth, J.F., Mackey, D.C., & Wasnick, J.D. (2013). Ch 38 *Morgan & Mikhail's Clinical Anesthesiology* (5th ed.). New York, NY: McGraw-Hill.

    Nagelhout, J.J., & Plaus, K.L. (2014) Ch 40 *Nurse Anesthesia* (5th ed.). St. Louis, MO: Elsevier.

59. Which principle is not included in radiation safety?

(A) Time

(B) Distance

(C) Shielding

(D) Temperature

Rationale: Time, distance, and shielding guide the need for anesthesia providers to avoid the hazards of radiation in the operating room. No relationship exists between the operating room temperature and radiation safety.

Ref: Butterworth, J.F., Mackey, D.C., & Wasnick, J.D. (2013). Ch 3 *Morgan & Mikhail's Clinical Anesthesiology* (5th ed.). New York, NY: McGraw-Hill.

60. What is a disadvantage of the Bain circuit?

(A) Increases circuit bulk

(B) Partial warming of inspiratory gas

(C) Kinking of the fresh gas inlet tube

(D) Requires low fresh gas flow

Rationale: A disadvantage of this circuit is the chance of kinking or disconnection of the fresh gas inlet. Periodic check of the inner tubing is set to prevent this complication.

Ref: Butterworth, J.F., Mackey, D.C., & Wasnick, J.D. (2013). Ch 3 *Morgan & Mikhail's Clinical Anesthesiology* (5th ed.). New York, NY: McGraw-Hill.

Nagelhout, J.J., & Plaus, K.L., (2014). Ch 15 *Nurse Anesthesia* (5th ed.). St. Louis, MO: Elsevier.

61. The E-cylinder oxygen gauge pressure reads 850 psi: How many liters are remaining presuming that the E-cylinder was full at 2,000 psi and 660 L?

(A) 300 L

(B) 660 L

(C) 240 L

(D) 280 L

Rationale: $\dfrac{Capacity\ L}{Service\ pressure\ psi} = \dfrac{Contents\ remaining\ L}{Gauge\ pressure\ psi}$

Ref: Butterworth, J.F., Mackey, D.C., & Wasnick, J.D. (2013). Ch 23 *Morgan & Mikhail's Clinical Anesthesiology* (5th ed.). New York, NY: McGraw-Hill.

Nagelhout, J.J., & Plaus, K.L., (2014). Ch 15 *Nurse Anesthesia* (5th ed.). St. Louis, MO: Elsevier.

62. How many liters of CO_2 per 100 g of absorbent can soda lime absorb?

(A) 23 L

(B) 32 L

(C) 44 L

(D) 18 L

Rationale: Soda lime is the more common absorbent and is capable of absorbing up to 23 L of CO_2 per 100 g of absorbent.

Ref: Butterworth, J.F., Mackey, D.C., & Wasnick, J.D. (2013). Ch 3 *Morgan & Mikhail's Clinical Anesthesiology* (5th ed.). New York, NY: McGraw-Hill.

Miller, R.D., & Pardo, M.C. (2011). *Basics of Anesthesia* (6th ed.). Philadelphia, PA: Elsevier.

63. What does the National Institute for Occupational Safety and Health (NIOSH) recommend for the room concentration of a halogenated agent when nitrous oxide is used?

(A) 25 ppm

(B) 2 ppm

(C) 0.5 ppm

(D) 2.5 ppm

Rationale: The National institute for Occupational Safety and Health (NIOSH) recommend limiting the room concentration of nitrous oxide to 25 ppm and halogenated agent to 2 ppm and 0.5 ppm when nitrous oxide is also used.

Ref: Butterworth, J.F., Mackey, D.C., & Wasnick, J.D. (2013). Ch 3 *Morgan & Mikhail's Clinical Anesthesiology* (5th ed.). New York, NY: McGraw-Hill.

Nagelhout, J.J., & Plaus, K.L., (2014). Ch 15 *Nurse Anesthesia* (5th ed.). St. Louis, MO: Elsevier.

64. Which selection pertains to a closed waste gas scavenging system with active scavenging?

(A) Must have a negative-pressure relief valve

(B) Must have both a negative and positive pressure relief valve

(C) Must have a positive-pressure relief valve

(D) Requires no pressure relief valves

Rationale: A closed waste gas scavenging system is closed to the outside atmosphere and requires negative and positive pressure relief valves that shield the patient from the negative pressure of the vacuum system and positive pressure from an impediment in the scavenging tubing.

Ref: Butterworth, J.F., Mackey, D.C., & Wasnick, J.D. (2013). Ch 3 *Morgan & Mikhail's Clinical Anesthesiology* (5th ed.). New York, NY: McGraw-Hill.

Nagelhout, J.J., & Plaus, K.L., (2014). Ch 15 *Nurse Anesthesia* (5th ed.). St. Louis, MO: Elsevier.

65. What is the approximate cylinder pressure delivered to the anesthesia machine?

    (A) 45 psi
    (B) 50 psi
    (C) 1,900 psi
    (D) 745 psi

    Rationale: The approximate cylinder pressure delivered to the anesthesia machine is 45 psi; 50 psi is pipeline pressure; 1,900 psi is the approximate psi for a full O_2 E-cylinder; and 745 is the psi for N_2O E-cylinder.
    Ref: Butterworth, J.F., Mackey, D.C., & Wasnick, J.D. (2013). Ch 3 *Morgan & Mikhail's Clinical Anesthesiology* (5th ed.). New York, NY: McGraw-Hill.
    Nagelhout, J.J., & Plaus, K.L., (2014). Ch 15 *Nurse Anesthesia* (5th ed.). St. Louis, MO: Elsevier.

66. How many liters per minute will the oxygen flush valve provide to the common gas outlet?

    (A) 10 L/min
    (B) 80-100 L/min
    (C) 20-30 L/min
    (D) 35-75 L/min

    Rationale: The oxygen flush valve provides a high flow of oxygen directly to the common gas outlet at 35-75 L/min.
    Ref: Butterworth, J.F., Mackey, D.C., & Wasnick, J.D. (2013). Ch 3 *Morgan & Mikhail's Clinical Anesthesiology* (5th ed.). New York, NY: McGraw-Hill.
    Nagelhout, J.J., & Plaus, K.L., (2014). Ch 15 *Nurse Anesthesia* (5th ed.). St. Louis, MO: Elsevier.

67. What is the outer diameter of the scavenger tubing?

    (A) 22- mm
    (B) 32- mm
    (C) 19- mm
    (D) 10- mm

    Rationale: The outer diameter of the scavenger tubing is 19- mm; the outer diameter for the common gas outlet is 22- mm.
    Ref: Butterworth, J.F., Mackey, D.C., & Wasnick, J.D. (2013). Ch 3 *Morgan & Mikhail's Clinical Anesthesiology* (5th ed.). New York, NY: McGraw-Hill.
    Miller, R.D., & Pardo, M.C. (2011). *Basics of Anesthesia* (6th ed.). Philadelphia, PA: Elsevier.

68. Which Mapleson circuit is most efficient for spontaneous ventilation?

    (A) Mapleson D
    (B) Mapleson A
    (C) Mapleson B
    (D) Mapleson C

    Rationale: Because the fresh gas flow is equal to minute ventilation, the Mapleson A circuit is the most efficient for spontaneous ventilation.
    Ref: Butterworth, J.F., Mackey, D.C., & Wasnick, J.D. (2013). Ch 3 *Morgan & Mikhail's Clinical Anesthesiology* (5th ed.). New York, NY: McGraw-Hill.
    Nagelhout, J.J., & Plaus, K.L., (2014). Ch 15 *Nurse Anesthesia* (5th ed.). St. Louis, MO: Elsevier.

69. What are the benefits of the Bain circuit?

    (A) Decreases the circuit bulk and retains heat and humidity
    (B) Decreases resistance
    (C) Decreases fresh gas flow
    (D) Scavenges waste gas

    Rationale: The Bain circuit incorporates the fresh gas inlet tubing inside the breathing tube, which decreases the circuit bulk and retains heat and humidity.
    Ref: Butterworth, J.F., Mackey, D.C., & Wasnick, J.D. (2013). Ch 3 *Morgan & Mikhail's Clinical Anesthesiology* (5th ed.). New York, NY: McGraw-Hill.
    Nagelhout, J.J., & Plaus, K.L., (2014). Ch 15 *Nurse Anesthesia* (5th ed.). St. Louis, MO: Elsevier.

70. What is the granule size commonly used in CO_2 absorbent?

    (A) 2-4 mesh
    (B) 6-8 mesh
    (C) 4-8 mesh
    (D) 1-2 mesh

    Rationale: Granule size is a compromise between the higher absorptive surface area of small granules and the lower resistance to gas flow of larger granules. The granule size commonly used in CO_2 absorbent is between 4 and 8 mesh.
    Ref: Butterworth, J.F., Mackey, D.C., & Wasnick, J.D. (2013). Ch 3 *Morgan & Mikhail's Clinical Anesthesiology* (5th ed.). New York, NY: McGraw-Hill.
    Nagelhout, J.J., & Plaus, K.L., (2014). Ch 15 *Nurse Anesthesia* (5th ed.). St. Louis, MO: Elsevier.

71. What does the American Society of Anesthesiologists' Closed Claims Project database identify as the most common single source of injury pertaining to the anesthesia gas machine?

    (A) Failure of the anesthesia delivery equipment
    (B) Faulty ventilator
    (C) Inaccurate calibration of the oxygen analyzer
    (D) Misconnect or disconnect of breathing circuit components

    Rationale: The breathing circuit was the most common single source of injury (39%). Nearly all damaging events were related to misconnect or disconnect. A misconnect was defined as a nonfunctional and unconventional configuration of breathing circuit components or attachments.
    Ref: Butterworth, J.F., Mackey, D.C., & Wasnick, J.D. (2013). Ch 3 *Morgan & Mikhail's Clinical Anesthesiology* (5th ed.). New York, NY: Lange Medical Books McGraw-Hill.
    Nagelhout, J.J., & Plaus, K.L., (2014). Ch 15 *Nurse Anesthesia* (5th ed.). St. Louis, MO: Elsevier.

72. What are three functions of the hanger yoke?

    (A) Shuts off nitrous oxide when oxygen pressure falls below 20 psi, provides a gas tight seal, and ensures unidirectional flow
    (B) Monitors inspired oxygen level, reduces pressure to 45-47 psi, and ensures unidirectional flow
    (C) Orients cylinders, provides a gas tight seal, and ensures unidirectional flow
    (D) Ensures at least 25% oxygen is given when using nitrous oxide, provides a gas tight seal, and ensures unidirectional flow

    Rationale: Part one of A refers to the oxygen shut off valve, parts one and two of B refer to the oxygen analyzer and the pressure regulator, part one of D refers to the hypoxic guard.
    Ref: Butterworth, J.F., Mackey, D.C., & Wasnick, J.D. (2013). Ch 23 *Morgan & Mikhail's Clinical Anesthesiology* (5th ed.). New York, NY: Lange Medical Books McGraw-Hill.
    Nagelhout, J.J., & Plaus, K.L., (2014). Ch 15 *Nurse Anesthesia* (5th ed.). St. Louis, MO: Elsevier Saunders.

73. Which oxygen analyzer works by using the oxygen molecules' unique attraction into magnetic fields?

    (A) Electrogalvanic cell
    (B) Polarographic electrode
    (C) Paramagnetic oxygen sensor
    (D) Fluorescence quenching

    Rationale: A creates its own electric current by using a lead anode and either a gold or silver anode. B creates its own electric current by using a silver anode and platinum cathode. D uses the fluorescence caused by a molecule emitting light in response to being energized.
    Ref: Butterworth, J.F., Mackey, D.C., & Wasnick, J.D. (2013). Ch 6 *Morgan & Mikhail's Clinical Anesthesiology* (5th ed.). New York, NY: McGraw-Hill.
    Nagelhout, J.J., & Plaus, K.L., (2014). Ch 14 *Nurse Anesthesia* (5th ed.). St. Louis, MO: Elsevier.

74. Which classification of breathing circuits has complete rebreathing?

    (A) Open
    (B) Semi-open
    (C) Semi-closed
    (D) Closed

    Rationale: Open and semi-open have no rebreathing; semi-closed has partial rebreathing.
    Ref: Nagelhout, J.J., & Plaus, K.L., (2014). Ch 15 *Nurse Anesthesia* (5th ed.). St. Louis, MO: Elsevier.

75. How many liters does an oxygen E-cylinder tank hold?

    (A) 660 L
    (B) 1,590 L
    (C) 625 L
    (D) 750 L

    Rationale: B is nitrous oxide; C is air.
    Ref: Butterworth, J.F., Mackey, D.C., & Wasnick, J.D. (2013). Ch 4 *Morgan & Mikhail's Clinical Anesthesiology* (5th ed.). New York, NY: McGraw-Hill.
    Nagelhout, J.J., & Plaus, K.L., (2014). Ch 15 *Nurse Anesthesia* (5th ed.). St. Louis, MO: Elsevier.

76. What are the appropriate measures to reduce the amount of oxygen consumed and prolong the duration of your backup oxygen supply when the oxygen supply fails?

    (A) Turn off the ventilator and ventilate manually through the circle system.
    (B) Increase oxygen flows to 5 L per minute.
    (C) Place the patient on pressure control ventilation.
    (D) Reduce tidal volume and increase respiratory rate on the ventilator.

Rationale: Most anesthesia machines utilize oxygen as the driving gas to power the ventilator. By reducing fresh oxygen flow rates and eliminating the use of the ventilator by allowing the patient to breathe spontaneously or ventilating via the reservoir bag, you will prolong the backup oxygen supply.

Ref: Nagelhout, J.J., & Plaus, K.L., (2014). Ch 15 *Nurse Anesthesia* (5th ed.). St. Louis, MO: Elsevier.

77. When the pressure gauge drops below 745 psig on a nitrous oxide E-cylinder at room temperature, approximately how much nitrous oxide is left in the tank?

    (A) 1,590 L
    (B) 660 L
    (C) 400 L
    (D) 625 L

Rationale: E-cylinder nitrous oxide tanks contain nitrous oxide in the liquid and gas state. The only accurate way to determine the amount of gas left in the tank is by weighing it. A full E-cylinder tank will hold 1,590 liters of nitrous oxide. When the liquid form is consumed and the tank pressure drops below 745 psig, the amount of nitrous oxide in the gas phase is about 400 liters.

Ref: Butterworth, J.F., Mackey, D.C., & Wasnick, J.D. (2013). Ch 4 *Morgan & Mikhail's Clinical Anesthesiology* (5th ed.). New York, NY: McGraw-Hill.

Nagelhout, J.J., & Plaus, K.L., (2014). Ch 15 *Nurse Anesthesia* (5th ed.). St. Louis, MO: Elsevier.

78. What is size of the transfer tubing in the scavenger system?

    (A) 22 mm
    (B) 20 mm
    (C) 19 mm
    (D) 9 mm

Rationale: Transfer tubing is 19 or 30 mm.

Ref: Butterworth, J.F., Mackey, D.C., & Wasnick, J.D. (2013). Ch 4 *Morgan & Mikhail's Clinical Anesthesiology* (5th ed.). New York, NY: Lange Medical Books McGraw-Hill.

Nagelhout, J.J., & Plaus, K.L., (2014). Ch 15 *Nurse Anesthesia* (5th ed.). St. Louis, MO: Elsevier Saunders.

79. What is the only piece of equipment that will ensure that oxygen is present in the pipelines or cylinder?

    (A) Oxygen analyzer
    (B) Hypoxic guard

    (C) Oxygen fail-safe device
    (D) Cylinder gauge

Rationale: Inspired oxygen analysis is the only method of ensuring the presence of oxygen in the pipeline or cylinder.

Ref: Butterworth, J.F., Mackey, D.C., & Wasnick, J.D. (2013). Ch 4 *Morgan & Mikhail's Clinical Anesthesiology* (5th ed.). New York, NY: McGraw-Hill.

Nagelhout, J.J., & Plaus, K.L., (2014). Ch 15 *Nurse Anesthesia* (5th ed.). St. Louis, MO: Elsevier.

80. What is the ideal value for the scavenging vacuum?

    (A) 10-15 L/min
    (B) 1-2 L/min
    (C) 2-5 L/min
    (D) 30-40 L/min

Rationale: This rate is adequate for periods of high fresh gas flow yet minimizes the risk of transmitting negative pressure to the breathing circuit during lower flow conditions.

Ref: Butterworth, J.F., Mackey, D.C., & Wasnick, J.D. (2013). Ch 4 *Morgan & Mikhail's Clinical Anesthesiology* (5th ed.). New York, NY: McGraw-Hill.

Nagelhout, J.J., & Plaus, K.L., (2014). Ch 15 *Nurse Anesthesia* (5th ed.). St. Louis, MO: Elsevier.

81. Which type of waste-gas scavenger interface requires negative and positive pressure relief valves?

    (A) Open interface
    (B) Passive closed interface
    (C) Active closed interface
    (D) Active open interface

Rationale: An active closed interface is closed to the outside atmosphere and requires negative and positive pressure relief valves that protect the patient from the negative pressure of the vacuum system and positive pressure from an obstruction in the disposal tubing.

Ref: Butterworth, J.F., Mackey, D.C., & Wasnick, J.D. (2013). Ch 4 *Morgan & Mikhail's Clinical Anesthesiology* (5th ed.). New York, NY: McGraw-Hill.

Nagelhout, J.J., & Plaus, K.L., (2014). Ch 15 *Nurse Anesthesia* (5th ed.). St. Louis, MO: Elsevier.

82. Which organization published a generic checkout procedure for anesthesia gas machines and breathing circuits?

    (A) American Association of Nurse Anesthetists (AANA)
    (B) Department of Transportation (DOT)

(C) Food and Drug Administration (FDA)

(D) American Society for Testing and Materials (ASTM)

Rationale: The Food and Drug Administration (FDA) published a generic checkout procedure for anesthesia gas machines and breathing circuits.

Ref: Butterworth, J.F., Mackey, D.C., & Wasnick, J.D. (2013). Ch 4 *Morgan & Mikhail's Clinical Anesthesiology* (5th ed.). New York, NY: McGraw-Hill.

Nagelhout, J.J., & Plaus, K.L., (2014). Ch 15 *Nurse Anesthesia* (5th ed.). St. Louis, MO: Elsevier.

83. What piece of equipment provides unidirectional flow to prevent retrograde flow of gases from the anesthesia machine to the pipeline or atmosphere?

(A) Pressure relief valve

(B) Pressure regulator valve

(C) Hypoxic guard

(D) Check valve

Rationale: The check valve provides unidirectional flow to prevent retrograde flow of gases from the anesthesia machine to the pipeline or atmosphere.

Ref: Butterworth, J.F., Mackey, D.C., & Wasnick, J.D. (2013). Ch 4 *Morgan & Mikhail's Clinical Anesthesiology* (5th ed.). New York, NY: McGraw-Hill.

Nagelhout, J.J., & Plaus, K.L., (2014). Ch 15 *Nurse Anesthesia* (5th ed.). St. Louis, MO: Elsevier.

84. After checking your oxygen E-cylinder on the back of the anesthesia machine, what is the next step?

(A) Keep open in case of pipeline failure.

(B) The oxygen E-cylinder is only for emergency so it does not matter if you leave it open or closed.

(C) Leave partly open.

(D) Close the cylinder.

Rationale: The oxygen E-cylinder should be closed because in the event pipeline pressure fails the anesthetist may not become aware until the emergency oxygen E-cylinders are empty.

Ref: Butterworth, J.F., Mackey, D.C., & Wasnick, J.D. (2013). Ch 4 *Morgan & Mikhail's Clinical Anesthesiology* (5th ed.). New York, NY: McGraw-Hill.

Nagelhout, J.J., & Plaus, K.L., (2014). Ch 15 *Nurse Anesthesia* (5th ed.). St. Louis, MO: Elsevier.

85. What circuit design incorporates a fresh gas inlet tube inside the breathing tube?

(A) Mapleson D

(B) Bain circuit

(C) Mapleson A

(D) Mapleson B

Rationale: The Bain circuit is a modification of the Mapleson D breathing system. The circuit contains a fresh gas inlet tube. Because of the modification, heat conservation, and humidity exist. The circuit is less bulky.

Ref: Butterworth, J.F., Mackey, D.C., & Wasnick, J.D. (2013). Ch 3 *Morgan & Mikhail's Clinical Anesthesiology* (5th ed.). New York, NY: McGraw-Hill.

Miller, R.D., & Pardo, M.C. (2011). Ch 15 *Basics of Anesthesia* (6th ed.). Philadelphia, PA: Elsevier.

86. Which of the following minimizes Phase I temperature loss?

(A) Warm blankets

(B) Forced air warming

(C) Heat and moisture exchanger

(D) Warm IV fluids

Rationale: To avoid the initial drop in body temperature (Phase I), pre-warm the patient with a forced-air warming blanket. To avoid heat loss during Phase II, all other warming methods in combination are useful.

Ref: Butterworth, J.F., Mackey, D.C., & Wasnick, J.D. (2013). Ch 52 *Morgan & Mikhail's Clinical Anesthesiology* (5th ed.). New York, NY: McGraw-Hill.

Nagelhout, J.J., & Plaus, K.L. (2014). Ch 50 *Nurse Anesthesia* (5th ed.). St. Louis, MO: Elsevier.

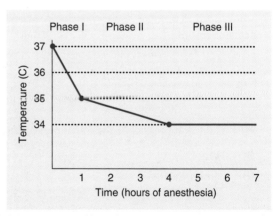

FIG. 2-8. Unintentional hypothermia during general anesthesia follows a typical pattern: a steep drop in core temperature during the first hour (phase one, redistribution), followed by a gradual decline during the next 3-4 h (phase two, heat loss), eventually reaching a steady state (phase three, equilibrium).

87. The formation of carbon monoxide by the degradation of volatile anesthetic by dry soda lime is greatest with which volatile anesthetic?

    (A) Desflurane
    (B) Isoflurane
    (C) Sevoflurane
    (D) Nitrous oxide

    Rationale: The drier the soda lime, the more aptly it will absorb and degrade volatile anesthetics. Volatile anesthetics can be broken down to carbon monoxide by dry absorbent to the extent that it is capable of causing clinically significant carbon monoxide poisoning. The formation of carbon monoxide is highest with desflurane.
    Ref: Butterworth, J.F., Mackey, D.C., & Wasnick, J.D. (2013). Ch 3 *Morgan & Mikhail's Clinical Anesthesiology* (5th ed.). New York, NY: McGraw-Hill.
    Nagelhout, J.J., & Plaus, K.L., (2014). Ch 15 *Nurse Anesthesia* (5th ed.). St. Louis, MO: Elsevier.

88. Compound A is one of the by-products of degradation of which volatile anesthetic?

    (A) Desflurane
    (B) Isoflurane
    (C) Sevoflurane
    (D) Nitrous oxide

    Rationale: Compound A is one of the byproducts of degradation of sevoflurane by absorbent. Higher concentrations of sevoflurane, prolonged exposure, and low-flow anesthetic technique seem to increase the formation of Compound A. Compound A has been shown to produce nephrotoxicity in animals.
    Ref: Butterworth, J.F., Mackey, D.C., & Wasnick, J.D. (2013). Ch 3 *Morgan & Mikhail's Clinical Anesthesiology* (5th ed.). New York, NY: McGraw-Hill.
    Nagelhout, J.J., & Plaus, K.L., (2014). Ch 15 *Nurse Anesthesia* (5th ed.). St. Louis, MO: Elsevier.

89. What is the end product of the soda lime reaction?

    (A) CO_2
    (B) Carbonic acid
    (C) Calcium carbonate
    (D) Ethyl violet

    Rationale: Soda lime contains hydroxide salts that are capable of neutralizing carbonic acid. Reaction end products include heat, water, and calcium carbonate.
    Ref: Butterworth, J.F., Mackey, D.C., & Wasnick, J.D. (2013). Ch 3 *Morgan & Mikhail's Clinical Anesthesiology* (5th ed.). New York, NY: McGraw-Hill.

    Nagelhout, J.J., & Plaus, K.L., (2014). Ch 15 *Nurse Anesthesia* (5th ed.). St. Louis, MO: Elsevier.

90. When should the LMA be removed?

    (A) When the patient moves
    (B) When the patient regains airway reflexes
    (C) When the surgery is completed
    (D) In the Post Anesthesia Care Unit

    Rationale: Because the LMA is not fully protective of phyarngeal secretions, risk of aspiration remains. For this reason ensure that the patient's airway reflexes have returned prior to removal.
    Ref: Butterworth, J.F., Mackey, D.C., & Wasnick, J.D. (2013). Ch 19 *Morgan & Mikhail's Clinical Anesthesiology* (5th ed.). New York, NY: McGraw-Hill.

91. Which Mapleson circuit is a modification of the Mapleson D?

    (A) Jackson-Reese
    (B) Mapleson A
    (C) Bain
    (D) Mapleson C

    Rationale: The Bain circuit is a coaxial adaptation of the Mapleson D system that incorporates the fresh gas inlet tubing inside the breathing tube. This modification decreases the circuit's bulkiness and preserves heat and humidity more effectively. A disadvantage of this circuit is the chance of kinking or detachment of the fresh gas inlet tubing.
    Ref: Butterworth, J.F., Mackey, D.C., & Wasnick, J.D. (2013). Ch 3 *Morgan & Mikhail's Clinical Anesthesiology* (5th ed.). New York, NY: McGraw-Hill.
    Nagelhout, J.J., & Plaus, K.L., (2014). Ch 15 *Nurse Anesthesia* (5th ed.). St. Louis, MO: Elsevier.

92. Which statement is true regarding the diameter-index safety system (DISS)?

    (A) The DISS prevents accidental connection of a wrong gas cylinder.
    (B) The DISS is attached to the machine via a hanger-yoke assembly Nitrous oxide- 2-5, air 1-5, and oxygen- 3-5.
    (C) The DISS prevents incorrect hose attachment nitrous oxide- 3-5, air 1-5, and oxygen- 2-5.
    (D) The DISS fittings for the oxygen inlet and the oxygen power outlet are different and cannot be interchanged.

Rationale: Oxygen, nitrous oxide, and air connect to the anesthesia machine from their central supply through a noninterchangeable diameter-index safety system (DISS) fitting that prevents incorrect hose attachment. The DISS fittings for the oxygen inlet and the oxygen power outlet are identical and should not be mistakenly interchanged.

Ref: Butterworth, J.F., Mackey, D.C., & Wasnick, J.D. (2013). Ch 4 *Morgan & Mikhail's Clinical Anesthesiology* (5th ed.). New York, NY: McGraw-Hill.

Nagelhout, J.J., & Plaus, K.L., (2014). Ch 15 *Nurse Anesthesia* (5th ed.). St. Louis, MO: Elsevier.

93. What is your greatest concern when inflating the pulmonary artery balloon?

    (A) Conduction abnormalities
    (B) Pulmonary artery rupture
    (C) Catheter knotting
    (D) Bacteremia

    Rationale: Each of the concerns is linked to complications associated with pulmonary artery catheters. Balloon overinflation and frequent wedge readings may be result in pulmonary artery rupture leading to death.

    Ref: Butterworth, J.F., Mackey, D.C., & Wasnick, J.D. (2013). Ch 6 *Morgan & Mikhail's Clinical Anesthesiology* (5th ed.). New York, NY: McGraw-Hill.

94. Following intubation you are unable to palpate the tracheal tube cuff in the sternal notch. The breathing bag compliance is decreased. Breath sounds are unilateral. Where is the endotracheal tube most likely positioned?

    (A) Hypopharynx
    (B) Esophagus
    (C) Supraglottic
    (D) Bronchus

    Rationale: Bronchial intubation results in unilateral breath sounds, falling pulse oximetry values, inability to feel the tracheal tube, and high peak inspiratory pressures.

    Ref: Butterworth, J.F., Mackey, D.C., & Wasnick, J.D. (2013). Ch 19 *Morgan & Mikhail's Clinical Anesthesiology* (5th ed.). New York, NY: McGraw-Hill.

CHAPTER 3

Basic Principles
Questions

1. When do symptoms of ischemic optic neuropathy that result in postoperative vision loss typically occur?

   (A) Immediately postoperatively
   (B) 2 hours postoperatively
   (C) 2 days postoperatively
   (D) 2 weeks postoperatively

2. During a general anesthetic you suspect an episode of malignant hyperthermia (MH). What will you do first?

   (A) Call the MHAUS hotline.
   (B) Administer dantrolene.
   (C) Inform the surgeon.
   (D) Turn off inhalational agents.

3. When is body temperature loss the greatest?

   (A) During the preoperative preparation
   (B) During the 1st hour in the operating room
   (C) During the 2nd and 3rd hours in the operating room
   (D) During the 4th hour in the operating room

4. For an awake fiberoptic intubation, anesthesia for the posterior 1/3 of the tongue, vallecula, anterior epiglottis, walls of the pharynx, and tonsils can be performed by injecting local anesthetic into which of the following structures?

   (A) Base of the frenulum
   (B) Palatoglossal arch
   (C) Thyroid membrane
   (D) Cricothyroid membrane

5. Which is an example of sensation without stimulus?

   (A) Temporal summation
   (B) Dynamic allodynia

   (C) Paresthesia
   (D) Analgesia

6. Which statement about stored blood is correct?

   (A) The amount of extracellular potassium transfused per unit is 10 mEq per unit.
   (B) Stored blood typically has a pH < 7.45.
   (C) Stored blood contains factors V and VIII.
   (D) Stored blood can contain as much as 150 mEq/L of potassium.

7. Which patients are at risk for aspiration?

   Select (3) three
   (A) Second trimester parturient
   (B) Gastroesophageal reflux
   (C) First trimester parturient
   (D) NPO >6 hours
   (E) Third trimester parturient

8. What percentage of the total body water is extracellular?

   (A) 67%
   (B) 33%
   (C) 25%
   (D) 100%

9. Which drugs are known triggers for malignant hyperthermia?

   Select (3) three
   (A) Halothane
   (B) Sevoflurane
   (C) Methohexital
   (D) Sodium thiopental
   (E) Succinylcholine

10. How is the brachial plexus formed?

    (A) Roots, divisions, trunks, cords, branches
    (B) Divisions, trunks, cords, branches
    (C) Cords, divisions, roots, branches
    (D) Trunks, divisions, cords, branches

11. Which laboratory test provides the most comprehensive assessment of coagulation in a patient with severe cirrhosis?

    (A) International normalized ratio
    (B) Prothrombin time
    (C) Partial thromboplastin time
    (D) Thromboelastography

12. Where does the spinal cord end in adults?

    (A) L1
    (B) L2
    (C) L3
    (D) L4

13. What volume of blood loss will decrease the hematocrit from 36-30% in a 7 year-old, 25 kg child?

    (A) 250 mL
    (B) 300 mL
    (C) 350 mL
    (D) 400 mL

14. Which cranial nerve (CN) provides sensation to the posterior 1/3 of the tongue?

    (A) CN I
    (B) CN V
    (C) CN IX
    (D) CN X

15. Which patients are more likely to experience complications when using a hypotensive technique?

    Select (2) two
    (A) Uncontrolled glaucoma
    (B) History of transient ischemic attack
    (C) Multiple sclerosis
    (D) Osteoarthritis

16. What is the smallest volume of infused ABO-incompatible donor blood that will cause an acute hemolytic reaction?

    (A) 40-60 mL
    (B) 25-30 mL
    (C) 10-15 mL
    (D) 1-3 mL

17. Which risk factors predispose patients to lower extremity neuropathy?

    Select (3) three
    (A) Hypertension
    (B) Obesity
    (C) Thin body habitus
    (D) Cigarette smoking
    (E) Diabetes

18. What is the mechanism of action of a transcutaneous electrical nerve stimulation (TENS) unit?

    (A) TENS stimulation of large diameter afferent nerve fibers competitively blocks pain signals from smaller fibers.
    (B) TENS stimulation of small diameter afferent nerve fibers competitively blocks pain signals from larger fibers.
    (C) TENS stimulation damages the small afferent fibers conducting the pain signals.
    (D) TENS stimulation induces a signal conduction interruption in large diameter fibers.

19. What are the primary adductors of the vocal cords?

    (A) Lateral cricoarytenoid muscles
    (B) Recurrent laryngeal nerve
    (C) Posterior cricoarytenoid muscles
    (D) External laryngeal nerve

20. Which group lists the Vitamin K-dependent clotting factors?

    (A) II, VII, IX, X
    (B) II, IV, IX, XII
    (C) III, VII, X, XI
    (D) I, VII, IX, XI

21. Which of the following chemical mediators is released from peripheral afferent C fibers resulting in dull pain?

    (A) Substance P
    (B) Glutamate
    (C) Histamine
    (D) Serotonin

22. To supplement a brachial plexus block to cover the anterior shoulder, the cervical plexus can be blocked at which of the following locations?

    (A) Anterior to the mastoid process
    (B) Posterior border of the sternocleidomastoid
    (C) At the interscalene groove
    (D) Posterior to the angle of the mandible

23. Following general endotracheal anesthesia, the patient is in respiratory distress and is unable to speak. What nerve(s) may be injured?

    (A) Unilateral recurrent laryngeal nerve
    (B) Bilateral superior laryngeal nerve
    (C) Unilateral superior laryngeal nerve
    (D) Bilateral vagus nerves

24. A patient's serum potassium level is 7.2 mEq/L. In which sequential order will cardiac manifestations of hyperkalemia progress?

    (A) Peaked T waves, loss of P wave, widened QRS complex, sine wave
    (B) Peaked T waves, widened QRS complex, loss of P wave, sine wave
    (C) Loss of R-wave amplitude, peaked T waves, widened QRS complex, sine wave
    (D) Prolonged P–R interval, peaked T waves, widened QRS complex, asystole

25. Which of the following is not a physiologic response to pain?

    (A) Increased peripheral vascular resistance
    (B) Decreased tidal volume
    (C) Increased platelet aggregation
    (D) Decreased urinary sphincter tone

26. What is the treatment of choice for hyponatremic patients with decreased total body sodium content?

    (A) 0.9% NS
    (B) D5. ½NS
    (C) 0.5 NS
    (D) 3% NS

27. What statement is false regarding nasal airways?

    (A) Nasal airways are 2-4 cm shorter than oral airways.
    (B) Thrombocytopenia is a contraindication.
    (C) Nasal airways are 2-4 cm longer than oral airways.
    (D) Basilar skull fracture is a contraindication.

28. A patient-controlled analgesia order is written. What is the lockout interval for morphine?

    (A) 8-20 minutes
    (B) 5-10 minutes
    (C) 10-15 minutes
    (D) 15-18 minutes

29. A patient taking duloxetine for chronic neuropathic pain is scheduled for a cholecystectomy. How is duloxetine classified?

    (A) Tricyclic antidepressant
    (B) Selective serotonin reuptake inhibitor
    (C) Serotonin-norepinephrine reuptake inhibitor
    (D) Nonselective serotonin reuptake inhibitor

30. What is the rationale for rapidly freezing plasma for the purpose of making fresh frozen plasma?

    (A) Rapid freezing prevents inactivation of factors VIII and I.
    (B) Rapid freezing prevents inactivation of factors V and VIII.
    (C) Rapid freezing prevents the inactivation of all the factors.
    (D) Rapid freezing prevents the inactivation of antithrombin III.

31. Which of the following is not a risk factor for developing cauda equine syndrome?

    (A) Lidocaine spinal anesthesia
    (B) Use of glucose to increase baricity of neuraxial anesthetics
    (C) Epidural anesthesia
    (D) Continuous spinal anesthesia (CSA)

32. How soon must fresh frozen plasma be transfused once thawed?

    (A) Within 4 hours
    (B) Within 8 hours
    (C) Within 12 hours
    (D) Within 24 hours

33. Preoxygenation results in how many minutes of oxygen reserve?

    (A) 1-3 minutes
    (B) 3-6 minutes
    (C) 5-8 minutes
    (D) >8 minutes

34. Which patient should receive a type and cross match instead of a type and screen prior to surgery?

    Select (3) three
    (A) A 48-year-old female scheduled for an endo-vascular stent of an aortic aneurysm
    (B) An obese 12-year-old male undergoing an emergency tonsillectomy
    (C) A 22-year-old male with a history of multiple blood transfusions
    (D) A pregnant Rh-positive patient with Rh-negative baby undergoing emergency surgery
    (E) An 80-year-old female scheduled a hip replacement with a positive type and screen

35. A 150-kg male patient has a serum sodium concentration of 110 mEq/L. How much sodium would be needed to bring the serum sodium to 125 mEq/L?

    (A) 750 mEq
    (B) 1,350 mEq
    (C) 2,400 mEq
    (D) 3,200 mEq

36. How much blood does a fully soaked laparotomy "lap" pad contain?

    (A) 10-20 mL
    (B) 25-50 mL
    (C) 50-100 mL
    (D) 100-150 mL

37. Six hours after a patient received a transfusion with 2 units of fresh frozen plasma and 1 unit of platelets, she presents with hypoxia, fever, and noncardiogenic pulmonary edema. What complication do you suspect?

    (A) Post-transfusion purpura
    (B) Transfusion-related acute lung injury
    (C) Delayed hemolytic reaction
    (D) Transfusion-related immunomodulation

38. A 44-year-old 50-kg male received 750 mL of fresh frozen plasma. What percent of normal would you expect his clotting factor concentration to achieve post transfusion?

    (A) 100%
    (B) 75%
    (C) 60%
    (D) 30%

39. For which infectious diseases is donor blood tested after it is collected, typed, and screened?

    (A) Hepatitis A, Hepatitis B, and Hepatitis C
    (B) Hepatitis B, Hepatitis C, and Hepatitis D
    (C) Hepatitis C, Syphilis, and Human Immunode-ficiency Virus
    (D) Hepatitis C, Cytomegalovirus (CMV), and Syphilis

40. Which is not an indication for cryoprecipitate administration?

    (A) Fibrinogen levels <80-100 mg/dL
    (B) Factor XIII deficiency
    (C) Antithrombin deficiency
    (D) Preoperative prophylaxis for patient with von Willebrand disease

41. Which factors are not complications associated with massive blood transfusion?

    Select (2) two
    (A) Serum K^+ 5.5
    (B) Core temperature 35.5 °C
    (C) Increased 2,3 DPG
    (D) Decreased 2,3 DPG
    (E) Ionized Ca^+ 1.25 mmol/L

42. What is the approximate half-life of serum albumin?

    (A) 12 hours
    (B) 6 days
    (C) 10 days
    (D) 21 days

43. Which of the following nerves must be separately blocked during an axillary approach to the brachial plexus?

    (A) Musculocutaneous
    (B) Ulnar
    (C) Medial brachial cutaneous
    (D) Median

44. What is the most effective initial treatment of symptomatic hypercalcemia?

    (A) Hydration with IV normal saline followed by furosemide
    (B) Thiazide followed by IV normal saline hydration
    (C) Hydration with IV normal saline followed by bisphosphonates
    (D) Glucocorticoids followed by IV normal saline hydration

45. Caudal anesthesia involves needle penetration of the sacrococcygeal ligament covering the sacral hiatus created by which unfused laminae?

    (A) S1 and S2
    (B) S2 and S3
    (C) S3 and S4
    (D) S4 and S5

46. A 154-lb female has a serum sodium level 120 mEq/L. In order to correct the sodium level to 128 mEq, how many milliequivalents of sodium are required?

    (A) 280 mEq
    (B) 336 mEq
    (C) 616 mEq
    (D) 739 mEq

47. C fibers transmit what type of sensation?

    (A) Proprioception
    (B) Touch-pressure
    (C) Somatic pain
    (D) Visceral pain

48. Which nerve provides sensory innervation to the lateral thigh?

    (A) Lateral femoral cutaneous
    (B) Saphenous
    (C) Femoral
    (D) Posterior femoral cutaneous

49. An axillary block is performed for a surgical procedure on the right forearm and hand. The patient begins to experience pain at the tip of the index finger during the procedure. An effective rescue block would involve injecting local into which of the following sites?

    (A) Antecubital space at the lateral aspect of the biceps tendon
    (B) Antecubital crease medial to the biceps insertion
    (C) One finger breadth proximal to the arcuate ligament
    (D) Immediately lateral to the flexor carpi ulnaris

50. Which of the following are associated with slow pain?

    Select (3) three
    (A) Myelinated Aδ primary efferents
    (B) Action potential 0.5-2 m/seconds
    (C) Myelinated Aδ primary afferents
    (D) Dull pain
    (E) Burning pain

51. A patient has pain on the dorsum of the foot and the lateral aspect of the knee. What nerve root is involved?

    (A) L3
    (B) L5
    (C) L4
    (D) S1

52. Which of the following patients is at greatest risk for postdural puncture headaches?

    (A) Obese
    (B) Elderly
    (C) Pregnant
    (D) Pediatric

53. While performing an axillary block utilizing the trans-arterial approach, a paresthesia is elicited after passing through the artery. Which nerve is posterior to the artery?

    (A) Ulnar
    (B) Radial
    (C) Median
    (D) Intercostobrachial

54. A patient receives large volumes of 0.9% normal saline during a case. What is the risk associated with this?

    (A) Hypochloremic alkalosis
    (B) Hyperchloremic alkalosis
    (C) Hypochloremic acidosis
    (D) Hyperchloremic acidosis

55. What causes hypocalcemia?

    Select (3) three
    (A) Hypoparathyroidism
    (B) Paget's disease
    (C) Fat embolism
    (D) Rapid infusion of 1,000 mL albumin
    (E) Biliary colic
    (F) Chronic immobilization

56. Which of the following local anesthetics should be avoided in a glucose-6-phosphate dehydrogenase (G_6PD) deficiency?

    (A) Ropivacaine
    (B) Etidocaine
    (C) Prilocaine
    (D) Tetracaine

57. You plan to use an intravenous regional technique for a hand surgery. What is your greatest concern?

    (A) Duration of the case
    (B) Using the dual tourniquet system
    (C) Tourniquet discomfort
    (D) Tourniquet failure

58. Removal of epidural catheters should be delayed for a minimum of how many hours following the administration of prophylactic low molecular weight heparin (LMWH)?

    (A) 1 hour
    (B) 10 hours

    (C) 3 hours
    (D) 6 hours

59. When performing an ankle block, which of the following nerves is located by identifying the groove formed proximally by the extensor hallucis longus tendon and the extensor digitorum longus tendon?

    (A) Saphenous
    (B) Deep peroneal
    (C) Posterior tibial
    (D) Sural

60. Which of the following terms is defined as perception of an ordinary non-noxious stimulus as pain?

    (A) Hyperalgesia
    (B) Allodynia
    (C) Hyperesthesia
    (D) Dysesthesia

61. What is your main anesthetic concern when caring for a patient taking anabolic steroids?

    (A) Myocardial infarction
    (B) Hepatotoxicity
    (C) Hypercoagulopathy
    (D) Stroke

62. Injecting local anesthetic at which site is associated with the greatest risk of systemic absorption?

    (A) Brachial plexus
    (B) Paracervical
    (C) Intercostal
    (D) Caudal

63. Which topical local anesthetics may cause methemoglobinemia?

    Select (2) two
    (A) Bupivacaine
    (B) Prilocaine
    (C) Mepivacaine
    (D) Benzocaine
    (E) Procaine

64. Which of the following factors has the greatest effect on the level of spinal anesthesia?

    (A) Age
    (B) Patient height
    (C) Position of patient during injection
    (D) Drug volume

65. How much blood could a 90-kg, adult female patient lose and still maintain a hematocrit of 30%, provided the preoperative hematocrit was 42%?

    (A) 702 mL
    (B) 2,106 mL
    (C) 2,457 mL
    (D) 5,850 mL

66. Interruption of pain impulses can be accomplished through the administration of intrathecal opioids. These opioids act by binding to which of the following sites?

    (A) Periaqueductal gray
    (B) Dorsal root ganglia
    (C) Anterior horn
    (D) Dorsal horn

67. Epidural morphine was administered for postoperative pain control. What is the duration of action?

    (A) 12-24 hours
    (B) 4-6 hours
    (C) 24-48 hours
    (D) 2-6 hours

68. A 20-kg child is scheduled for a urology procedure. What is the appropriate dose for a caudal anesthetic?

    (A) 10 mL
    (B) 5 mL
    (C) 3 mL
    (D) 25 mL

69. Which of the following peripheral nerve block(s) would provide the most effective analgesia for a total knee arthroplasty?

    (A) Femoral nerve block
    (B) Femoral nerve block and obturator nerve block
    (C) Sciatic nerve block and psoas block
    (D) Sciatic and popliteal block

70. Which mechanisms of action are common among nonsteroidal anti-inflammatory drugs?

    Select (2) two
    (A) Inhibition of cyclooxygenase
    (B) Inhibition of prostaglandin synthesis
    (C) Inhibition of lipoxygenase
    (D) Inhibition of leukotriene synthesis

71. What factor is not associated with postoperative pulmonary complications?

    (A) ASA III
    (B) Cigarette smoking
    (C) Aortic aneurysm repair
    (D) Surgery lasting 3 hours

72. Which muscle is likely to be unaffected by an axillary brachial plexus block?

    (A) Abductor pollicis brevis
    (B) Interosseous
    (C) Brachialis
    (D) Pronator teres

73. Which of the following does not define somatic nociceptive pain?

    (A) Transduction
    (B) Transmission
    (C) Thermal
    (D) Modulation

74. During an unremarkable spinal anesthetic a bilateral T2 level in a healthy parturient results in a cardiac arrest. Which of the following is most likely responsible?

    (A) Decreased preload
    (B) Effect of local anesthetic on the medulla
    (C) Blockade of the carotid sinus
    (D) Cardiogenic hypertensive chemoreflex

75. Which medications should be held on the day of surgery?

    Select (2) two
    (A) Oral hypoglycemic agents
    (B) Tricyclic antidepressants
    (C) Selective serotonin reuptake inhibitors
    (D) Beta-adrenergic blockers
    (E) Angiotensin-converting enzyme (ACE) inhibitors

76. What nerve injury results most often with the lithotomy position?

    (A) Common peroneal
    (B) Sciatic
    (C) Obturator
    (D) Saphenous

77. Which of the following explains the rapid onset of 2-chloroprocaine when used for epidural anesthesia?

    (A) It is activated by ester hydrolysis.
    (B) It is administered in high concentrations.
    (C) It has high potency and lipid solubility.
    (D) It has relatively low pKa.

78. A patient taking furosemide is scheduled for a total knee arthroscopy. What statement is true?

    (A) Continue in patients with chronic renal failure.
    (B) Discontinue.
    (C) Continue in patients with diabetes.
    (D) Discontinue in the elderly.

79. What discontinuation issues may result for patients who take angiotensin converting enzyme (ACE) inhibitors?

    (A) Potential clotting abnormalities
    (B) Cholinergic symptoms
    (C) Psychosis and agitation
    (D) Atrial fibrillation

80. What is the fluid deficit for a 13-kg patient fasting for 6 hours?

    (A) 46 mL/hr
    (B) 53 mL/hr
    (C) 138 mL/hr
    (D) 276 mL/hr

81. Which of the following elements in the postoperative note are not required by the Center for Medicare and Medicaid Services (CMS)?

    (A) Mental status
    (B) Temperature
    (C) Pain
    (D) Urine output

82. Which nerve is blocked by injection through the thyrohyoid membrane to anesthetize the area between the vocal cords and the epiglottis?

    (A) Hypoglossal
    (B) Recurrent laryngeal
    (C) Superior laryngeal
    (D) Glossopharyngeal

83. Tachycardia, euphoria, delirium, and excitement are noted when conducting the preoperative evaluation in the emergency department. Which of the following is probably not related to the symptoms?

    (A) Narcotics
    (B) Cocaine
    (C) Hallucinogens
    (D) Marijuana

84. Which of the following may cause prolonged sedation?

    Select (2) two
    (A) Echinacea
    (B) Ephedra
    (C) Garlic
    (D) Kava-kava
    (E) Valerian

85. Calculate the ideal body weight (BW) for a 6 feet, 90-kg male.

    (A) 80 kg
    (B) 177 kg
    (C) 72 kg
    (D) 145 kg

86. A morbidly obese male patient is scheduled for a bariatric surgery. Which of the following diagnostic tests should be ordered?

    Select (3) three
    (A) Chest X-ray
    (B) 12-lead EKG
    (C) Coagulation studies
    (D) HCG
    (E) Glucose tolerance test

87. A patient with two peripheral intravenous (PIV) lines is undergoing general endotracheal anesthesia (GETA) for an orthopedic procedure. A recent lab value reveals a serum potassium level of 2.9 mEq/L. Which intervention is appropriate for this patient?

    (A) Administer IV replacement K$^+$ in dextrose solutions.
    (B) Maintain ETCO^2 levels between 25-30 mmHg.
    (C) Reduce the rocuronium redose by 25-50%.
    (D) Administer IV replacement K$^+$ 20 mEq IV in 0.9% NS over 1 hour.

88. What is the primary innervation of the lumbar facet joint?

    (A) The spinal nerve at the level of the joint
    (B) The spinal nerve superior to the joint
    (C) Both the nerve at the joint level and the nerve immediately superior
    (D) Neither the superior nor inferior spinal nerve

89. What is the gold standard diagnostic test for obstructive sleep apnea?

    (A) Polysomnography
    (B) STOP–Bang Questionnaire
    (C) STOP questionnaire
    (D) Bang Questionnaire

90. A patient with rheumatoid arthritis is undergoing a total knee replacement. What is the recommended glucocorticoid dosing regimen?

    (A) Usual corticosteroid dose + hydrocortisone 25 mg
    (B) Usual corticosteroid dose + hydrocortisone 100 mg
    (C) Usual corticosteroid dose + hydrocortisone 150 mg
    (D) Usual corticosteroid dose + hydrocortisone 50 mg

91. Which diagnostic finding is consistent with intracranial hypertension?

    (A) MRI with a 0.5 cm midline brain shift
    (B) CT with a 0.5 cm midline brain shift
    (C) CT with contrast with a 0.4 cm midline brain shift
    D) MRI with a 0.4 cm midline brain shift

92. Which surgical procedures pose the lowest risk for myocardial infarction within 30 days of surgery?

    Select (3) three
    (A) Liver transplant
    (B) Breast reduction
    (C) Hysterectomy
    (D) Cataract
    (E) Prostatectomy

93. What is the most common cause of nonsurgical bleeding following massive blood transfusion?

    (A) Dilutional thrombocytopenia
    (B) Citrate toxicity
    (C) Dilution of factors V and X
    (D) Dilution of factors II and VIII

94. The patient weighs 120 kg. The Ideal Body Weight is 60 kg. What is the patient's classification?

    (A) Obese
    (B) Morbidly obese
    (C) Overweight
    (D) Moderate obesity

95. An adult patient's platelet count is 25,000/μL. After transfusing the patient with 2 units of apheresis platelets, what would you expect the platelet count to be?

    (A) 30,000-35,000/μL
    (B) 55,000-85,000/μL
    (C) 85,000-145,000/μL
    (D) 145,000-165,000/μL

96. During the preoperative interview the patient shares that he/she performs light housework, plays golf once a week, and walks to the grocery store to get the newspaper. What is his/her metabolic equivalent (METs)?

    (A) 1 MET
    (B) 2 METs
    (C) 3 METs
    (D) 4 METs

97. What AANA Standard guides the practice of providing post anesthesia report?

(A) Standard I

(B) Standard III

(C) Standard V

(D) Standard VII

98. Which statement about fresh frozen plasma (FFP) administration is correct?

Select (2) two

(A) Each unit of FFP will increase the level of each clotting factor by 2-3% in adults.

(B) The initial therapeutic dose is 10-15 mL/kg.

(C) It should be ABO-compatible.

(D) It must be Rh-compatible.

(E) The therapeutic goal is to achieve 80% of the normal coagulation factor concentration.

99. Which of the following are risk factors for postoperative nausea and vomiting?

Select (3) three

(A) Male

(B) History of motion sickness

(C) Opioids

(D) Strabismus surgery

(E) Cataract surgery

(F) Hypertension

100. Which of the following statements is true regarding airway blocks?

(A) Topical lidocaine may produce methemoglobinemia.

(B) 4% lidocaine is injected into the trachea upon inspiration.

(C) Nerve blocks of the airway pose risk for aspiration.

(D) Local anesthesia to the mouth and pharynx blocks nerve transmission from the superior laryngeal nerve.

101. A patient is admitted to the Post Anesthesia Care Unit with shallow, rapid respirations, diaphoresis, and tachycardia. What is the most likely cause?

(A) Delayed awakening

(B) Hypothermia

(C) Emergence delirium

(D) Inadequate oxygenation

102. The anesthesia plan includes using topical cocaine for nasal surgery. What is the maximum dose?

(A) 50 mg

(B) 200 mg

(C) 400 mg

(D) 40 mg

103. What factors are associated with hypotension in the Post Anesthesia Care Unit?

Select (2) two

(A) Hypervolemia

(B) Nausea

(C) Arrhythmias

(D) Pain

(E) Shivering

104. What constitutes the eutectic mixture of local anesthetic?

(A) Benzocaine and prilocaine

(B) Prilocaine and tetracaine

(C) Lidocaine and prilocaine

(D) Prilocaine and nesicaine

105. During postanesthesia recovery the patient is snoring and use of the accessory muscle for ventilation are noted. What is the most likely cause?

(A) Airway obstruction

(B) Hypoventilation

(C) Hypoxemia

(D) Bronchospasm

106. Gabapentin is most helpful in treating which type of pain?

(A) Acute somatic pain

(B) Deep visceral pain

(C) Neuropathic pain

(D) Chronic arthritic joint pain

107. When using eutectic mixture of lidocaine and prilocaine (EMLA) cream, what is the maximum total dose for children >20 kg?

(A) 20 g

(B) 10 g

(C) 2 g

(D) 1 g

108. Which peripheral nerve block provides complete anesthesia for ankle surgery?

(A) Femoral

(B) Sciatic

(C) Obturator

(D) Popliteal

109. Which nerve block results in the highest blood level of local anesthetic?

(A) Sciatic

(B) Intercostal

(C) Paravertebral

(D) Cervical plexus

110. What are the fluid requirements for redistribution and evaporative surgical fluid losses during a bowel resection?

(A) 0-2 mL/kg

(B) 2-4 mL/kg

(C) 4-8 mL/kg

(D) 10-14 mL/kg

111. Which airway block provides anesthesia below the vocal cords?

Select (2) two

(A) Superior laryngeal nerve block

(B) Transtracheal block

(C) Glossopharyngeal block

(D) Instilling local anesthetic onto the vocal cords

112. Which of the following form the lumbar plexus?

(A) L1–3 and T10

(B) L1–4 and T10

(C) L1–4 and T12

(D) L1–3 and T12

113. What results when placing a femoral block with nerve stimulation?

(A) Thigh adduction

(B) Quadriceps twitch

(C) Sciatic nerve block posterior approach

(D) Sciatic nerve block anterior approach

114. Which phrase describes radiculopathy?

(A) Abnormal sensation with or without a stimulus

(B) Pain linked to noxious stimulation

(C) Nerve distribution pain

(D) Abnormal function of nerve roots

115. Which of the following are pain modulating excitatory neurotransmitters?

Select (2) two

(A) Substance P

(B) Glycine

(C) GABA

(D) Glutamate

(E) Serotonin

116. Which of the following physiological effects result from acute pain stimulation?

Select (3) three

(A) Increased myocardial workload

(B) Decreased vital capacity

(C) Decreased gastric emptying

(D) Decreased platelet aggregation

(E) Increased intestinal motility

117. Vocal cord paralysis occurred following intubation. What is the most likely cause?

(A) Recurrent laryngeal nerve damage

(B) Epiglottic damage

(C) Esophageal damage

(D) Superior laryngeal nerve

118. A patient with a history of reflux and diabetes mellitus is scheduled for a bowel obstruction. Which of the following fasting guidelines apply?

(A) NPO for 8 hours

(B) Clear fluids up to 2 hours

(C) Light meal up to 6 hours

(D) NPO for 4 hours

119. A 40-year-old male with a history of well-controlled hypertension is scheduled for a carpal tunnel release. How will you classify the patient?

    (A) ASA IV
    (B) ASA III
    (C) ASA II
    (D) ASA I

120. During the preoperative airway exam, you visualize the soft palate, faces, and uvula. How would you classify the patient's airway?

    (A) Mallampati I
    (B) Mallampati III
    (C) Mallampati II
    (D) Mallampati IV

121. A patient's lab values reveal digoxin toxicity and hyperkalemia. Which option for treating for hyperkalemia will you need to avoid in this patient?

    (A) 10 units regular insulin with 30-50 gm dextrose 50% IV
    (B) 3-5 mL of 10% calcium chloride IV
    (C) 45 mEq sodium bicarbonate IV
    (D) 30 gm sodium polystyrene PR

122. A patient is scheduled for knee arthroscopy. The blood glucose is elevated along with the A_{1c}. What will you do first?

    (A) Notify the surgeon that the surgery will be delayed.
    (B) Proceed with the surgery.
    (C) Cancel the surgery.
    (D) Call the endocrinologist.

123. What is the primary intracellular cation?

    (A) Potassium
    (B) Sodium
    (C) Calcium
    (D) Chloride

124. What mechanism results in the greatest amount of heat loss in the operating room?

    (A) Convection
    (B) Evaporation
    (C) Radiation
    (D) Conduction

125. What is the average blood volume of an 80-kg male?

    (A) 5 L
    (B) 6 L
    (C) 5.2 L
    (D) 6.4 L

126. How much additional fluid will you administer to a patient undergoing a herniorrhaphy?

    (A) 4-8 mL/kg
    (B) 0-2 mL/kg
    (C) 2-4 mL/kg
    (D) 10 mL/kg

127. What statement is true regarding colloids?

    (A) Inexpensive
    (B) Increase plasma volume
    (C) Used for initial resuscitation
    (D) Used primarily for extracellular expansion

128. While receiving a blood transfusion during general anesthesia tachycardia and hypotension develop. What is the most likely cause?

    (A) Delayed hemolytic reaction
    (B) Anaphylactic reaction
    (C) Urticarial reaction
    (D) Acute hemolytic reaction

129. What statement is true regarding a patient who is awake in the supine position?

    (A) The blood pressure decreases due to autoregulation.
    (B) Venous return decreases.
    (C) Blood pressure remains relatively constant.
    (D) Sympathetic outflow increases.

130. What effect does the lithotomy position have on arterial pressure?

    (A) Lower than supine position
    (B) Higher than supine position
    (C) Lower than Trendelenburg
    (D) Lower than sitting position

131. A patient experiences low vision following a lumbar laminectomy in the prone position. What is the etiology?

(A) Decreased intracranial pressure

(B) Decreased venous pressure

(C) Increased cerebral blood flow

(D) Decreased ocular perfusion pressure

132. Where will you measure the blood pressure for patients undergoing surgery in the lateral decubitus position?

(A) Nondependent arm

(B) Both arms

(C) Dependent arm

(D) Right thigh

133. A sudden decreased SpO_2, blood pressure, and $ETCO_2$ occur during general anesthesia. A mill-wheel murmur exists. What is the most likely cause?

(A) Venous air embolism

(B) Pneumocephalus

(C) Fat embolism

(D) Cardiovascular accident

134. What nerve injury is most likely to occur when the arm is pronated?

(A) Brachial plexus

(B) Ulnar nerve

(C) Radial nerve

(D) Suprascapular nerve

135. In the supine position, what nerve injury is associated with arm abduction >90 degrees and lateral rotation of the head?

(A) Ulnar nerve

(B) Brachial plexus

(C) Radial nerve

(D) Suprascapular nerve

136. Following surgery in the lithotomy position the patient exhibits foot drop and the inability to extend the toes. What nerves are most likely injured?

(A) Sciatic and common peroneal

(B) Femoral and sciatic

(C) Common peroneal and femoral

(D) Obturator and sciatic

137. Which patient requires a preoperative chest X-ray?

(A) 55-year-old smoker undergoing a laparoscopic cholecystectomy

(B) 65-year-old chronic stable bronchitic undergoing a carpal tunnel release

(C) 60-year-old undergoing a transurethral resection of the prostate

(D) 50-year-old undergoing a mitral valve replacement

138. What is the average distance from the skin to the epidural space?

(A) 1 cm

(B) 1.5 cm

(C) 5 cm

(D) 7.5 cm

139. What statement is false regarding the lateral decubitus position?

(A) Rhabdomyolysis may occur.

(B) Flex the dependent arm <90 degrees.

(C) Pad the lateral aspect of the dependent leg.

(D) Pulmonary blood flow to the dependent lung decreases.

140. In what position is a venous air embolism (VAE) most likely to occur?

(A) Lateral decubitus

(B) Sitting

(C) Prone

(D) Trendelenburg

141. A T6 sensory level is identified following administration of a spinal anesthetic. At what level is the sympathetic block?

(A) T4

(B) T10

(C) T6

(D) T8

142. In which patient is spinal anesthesia contraindicated?

(A) 30-year-old taking daily garlic
(B) 50-year-old taking subcutaneous heparin injections
(C) 25-year-old taking NSAIDS
(D) 40-year-old who received thrombolytic therapy

143. What factor least affects the spread of spinal local anesthetic?

(A) Baricity
(B) Drug dosage
(C) Site of injection
(D) Drug volume

144. How do transient neurologic symptoms (TNS) differ from cauda equina syndrome?

(A) TNS persists for several weeks following surgery.
(B) Cauda equina syndrome disappears within 10 days following surgery.
(C) TNS symptoms spontaneously disappear.
(D) Cauda equina syndrome symptoms include severe radicular back pain.

145. What local anesthetic is linked to cauda equina syndrome?

(A) Ropivacaine
(B) Bupivacaine
(C) Tetracaine
(D) Lidocaine

146. Spinal anesthesia using tetracaine 12 mg is given for a patient undergoing a transurethral resection of the prostate. If you add epinephrine what is the longest anticipated duration?

(A) 0.5 hour
(B) 1 hour
(C) 2 hours
(D) 3 hours

147. Which clotting factor is the first to become inactivated shortly after a patient has begun warfarin therapy?

(A) IV
(B) V
(C) VII
(D) IX

148. Following administration of 15 mg spinal bupivacaine, the patient's heart rate and blood pressure fall precipitously. What is the cause?

(A) Sympathetic blockade
(B) Motor blockade
(C) Sensory blockade
(D) Sensory and motor blockade

149. A patient states that their feet are numb following administration of an epidural test dose. What is the most likely cause?

(A) Intravascular injection
(B) Local anesthetic toxicity
(C) Intrathecal injection
(D) Normal response to a test dose

150. Twenty-four hours following an epidural anesthetic the patient complains of occipital headache, nausea, vomiting, and double vision. What is the most likely cause?

(A) Neurologic injury
(B) Spinal hematoma
(C) Epidural hematoma
(D) Postdural puncture headache

151. What factor does not influence the spread of local anesthetic placed in the epidural space?

(A) Concentration
(B) Dose
(C) Site of injection
(D) Age

152. A patient is scheduled for a thoracotomy. A thoracic epidural is placed. What volume of local anesthetic will you use?

(A) 15 mL
(B) 10 mL
(C) 18 mL
(D) 20 mL

153. What is the best approach to avoiding cardiac arrest during spinal anesthesia?

(A) Decrease preload
(B) Give prophylactic ephedrine
(C) Increase preload
(D) Give prophylactic atropine

154. What patient is least likely to experience a postdural puncture headache?

- (A) 70-year-old male
- (B) 40-year-old male
- (C) 20-year-old female
- (D) 60-year-old female

155. What ultrasound frequency is used when placing an epidural or spinal?

- (A) 2-5 MHz
- (B) 5-10 MHz
- (C) 10-15 MHz
- (D) 20-25 MHz

156. Which statement is true regarding ultrasound for peripheral nerve blocks?

- (A) Structures that appear white on the ultrasound screen are hypoechoic.
- (B) Low frequencies are used for peripheral nerve blocks.
- (C) Structures that appear white on the ultrasound screen are hyperechoic.
- (D) High-frequency transducers offer a low resolution picture.

157. What is the innervation of the brachial plexus?

- (A) C5–C8 and T1
- (B) C4–C8
- (C) C4–C8 and T1
- (D) C5–C7 and T1–T2

158. What brachial plexus approach is indicated for a patient undergoing a shoulder surgery?

- (A) Supraclavicular
- (B) Infraclavicular
- (C) Interscalene
- (D) Axillary

159. Which would result from excessive pressure on the sciatic nerve by the piriformis muscle?

- (A) Chronic pain in the perineum with voiding difficulty
- (B) Anterior thigh pain and weakness upon standing
- (C) Gluteal pain with paresthesia in the posterior thigh
- (D) Lumbar vertebral pain exacerbated by flexion of the lower back

160. Which of the following is appropriate to use for intravenous regional anesthesia?

- (A) 0.5% lidocaine with epinephrine 50 mL
- (B) 5.0% lidocaine with epinephrine 40 mL
- (C) 0.5% lidocaine 50 mL
- (D) 0.5% bupivacaine 50 mL

161. For which medication is regional anesthesia an absolute contraindication?

- (A) Clopidogrel
- (B) Unfractionated heparin
- (C) Low-molecular-weight heparin
- (D) Thrombolytics

162. The patient received a Bier Block for hand surgery. The case was completed in 10 minutes. When will you deflate the tourniquet?

- (A) 10 minutes after the local anesthetic is injected.
- (B) 20 minutes after the local anesthetic is injected.
- (C) 30 minutes after the local anesthetic is injected.
- (D) 40 minutes after the local anesthetic is injected.

163. What statement is true regarding digital nerve blocks?

- (A) A small gauge needle is inserted at the distal aspect of the selected digit.
- (B) 2-3 mL of lidocaine with epinephrine is used.
- (C) A small gauge needle is inserted at the medial and lateral borders of the base of the selected digit.
- (D) 2-3 mL of lidocaine is used.

164. What is the definition of persistent postsurgical pain?

- (A) Pain resulting from outpatient surgery sufficient to require inpatient care
- (B) Pain for > 1-2 weeks following surgery
- (C) Pain for > 1-2 months following surgery
- (D) Pain for > 1 year following surgery

165. Where is local anesthetic injected in a radial block at the wrist?

    (A) Medial to the ulnar artery at the wrist
    (B) Lateral to the radial artery at the wrist
    (C) Medial to the radial artery at the wrist
    (D) Lateral to the ulnar artery at the wrist

166. Which nerve provides sensation to the anteromedial foot and medial lower leg?

    (A) Deep peroneal
    (B) Sural
    (C) Superficial peroneal
    (D) Saphenous

167. Calculate the Aldrete Score for a patient with the following criteria:

    SpO_2 >92% (room air); shallow breathing; blood pressure +/−20 mmHg of normal; arousable on calling, and moves all extremities.

168. What artery provides the majority of the blood supply to the anterior, lower 2/3 of the spinal cord?

    (A) Posterior spinal artery
    (B) Artery of Adamkiewicz
    (C) Posterior inferior cerebellar artery
    (D) Intercostal arteries

169. After placing a spinal anesthetic the sensory block is assessed at T8. Where is the most likely level of the motor block?

    (A) T4
    (B) T6
    (C) T10
    (D) T2

170. Which of the following characterize A-a nerve fibers?

    Select (3) three
    (A) Diameter 0.5-1 μm
    (B) Heavy myelination
    (C) Diameter 15-20 μm
    (D) Motor function
    (E) Light myelination
    (F) Pain and temperature

171. Following administration of spinal anesthesia the patient becomes hypotensive and bradycardic. What nerve fibers are affected?

    (A) T1–T4
    (B) T5–T6
    (C) T7–T8
    (D) T10–T12

172. Which clotting factor is not synthesized in the liver?

    (A) II
    (B) IV
    (C) VII
    (D) VIII

173. A 70-year-old patient with emphysema is undergoing an open cholecystectomy. What is the best anesthetic choice for this patient?

    (A) Spinal
    (B) Epidural
    (C) General
    (D) MAC

174. Which of the following are relative contraindications for regional anesthesia?

    Select (3) three
    (A) Uncooperative patient
    (B) Preexisting neurological deficits
    (C) Severe aortic stenosis
    (D) Patient refusal
    (E) Stenotic valvular disease

175. A patient who takes ticlopidine requests a spinal anesthetic for a total knee replacement. What is the waiting period for ticlopidine?

    (A) 7 days
    (B) 14 days
    (C) 48 hour
    (D) 8 hour

176. Where is Tuffier's line located?

    (A) L4
    (B) L2
    (C) L1
    (D) L3

177. What is the correct order of anatomical structure used when placing an epidural needle?

    (A) Skin, subcutaneous tissue, supraspinous ligament, interspinous ligament, ligamentum flavum, epidural space

    (B) Skin, subcutaneous tissue, interspinous ligament, supraspinous ligament, ligamentum flavum, epidural space

    (C) Skin, subcutaneous tissue, interspinous ligament, supraspinous ligament, ligamentum flavum, dura, subarachnoid space

    (D) Skin, subcutaneous tissue, interspinous ligament, supraspinous ligament, ligamentum flavum, dura, epidural space

178. Which statement is true of Aδ fibers?

    (A) Aδ fibers are myelinated, synapse in Rexed laminae I and V, and transmit primarily mechanical or thermal pain.

    (B) Aδ fibers are unmyelinated, synapse in Rexed laminae II and VII, and transmit primarily mechanical or thermal pain.

    (C) Aδ fibers are myelinated, synapse in Rexed laminae III and X, and transmit primarily mechanical or thermal pain.

    (D) Aδ fibers are unmyelinated, synapse in Rexed laminae IV and VI, and transmit primarily mechanical or thermal pain.

179. Which laminae receive input from C fibers?

    (A) III, IV, VI
    (B) I, VI, X
    (C) II, VII, IX
    (D) I, II, V

180. How would postoperative pain localized to the site of skin incision be classified?

    (A) Visceral pain
    (B) Deep somatic pain
    (C) Superficial somatic pain
    (D) Referred pain

181. Referred pain from the diaphragm can be expected in which dermatome?

    (A) C4
    (B) C7

    (C) T4
    (D) T7

182. What is the surface landmark of the fourth cervical cutaneous dermatome?

    (A) Anterior neck
    (B) Shoulder
    (C) Biceps
    (D) Xiphoid

183. Which act to diminish pain signals?

    Select (2) two
    (A) Glutamate
    (B) Enkephalin
    (C) Substance P
    (D) ß-Endorphin

184. What complication is associated with using 6% hetastarch in volumes > 20 mL/kg?

    (A) Interference with blood typing
    (B) Coagulopathy
    (C) Kidney failure
    (D) Anaphylaxis

185. Which portion of the spinal cord is most associated with transmission of pain signals?

    (A) Dorsal horn
    (B) Central canal
    (C) Ventral horn
    (D) Pia mater

186. Which of the following does not relieve pain by decreasing inflammation?

    (A) Acetaminophen
    (B) Ketorolac
    (C) Ibuprofen
    (D) Celecoxib

187. Which are mechanisms of action for gabapentin?

    Select (2) two
    (A) GABA agonist effect
    (B) Calcium channel blockade
    (C) Excitatory neurotransmitter inhibition
    (D) Inhibition of prostaglandin synthesis

188. Which of these analgesic agents is a GABA agonist?

(A) Baclofen

(B) Pregabalin

(C) Dexmedetomidine

(D) Celecoxib

189. What is the most common level of approach to perform a stellate ganglion block?

(A) C3

(B) C4

(C) C5

(D) C6

190. What are mechanisms of action for duloxetine?

Select (2) two

(A) Monoamine oxidase inhibition

(B) Serotonin reuptake inhibition

(C) α_2 receptor agonist effect

(D) Norepinephrine reuptake inhibition

191. Which is an α_2 agonist?

(A) Carbamazepine

(B) Tapentadol

(C) Phenytoin

(D) Tizanidine

192. Which route of administration of fentanyl is subject to the hepatic first-pass effect?

(A) Transdermal patch

(B) Intravenous injection

(C) Sublingual spray

(D) Oral tablet

193. What would be the correct classification of hyperalgesia with sympathetic dysfunction following a traumatic injury that included direct nerve damage persisting beyond the standard healing period in the absence of other conditions that may be responsible for the pain?

(A) Complex regional pain syndrome type I

(B) Reflex sympathetic dystrophy

(C) Complex regional pain syndrome type II

(D) Persistent allodynia

194. Following placement of a stellate ganglion block the patient becomes hoarse. What has occurred?

(A) Phrenic nerve block

(B) Recurrent laryngeal nerve block

(C) Subdural injection

(D) Pneumothorax

195. Which are appropriate for inclusion in an epidural steroid injection?

Select (3) three

(A) Saline

(B) Methylprednisolone acetate

(C) Triamcinolone diacetate

(D) Fentanyl

196. Which steroid has the smallest particulate size?

(A) Methylprednisolone acetate

(B) Triamcinolone diacetate

(C) Dexamethasone sodium phosphate

(D) Betamethasone

197. What is the maximal volume of solution that can be safely injected into the lumbar facet joint?

(A) 1 mL

(B) 2 mL

(C) 3 mL

(D) 4 mL

198. Which is an indication for a celiac plexus block?

(A) Post-traumatic hypoperfusion of the arm

(B) Lower extremity vascular insufficiency

(C) Intractable lumbar pain

(D) Pain resulting from pancreatic malignancy

199. Which class of nerve fiber will be the site of therapeutic stimulation for a transcutaneous electrical nerve stimulation (TENS) unit?

(A) Aδ fibers

(B) C fibers

(C) Aβ fibers

(D) B fibers

200. When selecting a needle for spinal anesthesia, which type is most likely to cause a postdural puncture headache?

(A) 20-g Quincke

(B) 22-g Whitacre

(C) 22-g Sprotte

(D) 22-g Quincke

201. An adult patient with moderate aortic regurgitation receives a spinal anesthetic. A blood pressure drop to 68/42 is treated with 100 μg of phenylephrine. How will this dose impact the patient's underlying disease state?

(A) It will improve the regurgitation.

(B) It will exacerbate the regurgitation.

(C) It will have no impact on the regurgitation.

(D) Phenylephrine is contraindicated in this patient.

202. Which estimated blood volume is correctly paired with its age group?

(A) Preterm neonate: 85 mL/kg

(B) 6-month old: 90 mL/kg

(C) Adult male: 80 mL/kg

(D) Adult female: 65 mL/kg

203. How will the symptoms of an acute hemolytic transfusion reaction manifest in a patient under general anesthesia?

(A) Fever, unexplained tachycardia, hypotension and diffuse oozing in surgical field

(B) Nausea, fever, flank pain, unexplained tachycardia, and hypotension

(C) Hemoglobinuria, chest and flank pain, fever, and hypotension

(D) Hypertension, unexplained tachycardia, fever, erythema, and hives

204. An injection of 0.5% ropivacaine is placed into the brachial plexus via the interscalene approach. Which of the following is most likely to be spared?

(A) Sensation of the radial side of the forearm

(B) Sensation of the medial upper arm

(C) Sensation of half of the fourth and all of the fifth fingers

(D) Sensation of the palmar surface of the first three fingers

205. How does an opioid inhibit postsynaptic nociceptive signal transmission?

Select (2) two

(A) Hyperpolarization

(B) Excitation

(C) Opening calcium channels

(D) Opening potassium channels

206. When administering a spinal anesthetic, which nerve roots are easily blocked?

(A) Smaller, unmyelinated

(B) Larger, myelinated

(C) Smaller, myelinated

(D) Larger, unmyelinated

207. Which corticosteroid has the most potent glucocorticoid activity?

(A) Hydrocortisone

(B) Prednisone

(C) Methylprednisolone

(D) Dexamethasone

208. Where does the spinal cord end in a 5-year-old?

(A) L1

(B) L2

(C) L3

(D) L4

209. When is a type and screen preferable to a type and cross match?

(A) The probability of transfusing blood is low

(B) The probability of transfusing blood is high

(C) The patient has high risk for alloimmunization

(D) The patient has a history of a positive antibody screen

Answers and Explanations: Basic Principles

1. When do symptoms of ischemic optic neuropathy that result in postoperative vision loss typically occur?

   (A) Immediately postoperatively
   (B) 2 hours postoperatively
   (C) 2 days postoperatively
   (D) 2 weeks postoperatively

   Rationale: Symptoms typically start following emergence from anesthesia, but may occur up to 12 days following surgery.

   Ref: Butterworth, J.F., Mackey, D.C., & Wasnick, J.D. (2013). Ch 54 *Morgan & Mikhail's Clinical Anesthesiology* (5th ed.). New York, NY: McGraw-Hill.

2. During a general anesthetic you suspect an episode of malignant hyperthermia (MH). What will you do first?

   (A) Call the MHAUS hotline.
   (B) Administer dantrolene.
   (C) Inform the surgeon.
   (D) Turn off inhalational agents.

   Rationale: When suspicion of an episode of malignant hyperthermia exists, each of the responses is in order; however, turning off the inhalational agents is the first priority.

   Ref: Butterworth, J.F., Mackey, D.C., & Wasnick, J.D. (2013). Ch 52 *Morgan & Mikhail's Clinical Anesthesiology* (5th ed.). New York, NY: McGraw-Hill.

   Longnecker, D.E., Brown, D.L., Newman, M.F., & Zapol, W.M. (2012). Ch 87 *Anesthesiology* (2nd ed.). New York, NY: McGraw-Hill.

3. When is body temperature loss the greatest?

   (A) During the preoperative preparation
   (B) During the 1st hour in the operating room
   (C) During the 2nd and 3rd hours in the operating room
   (D) During the 4th hour in the operating room

> **BOX 3-1**
>
> **Management of Patient with Highly Suspicious Episode of MH**
>
> I. Discontinue all potent inhalational agents and succinylcholine. Maintain anesthesia with total intravenous, nontriggering anesthetics.
> II. Increase minute ventilation to at least 10 L/min to flush out volatile anesthetics and to lower $ETCO_2$. Administer 100% oxygen. Insert activated charcoal filters into the inspiratory and expiratory limbs of the breathing circuit. Consider switching to a freestanding ventilator as soon as possible.
> III. Inform the surgeon to expedite or abort the procedure, if possible, and obtain assistance from MHAUS Hotline (1-800-644-9737) for acute crisis.
> IV. Administer IV dantrolene, 2.5 mg/kg. Be prepared to repeat this dose until the patient responds with a decrease in $ETCO_2$, rigidity, or heart rate.
> V. Obtain blood gas analysis to determine if bicarbonate therapy is indicated. Place central or arterial catheter for serial blood gas and CK measurements.
> VI. Begin cooling measures if the patient is hyperthermic. Efforts to cool the patient must correspond with the extent of temperature elevation. Patients can be cooled by decreasing room temperature, surface cooling with ice, or using cold solutions for gastric, bladder, and rectal lavage.
> VII. Hyperkalemia is common and is treated with insulin and glucose. In adults use 10 units of regular insulin in 1000 mL of $D_{10}W$ (10% aqueous dextrose solution). Serum potassium and glucose levels must be monitored.
> VIII. Measure baseline CK and serial CKs every 6 hours until CK plateaus.

Rationale: The greatest amount of heat loss occurs during the 1st hour in the operating room (0.5-1.5C). Thereafter temperature decline is gradual and then plateaus.

Ref: Butterworth, J.F., Mackey, D.C., & Wasnick, J.D. (2013). Ch 52 *Morgan & Mikhail's Clinical Anesthesiology* (5th ed.). New York, NY: McGraw-Hill.

Longnecker, D.E., Brown, D.L., Newman, M.F., & Zapol, W.M. (2012). Ch 88 *Anesthesiology* (2nd ed.). New York, NY: McGraw-Hill.

4. For an awake fiberoptic intubation, anesthesia for the posterior 1/3 of the tongue, vallecula, anterior epiglottis, walls of the pharynx, and tonsils can be performed by injecting local anesthetic into which of the following structures?

   (A) Base of the frenulum
   (B) Palatoglossal arch
   (C) Thyroid membrane
   (D) Cricothyroid membrane

   Rationale: Innervation of the airway related to an awake fiber optic intubation is through two neural pathways: the glossopharyngeal nerve cephalad to the epiglottis and vagal braches (superior laryngeal and recurrent laryngeal nerves) distal to the epiglottis. Sensation to the mucosa of the palatine tonsils, soft palate, and sensory branch to the posterior 1/3 of the tongue are provided by the tonsillar nerves (branches of the glossopharyngeal nerve). Blockade of these nerves facilitates intubation by blocking the gag reflex. A submucosal injection can be performed at the cephalad portion of the posterior tonsillar pillars at the palatoglossal arch.
   Ref: Butterworth, J.F., Mackey, D.C., & Wasnick, J.D. (2013). Ch 19 *Morgan & Mikhail's Clinical Anesthesiology* (5th ed.). New York, NY: McGraw-Hill.
   Hadzic, A. (2007). Ch 19 *Textbook of Regional Anesthesia and Acute Pain Management*. New York, NY: McGraw Hill Medical.

5. Which is an example of sensation without stimulus?

   (A) Temporal summation
   (B) Dynamic allodynia
   (C) Paresthesia
   (D) Analgesia

   Rationale: Paresthesia is the spontaneous perception of an abnormal sensation.
   Ref: Butterworth, J.F., Mackey, D.C., & Wasnick, J.D. (2013). Ch 47 *Morgan & Mikhail's Clinical Anesthesiology* (5th ed.). New York, NY: McGraw-Hill.
   Longnecker, D.E., Brown, D.L., Newman, M.F., & Zapol, W.M. (eds.) (2012). Ch 89 *Anesthesiology* (2nd ed.). New York, NY: McGraw-Hill.

6. Which statement about stored blood is correct?

   (A) The amount of extracellular potassium transfused per unit is 10 mEq per unit.
   (B) Stored blood typically has a pH < 7.45.
   (C) Stored blood contains factors V and VIII.
   (D) Stored blood can contain as much as 150 mEq/L of potassium.

   Rationale: The amount of extracellular potassium transfused per unit is usually < 4 mEq per unit. Stored blood is acidic due to the citric acid anticoagulant and accumulation of lactic acid. Stored blood does not contain factors V and VIII and stored blood can contain as much as 17 mEq/L of potassium.
   Ref: Butterworth, J.F., Mackey, D.C., & Wasnick, J.D. (2013). Ch 51 *Morgan & Mikhail's Clinical Anesthesiology* (5th ed.). New York, NY: McGraw-Hill.
   Nagelhout, J.J., & Plaus, K.L. (2014). Ch 20 *Nurse Anesthesia* (5th ed.). St. Louis, MO: Elsevier.

7. Which patients are at risk for aspiration?

   Select (3) three
   (A) Second trimester parturient
   (B) Gastroesophageal reflux
   (C) First trimester parturient
   (D) NPO >6 hrs
   (E) Third trimester parturient

   Rationale: Patients at greatest risk for aspiration include the 2nd and 3rd trimester parturients, patients with gastroesophageal reflux disease, and those who consumed solid food <6 hours prior to surgery.
   Ref: Butterworth, J.F., Mackey, D.C., & Wasnick, J.D. (2013). Ch 18 *Morgan & Mikhail's Clinical Anesthesiology* (5th ed.). New York, NY: McGraw-Hill.

8. What percentage of the total body water is extracellular?

   (A) 67%
   (B) 33%
   (C) 25%
   (D) 100%

   Rationale: Extracellular fluid (interstitial and intravascular) contains approximately 30% of the total body water. The intracellular compartment is approximately 67% of the total body water.

TABLE 3-1. Body fluid compartments (based on average 70-kg male).

Compartment	Fluid as Percent Body Weight (%)	Total Body Water (%)	Fluid Volume (L)
Intracellular	40	67	28
Extracellular			
Interstitial	15	25	10.5
Intravascular	5	8	3.5
Total	60	100	42

Ref: Butterworth, J.F., Mackey, D.C., & Wasnick, J.D. (2013). Ch 49 *Morgan & Mikhail's Clinical Anesthesiology* (5ᵗʰ ed.). New York, NY: McGraw-Hill.

Nagelhout, J.J., & Plaus, K.L. (2014). Ch 20 *Nurse Anesthesia* (5ᵗʰ ed.). St. Louis, MO: Elsevier.

9. Which drugs are known triggers for malignant hyperthermia?

    Select (3) three

    (A) Halothane

    (B) Sevoflurane

    (C) Methohexital

    (D) Sodium thiopental

    (E) Succinylcholine

    Rationale: All inhalation general anesthetics and depolarizing muscle relaxants trigger malignant hyperthermia. Barbiturates are considered safe anesthetic agents.

Ref: Butterworth, J.F., Mackey, D.C., & Wasnick, J.D. (2013). Ch 52 *Morgan & Mikhail's Clinical Anesthesiology* (5ᵗʰ ed.). New York, NY: McGraw-Hill.

Longnecker, D.E., Brown, D.L., Newman, M.F., & Zapol, W.M. (2012). *Anesthesiology* (2ⁿᵈ ed.). New York, NY: McGraw-Hill.

10. How is the brachial plexus formed?

    (A) Roots, divisions, trunks, cords, branches

    (B) Divisions, trunks, cords, branches

    (C) Cords, divisions, roots, branches

    (D) Trunks, divisions, cords, branches

    Rationale: Nerve roots leaving the intervertebral foramina join to form trunks, divisions, cords, and branches.

Ref: Butterworth, J.F., Mackey, D.C., & Wasnick, J.D. (2013). Ch 46 *Morgan & Mikhail's Clinical Anesthesiology* (5ᵗʰ ed.). New York, NY: McGraw-Hill.

Miller, R.D., & Pardo, M.C. (2011). Ch 18 *Basics of Anesthesia* (6ᵗʰ ed.). Philadelphia, PA: Elsevier.

Nagelhout, J.J., & Plaus, K.L. (2014). Ch 45 *Nurse Anesthesia* (5ᵗʰ ed.). St. Louis, MO: Elsevier.

11. Which laboratory test provides the most comprehensive assessment of coagulation in a patient with severe cirrhosis?

    (A) International normalized ratio

    (B) Prothrombin time

    (C) Partial thromboplastin time

    (D) Thromboelastography

Rationale: Thromboelastography allows assessment of the initial clotting process through fibrinolysis which is more comprehensive than an isolated measure of clotting time.

Ref: Butterworth, J.F., Mackey, D.C., & Wasnick, J.D. (2013). Ch 33 *Morgan & Mikhail's Clinical Anesthesiology* (5ᵗʰ ed.). New York, NY: McGraw-Hill.

Miller, R.D. Eriksson, L.I., Fleisher, L.A., Wiener-Kronish, J.P., & Young, W.L. (Eds.). (2010). Ch 56 *Miller's Anesthesia* (7ᵗʰ ed.). Philadelphia, PA: Elsevier.

12. Where does the spinal cord end in adults?

    (A) L1

    (B) L2

    (C) L3

    (D) L4

    Rationale: In adults the spinal cord ends at L1 and in some adults to L2. In children the cord ends at L3.

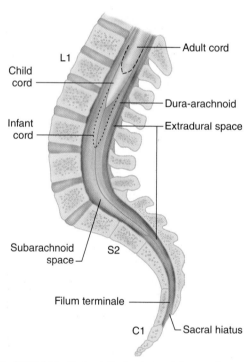

FIG. 3-1. Sagittal view through the lumbar vertebrae and sacrum. Note the end of the spinal cord rises with development from approximately L3 to L1. The dural sac normally ends at S2.

Ref: Butterworth, J.F., Mackey, D.C., & Wasnick, J.D. (2013). Ch 45 *Morgan & Mikhail's Clinical Anesthesiology* (5ᵗʰ ed.). New York, NY: McGraw-Hill.

Nagelhout, J.J., & Plaus, K.L. (2014). Ch 44 *Nurse Anesthesia* (5ᵗʰ ed.). St. Louis, MO: Elsevier.

13. What volume of blood loss will decrease the hematocrit from 36-30% in a 7 year-old, 25 kg child?

(A) 250 mL

(B) 300 mL

(C) 350 mL

(D) 400 mL

Rationale: The amount of blood loss that causes the hematocrit to decrease from 36-30% in this patient can be calculated as follows:

Estimated blood volume in an older child is ~70 mL/kg. 70 mL/kg × 25 kg = 1750 mL EBV. The Maximal blood loss formula is: $ABL = \dfrac{EBV\,(Hs - Hf)}{Hs}$ where ABL = allowable blood loss, EBV = estimated total blood volume, Hs = starting hematocrit, Hf = final hematocrit. The solution is ~292 mL, option B is the closest answer.

Ref: Butterworth, J.F., Mackey, D.C., & Wasnick, J.D. (2013). Ch 82 *Morgan & Mikhail's Clinical Anesthesiology* (5th ed.). New York, NY: McGraw-Hill.

Barash, P.G., Cullen, B.F., Stoelting, R.K., Calahan, M.K., & Stock, M.C. (2009). Ch 45 *Clinical Anesthesia* (6th ed.). Philadelphia, PA: Lippincott Williams & Wilkins.

14. Which cranial nerve (CN) provides sensation to the posterior one-third of the tongue?

(A) CN I

(B) CN V

(C) CN IX

(D) CN X

Rationale: CN I (olfactory) provides innervation to the nasal mucosa; the superior and inferior surfaces of the hard and soft palate are innervated by fibers of CN V (trigeminal). CN IX (glossopharyngeal) innervates the posterior 1/3 of the tongue, whereas the lingual nerve provides sensation to the anterior 2/3 of the tongue. Areas of sensation below the epiglottis are innervated by CN X (vagus).

Ref: Butterworth, J.F., Mackey, D.C., & Wasnick, J.D. (2013). Ch 18 *Morgan & Mikhail's Clinical Anesthesiology* (5th ed.). New York, NY: McGraw-Hill.

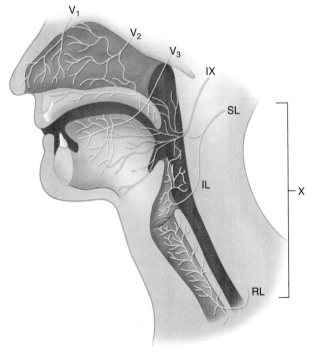

V₁ Ophthalmic division of trigeminal nerve (anterior ethmoidal nerve)

V₂ Maxillary division of trigeminal nerve (sphenopalatine nerves)

V₃ Mandibular division of trigeminal nerve (lingual nerve)

IX Glossopharyngeal nerve

X Vagus nerve
  SL Superior laryngeal nerve
  IL Internal laryngeal nerve
  RL Recurrent laryngeal nerve

FIG. 3-2. Sensory nerve supply of the airway.

15. Which patients are more likely to experience complications when using a hypotensive technique?

    Select (2) two

    (A) Uncontrolled glaucoma
    (B) History of transient ischemic attack
    (C) Multiple sclerosis
    (D) Osteoarthritis

    Rationale: Patients with cerebrovascular, cardiac, hepatic, uncontrolled glaucoma, and renal disease are not the best candidates for hypotensive anesthesia. Hypotensive anesthesia is relatively contraindicated. Complications including blindness, cardiac (myocardial infarction), stroke, and renal dysfunction (acute tubular necrosis) are possible outcomes.
    Ref: Butterworth, J.F., Mackey, D.C., & Wasnick, J.D. (2013). Ch 33 *Morgan & Mikhail's Clinical Anesthesiology* (5th ed.). New York, NY: McGraw-Hill.

16. What is the smallest volume of infused ABO-incompatible donor blood that will cause an acute hemolytic reaction?

    (A) 40-60 mL
    (B) 25-30 mL
    (C) 10-15 mL
    (D) 1-3 mL

    Rationale: Acute hemolytic reactions may occur after infusion with as little as 10-15 mL of ABO-incompatible blood and may result in death for 20-60% of patients.
    Ref: Butterworth, J.F., Mackey, D.C., & Wasnick, J.D. (2013). Ch 51 *Morgan & Mikhail's Clinical Anesthesiology* (5th ed.). New York, NY: McGraw-Hill.
    Nagelhout, J.J., & Plaus, K.L. (2014). Ch 20 *Nurse Anesthesia* (5th ed.). St. Louis, MO: Elsevier.

17. Which risk factors predispose patients to lower extremity neuropathy?

    Select (3) three

    (A) Hypertension
    (B) Obesity
    (C) Thin body habitus
    (D) Cigarette smoking
    (E) Diabetes

    Rationale: Surgeries longer than 2 hours, positioning that involves the peroneal nerve, hypotension, elderly and vascular diseases are risk factors predisposing patients to lower extremity neuropathy.

Ref: Butterworth, J.F., Mackey, D.C., & Wasnick, J.D. (2013). Ch 54 *Morgan & Mikhail's Clinical Anesthesiology* (5th ed.). New York, NY: McGraw-Hill.

18. What is the mechanism of action of a transcutaneous electrical nerve stimulation (TENS) unit?

    (A) TENS stimulation of large diameter afferent nerve fibers competitively blocks pain signals from smaller fibers.
    (B) TENS stimulation of small diameter afferent nerve fibers competitively blocks pain signals from larger fibers.
    (C) TENS stimulation damages the small afferent fibers conducting the pain signals.
    (D) TENS stimulation induces a signal conduction interruption in large diameter fibers.

    Rationale: TENS is an application of gate theory; stimulation and activation of large fibers introduces a competing stimulus to counteract pain signals carried along smaller afferent fibers.
    Ref: Butterworth, J.F., Mackey, D.C., & Wasnick, J.D. (2013). Ch 47 *Morgan & Mikhail's Clinical Anesthesiology* (5th ed.). New York, NY: McGraw-Hill.

19. What are the primary adductors of the vocal cords?

    (A) Lateral cricoarytenoid muscles
    (B) Recurrent laryngeal nerve
    (C) Posterior cricoarytenoid muscles
    (D) External laryngeal nerve

    Rationale: The primary *abductors* of the vocal cords are the posterior cricoarytenoid muscles. The recurrent laryngeal nerve innervates the muscles of the larynx. The external laryngeal nerve innervates the cricothyroid muscle.
    Ref: Butterworth, J.F., Mackey, D.C., & Wasnick, J.D. (2013). Ch 18 *Morgan & Mikhail's Clinical Anesthesiology* (5th ed.). New York, NY: McGraw-Hill.

20. Which group lists the Vitamin K-dependent clotting factors?

    (A) II, VII, IX, X
    (B) II, IV, IX, XII
    (C) III, VII, X, XI
    (D) I, VII, IX, XI

    Rationale: Vitamin K-dependent factors include factors II, VII, IX, and X. They require vitamin K for completion of their synthesis in the liver. In the absence of vitamin K, these 4 clotting factors are produced in normal amounts but are nonfunctional.

Ref: Butterworth, J.F., Mackey, D.C., & Wasnick, J.D. (2013). Ch 32 *Morgan & Mikhail's Clinical Anesthesiology* (5th ed.). New York, NY: McGraw-Hill.

Barash, P.G., Cullen, B.F., Stoelting, R.K., Calahan, M.K., & Stock, M.C. (2009). Ch 16 *Clinical Anesthesia* (6th ed.). Philadelphia, PA: Lippincott Williams & Wilkins.

21. Which of the following chemical mediators is released from peripheral afferent C fibers resulting in dull pain?

    (A) Substance P
    (B) Glutamate
    (C) Histamine
    (D) Serotonin

    Rationale: Glutamate results in fast sharp pain via Aδ and C nerve fibers. Edema and vasodilatation result from the release of histamine via substance P. Platelets release serotonin following tissue injury reacting with multiple receptors.

    Ref: Butterworth, J.F., Mackey, D.C., & Wasnick, J.D. (2013). Ch 47 *Morgan & Mikhail's Clinical Anesthesiology* (5th ed.). New York, NY: McGraw-Hill.

    Nagelhout, J.J., & Plaus, K.L. (2014). Ch 51 *Nurse Anesthesia* (5th ed.). St. Louis, MO: Elsevier.

22. To supplement a brachial plexus block to cover the anterior shoulder, the cervical plexus can be blocked at which of the following locations?

    (A) Anterior to the mastoid process
    (B) Posterior border of the sternocleidomastoid
    (C) At the interscalene groove
    (D) Posterior to the angle of the mandible

    Rationale: Areas of the anterior shoulder are supplied by the superficial cervical plexus, which passes through the platysma at the posterior sternocleidomastoid (SCM) giving off superficial and deep branches. The superficial cervical plexus innervates the skin and the superficial structures of the head, neck, and shoulders. It lies in the plane just behind the SCM and can be blocked with a field block at that location.

    Ref: Butterworth, J.F., Mackey, D.C., & Wasnick, J.D. (2013). Ch 46 *Morgan & Mikhail's Clinical Anesthesiology* (5th ed.). New York, NY: McGraw-Hill.

    Hadzic, A. (2007). Ch 23 *Textbook of Regional Anesthesia and Acute Pain Management*. New York, NY: McGraw-Hill.

23. Following general endotracheal anesthesia, the patient is in respiratory distress and is unable to speak. What nerve(s) may be injured?

    (A) Unilateral recurrent laryngeal nerve
    (B) Bilateral superior laryngeal nerve
    (C) Unilateral superior laryngeal nerve
    (D) Bilateral vagus nerves

    Rationale: Injury to the superior laryngeal nerve may result in vocal fatigue and hoarseness. Unilateral vagal and recurrent laryngeal nerve damage also results in hoarseness. Bilateral vagus nerve injury results in aphonia.

TABLE 3-2. The effects of laryngeal nerve injury on the voice.

Nerve	Effect of Nerve Injury
Superior laryngeal nerve	
Unilateral	Minimal effects
Bilateral	Hoarseness, tiring of voice
Recurrent laryngeal nerve	
Unilateral	Hoarseness
Bilateral	
Acute	Stridor, respiratory distress
Chronic	Aphonia
Vagus nerve	
Unilateral	Hoarseness
Bilateral	Aphonia

Ref: Butterworth, J.F., Mackey, D.C., & Wasnick, J.D. (2013). Ch 18 *Morgan & Mikhail's Clinical Anesthesiology* (5th ed.). New York, NY: McGraw-Hill.

24. A patient's serum potassium level is 7.2 mEq/L. In which sequential order will cardiac manifestations of hyperkalemia progress?

    (A) Peaked T waves, loss of P wave, widened QRS complex, sine wave
    (B) Peaked T waves, widened QRS complex, loss of P wave, sine wave
    (C) Loss of R-wave amplitude, peaked T waves, widened QRS complex, sine wave
    (D) Prolonged P–R interval, peaked T waves, widened QRS complex, asystole

    Rationale: ECG changes associated with severe hyperkalemia characteristically progress sequentially in the following order: First, peaked T waves, next a widening of the QRS complex, followed by a progression of the P-R interval, then a loss of P wave, then a loss of R wave amplitude, ST-segment depression (sometimes elevation), and, finally, a sine wave that will ultimately change into ventricular fibrillation and asystole.

Ref: Butterworth, J.F., Mackey, D.C., & Wasnick, J.D. (2013). Ch 49 *Morgan & Mikhail's Clinical Anesthesiology* (5th ed.). New York, NY: McGraw-Hill.

Barash, P.G., Cullen, B.F., Stoelting, R.K., Calahan, M.K., & Stock, M.C. (2009). Ch 14 *Clinical Anesthesia* (6th ed.). Philadelphia, PA: Lippincott Williams & Wilkins.

25. Which of the following is not a physiologic response to pain?

    (A) Increased peripheral vascular resistance
    (B) Decreased tidal volume
    (C) Increased platelet aggregation
    (D) Decreased urinary sphincter tone

    Rationale: Pain results in increased urinary sphincter tone.
    Ref: Nagelhout, J.J., & Plaus, K.L. (2014). Ch 51 *Nurse Anesthesia* (5th ed.). St. Louis, MO: Elsevier.

26. What is the treatment of choice for hyponatremic patients with decreased total body sodium content?

    (A) 0.9% NS
    (B) D5. ½NS
    (C) 0.5 NS
    (D) 3% NS

    Rationale: Isotonic saline is the treatment of choice for hyponatremic patients with decreased total body sodium content. This is sometimes called hypovolemic hypotonic hyponatremia. B is hypertonic; C is hypotonic; and D is hypertonic.
    Ref: Butterworth, J.F., Mackey, D.C., & Wasnick, J.D. (2013). Ch 49 *Morgan & Mikhail's Clinical Anesthesiology* (5th ed.). New York, NY: McGraw-Hill.

    Nagelhout, J.J., & Plaus, K.L. (2014). Ch 20 *Nurse Anesthesia* (5th ed.). St. Louis, MO: Elsevier.

27. What statement is false regarding nasal airways?

    (A) Nasal airways are 2-4 cm shorter than oral airways.
    (B) Thrombocytopenia is a contraindication.
    (C) Nasal airways are 2-4 cm longer than oral airways.
    (D) Basilar skull fracture is a contraindication.

    Rationale: Any condition leading to nasal bleeding is a relative contraindication to the use of nasal airways. Use of a nasal airway in conditions of the skull including basilar fractures may result in malposition of the airway. Nasal airways are longer than oral airways.

Ref: Butterworth, J.F., Mackey, D.C., & Wasnick, J.D. (2013). Ch 18 *Morgan & Mikhail's Clinical Anesthesiology* (5th ed.). New York, NY: McGraw-Hill.

28. A patient-controlled analgesia order is written. What is the lockout interval for morphine?

    (A) 8-20 minutes
    (B) 5-10 minutes
    (C) 10-15 minutes
    (D) 15-18 minutes

    Rationale: The lockout interval for morphine and hydromorphone is 5-10 minutes; 8-20 minutes for methadone; and 4-10 minutes for fentanyl.
    Ref: Nagelhout, J.J., & Plaus, K.L. (2014). Ch 51 *Nurse Anesthesia* (5th ed.). St. Louis, MO: Elsevier.

29. A patient taking duloxetine for chronic neuropathic pain is scheduled for a cholecystectomy. How is duloxetine classified?

    (A) Tricyclic antidepressant
    (B) Selective serotonin reuptake inhibitor
    (C) Serotonin-norepinephrine reuptake inhibitor
    (D) Nonselective serotonin reuptake inhibitor

    Rationale: Selective-norepinephrine reuptake inhibitors commonly used for chronic neuropathic pain include venlafaxine, duloxetine, and milnacipran.
    Ref: Nagelhout, J.J., & Plaus, K.L. (2014). Ch 51 *Nurse Anesthesia* (5th ed.). St. Louis, MO: Elsevier.

30. What is the rationale for rapidly freezing plasma for the purpose of making fresh frozen plasma?

    (A) Rapid freezing prevents inactivation of factors VIII and I.
    (B) Rapid freezing prevents inactivation of factors V and VIII.
    (C) Rapid freezing prevents the inactivation of all the factors.
    (D) Rapid freezing prevents the inactivation of antithrombin III.

    Rationale: Plasma is rapidly frozen to help prevent inactivation of the labile coagulation factors, factors V and VIII.
    Ref: Butterworth, J.F., Mackey, D.C., & Wasnick, J.D. (2013). Ch 51 *Morgan & Mikhail's Clinical Anesthesiology* (5th ed.). New York, NY: McGraw-Hill.

    Barash, P.G., Cullen, B.F., Stoelting, R.K., Calahan, M.K., & Stock, M.C. (2009). Ch 16 *Clinical Anesthesia* (6th ed.). Philadelphia, PA: Lippincott Williams & Wilkins.

31. Which of the following is not a risk factor for developing cauda equine syndrome?

    (A) Lidocaine spinal anesthesia

    (B) Use of glucose to increase baricity of neuraxial anesthetics

    (C) Epidural anesthesia

    (D) Continuous spinal anesthesia (CSA)

    Rationale: Injuries have occurred with CSA most likely because of increased anesthetic doses administered to compensate for an inadequate block. Toxicity can occur with accidental intrathecal injection through what was intended to be an epidural injection. Most cases of cauda equine syndrome due to local anesthetic neurotoxicity have occurred with the use of lidocaine. Recent cases of cauda equine syndrome have been associated with markedly hyperbaric solutions. Despite this, there is no evidence to suggest that hyperbaric solutions are responsible.

    Ref: Butterworth, J.F., Mackey, D.C., & Wasnick, J.D. (2013). Ch 45 *Morgan & Mikhail's Clinical Anesthesiology* (5th ed.). New York, NY: McGraw-Hill.

    Hadzic, A. (2007). Ch 13 *Textbook of Regional Anesthesia and Acute Pain Management.* New York, NY: McGraw-Hill.

32. How soon must fresh frozen plasma be transfused once thawed?

    (A) Within 4 hours

    (B) Within 8 hours

    (C) Within 12 hours

    (D) Within 24 hours

    Rationale: Once fresh frozen plasma has been thawed, it must be given within 24 hours to avoid wastage.

    Ref: Butterworth, J.F., Mackey, D.C., & Wasnick, J.D. (2013). Ch 51 *Morgan & Mikhail's Clinical Anesthesiology* (5th ed.). New York, NY: McGraw-Hill.

    Barash, P.G., Cullen, B.F., Stoelting, R.K., Calahan, M.K., & Stock, M.C. (2009). Ch 16 *Clinical Anesthesia* (6th ed.). Philadelphia, PA: Lippincott Williams & Wilkins.

33. Preoxygenation results in how many minutes of oxygen reserve?

    (A) 1-3 minutes

    (B) 3-6 minutes

    (C) 5-8 minutes

    (D) >8 minutes

    Rationale: Preoxygenation affords approximately 5-8 minutes of oxygen reserve.

    Ref: Butterworth, J.F., Mackey, D.C., & Wasnick, J.D. (2013). Ch 19 *Morgan & Mikhail's Clinical Anesthesiology* (5th ed.). New York, NY: McGraw-Hill.

34. Which patient should receive a type and cross match instead of a type and screen prior to surgery?

    Select (3) three

    (A) A 48-year-old female scheduled for an endovascular stent of an aortic aneurysm

    (B) An obese 12-year-old male undergoing an emergency tonsillectomy

    (C) A 22-year-old male with a history of multiple blood transfusions

    (D) A pregnant Rh-positive patient with Rh-negative baby undergoing emergency surgery

    (E) An 80-year-old female scheduled a hip replacement with a positive type and screen

    Rationale: Type and cross matches are often performed before the need to transfuse but only when the patient's antibody screen is positive or high risk for a positive screen (C), when the probability of transfusion is high (A and E), or when the patient is considered at risk for alloimmunization.

    Ref: Butterworth, J.F., Mackey, D.C., & Wasnick, J.D. (2013). Ch 51 *Morgan & Mikhail's Clinical Anesthesiology* (5th ed.). New York, NY: McGraw-Hill.

    Barash, P.G., Cullen, B.F., Stoelting, R.K., Calahan, M.K., & Stock, M.C. (2009). Ch 16 *Clinical Anesthesia* (6th ed.). Philadelphia, PA: Lippincott Williams & Wilkins.

35. A 150-kg male patient has a serum sodium concentration of 110 mEq/L. How much sodium would be needed to bring the serum sodium to 125 mEq/L?

    (A) 750 mEq

    (B) 1,350 mEq

    (C) 2,400 mEq

    (D) 3,200 mEq

    Rationale: Using the sodium deficit formula, the answer will be 1,350 mEq. The sodium deficit equation is the following: Sodium deficit (mEq) = ([Na] goal − [Na] plasma) × TBW; TBW = body weight (in kg) × 60%.

    Ref: Butterworth, J.F., Mackey, D.C., & Wasnick, J.D. (2013). Ch 49 *Morgan & Mikhail's Clinical Anesthesiology* (5th ed.). New York, NY: McGraw-Hill.

    Nagelhout, J.J., & Plaus, K.L. (2014). Ch 20 *Nurse Anesthesia* (5th ed.). St. Louis, MO: Elsevier.

36. How much blood does a fully soaked laparotomy "lap" pad contain?

(A) 10-20 mL

(B) 25-50 mL

(C) 50-100 mL

(D) 100-150 mL

Rationale: A fully soaked lap pad holds 100-150 ml of blood whereas a fully soaked 4×4 sponge holds approximately 10 mL.

Ref: Butterworth, J.F., Mackey, D.C., & Wasnick, J.D. (2013). Ch 51 *Morgan & Mikhail's Clinical Anesthesiology* (5th ed.). New York, NY: McGraw-Hill.

37. Six hours after a patient received transfusion with 2 units of fresh frozen plasma and 1 unit of platelets, she presents with hypoxia, fever, and noncardiogenic pulmonary edema. What complication do you suspect?

(A) Post-transfusion purpura

(B) Transfusion-related acute lung injury

(C) Delayed hemolytic reaction

(D) Transfusion-related immunomodulation

Rationale: Transfusion-related acute lung injury (TRALI) presents as hypoxia, often acute; fever and noncardiogenic pulmonary edema within 6 hours of a blood product transfusion, especially fresh frozen plasma or platelets. A would occur from development of platelet alloantibodies and noted in the precipitous platelet count drop 5-10 days after transfusion. Because TRALI is a type of nonhemolytic reaction, C is incorrect. D would manifest as diminished immunoresposiveness and inflammation promotion.

Ref: Butterworth, J.F., Mackey, D.C., & Wasnick, J.D. (2013). Ch 51 *Morgan & Mikhail's Clinical Anesthesiology* (5th ed.). New York, NY: McGraw-Hill.

Barash, P.G., Cullen, B.F., Stoelting, R.K., Calahan, M.K., & Stock, M.C. (2009). Ch 16 *Clinical Anesthesia* (6th ed.). Philadelphia, PA: Lippincott Williams & Wilkins.

38. A 44-year-old 50-kg male received 750 mL of fresh frozen plasma. What percent of normal would you expect his clotting factor concentration to achieve post transfusion?

(A) 100%

(B) 75%

(C) 60%

(D) 30%

Rationale: The initial therapeutic dose of fresh frozen plasma (FFP) is usually 10-15 mL/kg. The final goal of FFP administration is to achieve 30% of the normal coagulation factor concentration.

Ref: Butterworth, J.F., Mackey, D.C., & Wasnick, J.D. (2013). Ch 51 *Morgan & Mikhail's Clinical Anesthesiology* (5th ed.). New York, NY: McGraw-Hill.

Barash, P.G., Cullen, B.F., Stoelting, R.K., Calahan, M.K., & Stock, M.C. (2009). Ch 16 *Clinical Anesthesia* (6th ed.). Philadelphia, PA: Lippincott Williams & Wilkins.

39. For which infectious diseases is donor blood tested after it is collected, typed, and screened?

(A) Hepatitis A, Hepatitis B, and Hepatitis C

(B) Hepatitis B, Hepatitis C, and Hepatitis D

(C) Hepatitis C, Syphilis, and Human Immunodeficiency Virus

(D) Hepatitis C, Cytomegalovirus (CMV), and Syphilis

Rationale: Once donor blood is collected, it is typed, screened for antibodies, and tested for hepatitis B, hepatitis C, syphilis, and human immunodeficiency virus (HIV).

Ref: Butterworth, J.F., Mackey, D.C., & Wasnick, J.D. (2013). Ch 51 *Morgan & Mikhail's Clinical Anesthesiology* (5th ed.). New York, NY: McGraw-Hill.

Nagelhout, J.J., & Plaus, K.L. (2014). Ch 20 *Nurse Anesthesia* (5th ed.). St. Louis, MO: Elsevier.

40. Which is not an indication for cryoprecipitate administration?

(A) Fibrinogen levels <80-100 mg/dL

(B) Factor XIII deficiency

(C) Antithrombin deficiency

(D) Preoperative prophylaxis for patient with von Willebrand disease

Rationale: Cryoprecipitate contains factor VIII, von Willebrand factor (vWF), fibrinogen, fibronectin, and factor XIII. Although factor-specific concentrates can be administered for patients with hemophilia and von Willebrand disease, it remains an indication for cryoprecipitate administration. Cryoprecipitate is typically administered for documented or suspected fibrinogen levels < 80-100 mg/dL. Antithrombin deficiency is an indication for fresh frozen plasma administration.

Ref: Barash, P.G., Cullen, B.F., Stoelting, R.K., Calahan, M.K., & Stock, M.C. (2009). Ch 16 *Clinical Anesthesia* (6th ed.). Philadelphia, PA: Lippincott Williams & Wilkins.

Miller, R., Fleisher, L., Wiener-Krunish, J., Young, W., & Eriksson, L. Ch 55 *Miller's Anesthesia* (7th ed.). Philadelphia, PA: Elsevier.

41. Which factors are not complications associated with massive blood transfusion?

Select (2) two

(A) Serum K$^+$ 5.5

(B) Core temperature 35.5 °C

(C) Increased 2,3 DPG

(D) Decreased 2,3 DPG

(E) Ionized Ca$^+$ 1.25 mmol/L

Rationale: Decreased 2,3 DPG is a complication associated with massive transfusion, not increased 2,3 DPG. Hypocalcemia is also associated with massive transfusion. This ionized calcium value is normal. Hyperkalemia (A), hypothermia (B), and decreased 2,3 DPG (D) are all complications of massive blood transfusion.

Ref: Butterworth, J.F., Mackey, D.C., & Wasnick, J.D. (2013). Ch 51 & 49 *Morgan & Mikhail's Clinical Anesthesiology* (5th ed.). New York, NY: McGraw-Hill.

Nagelhout, J.J., & Plaus, K.L. (2014). Ch 20 *Nurse Anesthesia* (5th ed.). St. Louis, MO: Elsevier.

42. What is the approximate half-life of serum albumin?

(A) 12 hours

(B) 6 days

(C) 10 days

(D) 21 days

Rationale: The half-life of serum albumin is approximately 14-21 days, which is why it is not a reliable indicator of acute liver disease.

Ref: Butterworth, J.F., Mackey, D.C., & Wasnick, J.D. (2013). Ch 32 *Morgan & Mikhail's Clinical Anesthesiology* (5th ed.). New York, NY: McGraw-Hill.

Barash, P.G., Cullen, B.F., Stoelting, R.K., Calahan, M.K., & Stock, M.C. (2009). Ch 48 *Clinical Anesthesia* (6th ed.). Philadelphia, PA: Lippincott Williams & Wilkins

43. Which of the following nerves must be separately blocked during an axillary approach to the brachial plexus?

(A) Musculocutaneous

(B) Ulnar

(C) Medial brachial cutaneous

(D) Median

Rationale: During the axillary approach to the brachial plexus, the block is performed in the axilla, where large terminal branches have formed. At this point the musculocutaneous nerve (MCN) lies deep within the coracobrachialis, having already left the sheath. A separate block is therefore essential to complete forearm and wrist anesthesia. The MCN can be blocked by redirecting the needle, after completing the axillary block, superiorly and posterior to inject within the coracobrachialis.

Ref: Butterworth, J.F., Mackey, D.C., & Wasnick, J.D. (2013). Ch 46 *Morgan & Mikhail's Clinical Anesthesiology* (5th ed.). New York, NY: McGraw-Hill.

Hadzic, A. (2012). Ch 28 Hadzic's *Peripheral Nerve Blocks and Anatomy for Ultrasound-Guided Regional Anaesthesia* (2nd ed.). New York, NY: McGraw-Hill.

44. What is the most effective initial treatment of symptomatic hypercalcemia?

(A) Hydration with IV normal saline followed by furosemide

(B) Thiazide followed by IV normal saline hydration

(C) Hydration with IV normal saline followed by bisphosphonates

(D) Glucocorticoids followed by IV normal saline hydration

Rationale: The most effective initial treatment for symptomatic hypercalcemia is hydration with normal saline followed by a loop diuretic to accelerate calcium excretion. Additional therapy would include administering calcitonin or bisphosphonates. Glucocorticoids would be warranted treatment in the case of Vitamin D-induced hypercalcemia, but it would not be the most effective initial treatment.

Ref: Butterworth, J.F., Mackey, D.C., & Wasnick, J.D. (2013). Ch 49 *Morgan & Mikhail's Clinical Anesthesiology* (5th ed.). New York, NY: McGraw-Hill.

Nagelhout, J.J., & Plaus, K.L. (2014). Ch 20 *Nurse Anesthesia* (5th ed.). St. Louis, MO: Elsevier.

45. Caudal anesthesia involves needle penetration of the sacrococcygeal ligament covering the sacral hiatus created by which unfused laminae?

(A) S1 and S2

(B) S2 and S3

(C) S3 and S4

(D) S4 and S5

Rationale: Caudal anesthesia involves needle penetration of the sacrococcygeal ligament covering the sacral hiatus created by unfused S4 and S5 laminae.

Ref: Butterworth, J.F., Mackey, D.C., & Wasnick, J.D. (2013). Ch 45 *Morgan & Mikhail's Clinical Anesthesiology* (5th ed.). New York, NY: McGraw-Hill.

Hadzic, A. (2012). Ch 15 Hadzic's *Peripheral Nerve Blocks and Anatomy for Ultrasound-Guided Regional Anaesthesia* (2nd ed.). New York, NY: McGraw-Hill.

46. A 154-lb female has a serum sodium level 120 mEq/L. In order to correct the sodium level to 128 mEq, how many milliequivalents of sodium are required?

    (A) 280 mEq
    (B) 336 mEq
    (C) 616 mEq
    (D) 739 mEq

    Rationale: Here is the formula: Sodium deficit = TBW × (desired [Na$^+$] − present [Na$^+$])

    Step 1: Convert 154 lbs-70 kilograms by dividing by 2.2.

    Step 2: Determine that total body water (TBW) for a female is 50%.

    Step 3: Plug variables into formula: 70 × .50 × [128-120] = 280 mEq.

    B is derived if TBW was calculated using 60% of body weight for males.

    C is derived if TBW was calculated using 50% of body weight for females but without converting pounds to kg.

    D is derived if TBW was calculated using 60% of body weight for males and without converting pounds to kg.

    Ref: Butterworth, J.F., Mackey, D.C., & Wasnick, J.D. (2013). Ch 49 *Morgan & Mikhail's Clinical Anesthesiology* (5th ed.). New York, NY: Lange Medical Books McGraw-Hill.
    Nagelhout, J.J., & Plaus, K.L. (2014). Ch 20 *Nurse Anesthesia* (5th ed.). St. Louis, MO: Elsevier.

47. C fibers transmit what type of sensation?

    (A) Proprioception
    (B) Touch-pressure
    (C) Somatic pain
    (D) Visceral pain

    Rationale: C fibers transmit visceral pain. They are unmyelinated and slow transmitting. Sensation is aching, poorly localized and usually from a hallow viscus.
    Ref: Butterworth, J.F., Mackey, D.C., & Wasnick, J.D. (2013). Ch 47 *Morgan & Mikhail's Clinical Anesthesiology* (5th ed.). New York, NY: McGraw-Hill.
    Hadzic, A. (2007). Ch 53 *Textbook of Regional Anesthesia and Acute Pain Management*. New York, NY: McGraw-Hill.

48. Which nerve provides sensory innervation to the lateral thigh?

    (A) Lateral femoral cutaneous
    (B) Saphenous
    (C) Femoral
    (D) Posterior femoral cutaneous

    Rationale: The saphenous nerve provides innervation below the knee. The femoral nerve and its branches innervate the anterior thigh, hip, medial leg, and ankle. The posterior femoral cutaneous nerve innervates the posterior thigh.
    Ref: Butterworth, J.F., Mackey, D.C., & Wasnick, J.D. (2013). Ch 46 *Morgan & Mikhail's Clinical Anesthesiology* (5th ed.). New York, NY: McGraw-Hill.
    Nagelhout, J.J., & Plaus, K.L. (2014). Ch 45 *Nurse Anesthesia* (5th ed.). St. Louis, MO: Elsevier.

49. An axillary block is performed for a surgical procedure on the right forearm and hand. The patient begins to experience pain at the tip of the index finger during the procedure. An effective rescue block would involve injecting local into which of the following sites?

    (A) Antecubital space at the lateral aspect of the biceps tendon
    (B) Antecubital crease medial to the biceps insertion
    (C) One finger breadth proximal to the arcuate ligament
    (D) Immediately lateral to the flexor carpi ulnaris

    Rationale: Sensation for the distal 1st three fingers is provided by the median nerve. A median nerve rescue block can be performed either at the antecubital crease, medial to the biceps insertion or at the wrist medial and deep to the palmaris longus tendon.
    Ref: Butterworth, J.F., Mackey, D.C., & Wasnick, J.D. (2013). Ch 46 *Morgan & Mikhail's Clinical Anesthesiology* (5th ed.). New York, NY: McGraw-Hill.
    Hadzic, A. (2007). Ch 28 *Textbook of Regional Anesthesia and Acute Pain Management*. New York, NY: McGraw-Hill.

50. Which of the following are associated with slow pain?

    Select (3) three
    (A) Myelinated Aδ primary efferents
    (B) Action potential 0.5-2 m/seconds
    (C) Myelinated Aδ primary afferents
    (D) Dull pain
    (E) Burning pain

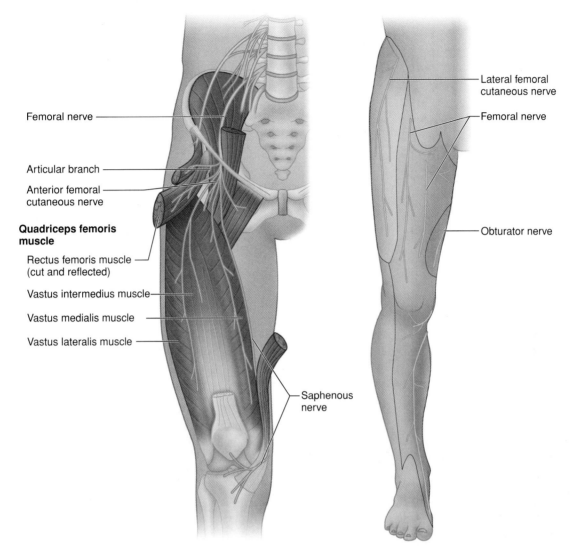

FIG. 3-3. The femoral nerve provides sensory innervation to the hip and thigh, and to the medial leg via its terminal branch, the saphenous nerve.

Rationale: Sharp fast pain is characterized by action potentials conducted between 6 and 30 m/sec via the myelinated Aδ primary afferent neurons. In contrast, dull, burning, throbbing, or aching pain characterizes slow pain with conduction velocities of 0.5-2 m/sec via C fibers.

Ref: Butterworth, J.F., Mackey, D.C., & Wasnick, J.D. (2013). Ch 47 *Morgan & Mikhail's Clinical Anesthesiology* (5th ed.). New York, NY: McGraw-Hill.

Nagelhout, J.J., & Plaus, K.L. (2014). Ch 51 *Nurse Anesthesia* (5th ed.). St. Louis, MO: Elsevier.

51. A patient has pain on the dorsum of the foot and the lateral aspect of the knee. What nerve root is involved?

(A) L3
(B) L5
(C) L4
(D) S1

Rationale: L5 provides sensation to the lateral aspect of the knee and leg as well as the dorsum of the foot.

Ref: Butterworth, J.F., Mackey, D.C., & Wasnick, J.D. (2013). Ch 19 *Morgan & Mikhail's Clinical Anesthesiology* (5th ed.). New York, NY: McGraw-Hill.

Hadzic, A. (2007). Ch 19 *Textbook of Regional Anesthesia and Acute Pain Management*. New York, NY: McGraw-Hill.

52. Which of the following patients is at greatest risk for postdural puncture headaches?

(A) Obese
(B) Elderly
(C) Pregnant
(D) Pediatric

Rationale: Postdural puncture headache is strongly related to young, female parturients.

Ref: Butterworth, J.F., Mackey, D.C., & Wasnick, J.D. (2013). Ch 41 *Morgan & Mikhail's Clinical Anesthesiology* (5th ed.). New York, NY: McGraw-Hill.
Hadzic, A. (2007). Ch 14 *Textbook of Regional Anesthesia and Acute Pain Management*. New York, NY: McGraw-Hill.

53. While performing an axillary block utilizing the transarterial approach, a paresthesia is elicited after passing through the artery. Which nerve is posterior to the artery?

(A) Ulnar
(B) Radial
(C) Median
(D) Intercostobrachial

Rationale: The radial nerve lies posterior to the axillary artery, and it is anesthetized when injecting posterior to the artery.

Ref: Butterworth, J.F., Mackey, D.C., & Wasnick, J.D. (2013). Ch 46 *Morgan & Mikhail's Clinical Anesthesiology* (5th ed.). New York, NY: McGraw-Hill.
Hadzic, A. (2007). Ch 28 *Textbook of Regional Anesthesia and Acute Pain Management*. New York, NY: McGraw-Hill.

54. A patient receives large volumes of 0.9% normal saline during a case. What is the risk associated with this?

(A) Hypochloremic alkalosis
(B) Hyperchloremic alkalosis
(C) Hypochloremic acidosis
(D) Hyperchloremic acidosis

Rationale: When large volumes of normal saline are given, a dilutional hyperchloremic metabolic acidosis with normal anion gap is produced due to the high sodium and chloride content. As serum chloride concentration increases, plasma bicarbonate concentration decreases.

Ref: Butterworth, J.F., Mackey, D.C., & Wasnick, J.D. (2013). Ch 51 *Morgan & Mikhail's Clinical Anesthesiology* (5th ed.). New York, NY: McGraw-Hill.
Barash, P.G., Cullen, B.F., Stoelting, R.K., Calahan, M.K., & Stock, M.C. (2009). Ch 14 *Clinical Anesthesia* (6th ed.). Philadelphia, PA: Lippincott Williams & Wilkins.

55. What causes hypocalcemia?

Select (3) three
(A) Hypoparathyroidism
(B) Paget's disease
(C) Fat embolism
(D) Rapid infusion of 1,000 mL albumin
(E) Biliary colic
(F) Chronic immobilization

Rationale: Low PTH levels, fat embolism, and rapid infusion of large volumes of blood preservative with citrate ions (including albumin) cause hypocalcemia.

Ref: Butterworth, J.F., Mackey, D.C., & Wasnick, J.D. (2013). Ch 49 *Morgan & Mikhail's Clinical Anesthesiology* (5th ed.). New York, NY: McGraw-Hill.
Barash, P.G., Cullen, B.F., Stoelting, R.K., Calahan, M.K., & Stock, M.C. (2009). Ch 14 *Clinical Anesthesia* (6th ed.). Philadelphia, PA: Lippincott Williams & Wilkins.

56. Which of the following local anesthetics should be avoided in a glucose-6-phosphate dehydrogenase (G_6PD) deficiency?

(A) Ropivacaine
(B) Etidocaine
(C) Prilocaine
(D) Tetracaine

Rationale: Both prilocaine and lidocaine have been associated with red cell hemolysis in patients with G_6PD deficiency. The enzyme G_6PD, catalyzes the initial step in the hexose monophosphate shunt which protects red blood cells against oxidative injury by producing NADPH. Hemolysis is triggered when older red blood cells that are deficient in the enzyme are destroyed when exposed to drugs such as prilocaine with high redox potential.

Ref: Butterworth, J.F., Mackey, D.C., & Wasnick, J.D. (2013). Ch 51 *Morgan & Mikhail's Clinical Anesthesiology* (5th ed.). New York, NY: McGraw-Hill.

57. You plan to use an intravenous regional technique for a hand surgery. What is your greatest concern?

   (A) Duration of the case
   (B) Using the dual tourniquet system
   (C) Tourniquet discomfort
   (D) Tourniquet failure

   Rationale: A large volume of local anesthetic from the periphery to the central circulation represents the most serious concern associated with intravenous regional anesthesia. The other variables pose challenges, but are readily remedied.
   Ref: Butterworth, J.F., Mackey, D.C., & Wasnick, J.D. (2013). Ch 46 *Morgan & Mikhail's Clinical Anesthesiology* (5th ed.). New York, NY: McGraw-Hill.
   Miller, R.D., & Pardo, M.C. (2011). Ch 18 *Basics of Anesthesia* (6th ed.). Philadelphia, PA: Elsevier.
   Nagelhout, J.J., & Plaus, K.L. (2014). Ch 45 *Nurse Anesthesia* (5th ed.). St. Louis, MO: Elsevier.

58. Removal of epidural catheters should be delayed for a minimum of how many hours following the administration of prophylactic low molecular weight heparin (LMWH)?

   (A) 1 hour
   (B) 10 hours
   (C) 3 hours
   (D) 6 hours

   Rationale: Because of the risk of spinal hematomas, epidural catheters should be removed 2 hours prior to the first dose of LMWH. If already present, epidural catheters should be removed greater than 10 hours after the last dose of LMWH.
   Ref: Butterworth, J.F., Mackey, D.C., & Wasnick, J.D. (2013). Ch 45 *Morgan & Mikhail's Clinical Anesthesiology* (5th ed.). New York, NY: McGraw-Hill.
   Hadzic, A. (2007). Ch 70 *Textbook of Regional Anesthesia and Acute Pain Management*. New York, NY: McGraw-Hill.

59. When performing an ankle block, which of the following nerves is located by identifying the groove formed proximally by the extensor hallucis longus tendon and the extensor digitorum longus tendon?

   (A) Saphenous
   (B) Deep peroneal
   (C) Posterior tibial
   (D) Sural

   Rationale: The deep peroneal nerve passes lateral to the anterior tibial artery, extensor hallucis longus, and tibialis anterior tendons and medial to the extensor digitorum longus tendon. It is easily accessible as it becomes more superficial to travel with the dorsalis pedis artery. It is located by identifying the groove formed proximally by the extensor hallicus longus tendon and the extensor digitorum longus tendon. This groove can be identified by having the patient extend the great toe, making the extensor hallucis longus tendon more prominent.
   Ref: Butterworth, J.F., Mackey, D.C., & Wasnick, J.D. (2013). Ch 46 *Morgan & Mikhail's Clinical Anesthesiology* (5th ed.). New York, NY: McGraw-Hill.
   Hadzic, A. (2007). Ch 39 *Textbook of Regional Anesthesia and Acute Pain Management*. New York, NY: McGraw-Hill.

60. Which of the following terms is defined as perception of an ordinary non-noxious stimulus as pain?

   (A) Hyperalgesia
   (B) Allodynia
   (C) Hyperesthesia
   (D) Dysesthesia

   Rationale: Allodynia is a perception of an ordinary non-noxious stimulus as pain.
   Ref: Butterworth, J.F., Mackey, D.C., & Wasnick, J.D. (2013). Ch 47 *Morgan & Mikhail's Clinical Anesthesiology* (5th ed.). New York, NY: Lange Medical Books McGraw-Hill.
   Hadzic, A. (2007). Ch 76 *Textbook of Regional Anesthesia and Acute Pain Management*. New York, NY: McGraw-Hill.

61. What is your main anesthetic concern when caring for a patient taking anabolic steroids?

   (A) Myocardial infarction
   (B) Hepatotoxicity
   (C) Hypercoagulopathy
   (D) Stroke

   Rationale: Each of the responses may be linked to the use of anabolic steroids. Hepatotoxicity poses direct implications for the anesthetic plan specifically regarding medications metabolized by the liver.
   Ref: Nagelhout, J.J., & Plaus, K.L. (2014). Ch 19 *Nurse Anesthesia* (5th ed.). St. Louis, MO: Elsevier.

62. Injecting local anesthetic at which site is associated with the greatest risk of systemic absorption?

    (A) Brachial plexus
    (B) Paracervical
    (C) Intercostal
    (D) Caudal

    Rationale: Intercostal nerve blocks result in the highest blood levels of any block in the body. In general, more vascular locations result in greater risk of systemic absorption. The risk declines as follows: Intercostal > caudal > paracervical > epidural > brachial plexus > sciatic > subcutaneous.

    Ref: Butterworth, J.F., Mackey, D.C., & Wasnick, J.D. (2013). Ch 16 *Morgan & Mikhail's Clinical Anesthesiology* (5th ed.). New York, NY: McGraw-Hill.
    Hadzic, A. (2007). Ch 44 *Textbook of Regional Anesthesia and Acute Pain Management*. New York, NY: McGraw-Hill.

63. Which topical local anesthetics may cause methemoglobinemia?

    Select (2) two
    (A) Bupivacaine
    (B) Prilocaine
    (C) Mepivacaine
    (D) Benzocaine
    (E) Procaine

    Rationale: Clinically significant methemoglobinemia may result when using topical prilocaine and benzocaine. Bupivacaine, mepivacaine, and procaine are not topical anesthetics.

    Ref: Butterworth, J.F., Mackey, D.C., & Wasnick, J.D. (2013). Ch 16 *Morgan & Mikhail's Clinical Anesthesiology* (5th ed.). New York, NY: McGraw-Hill.
    Nagelhout, J.J., & Plaus, K.L. (2014). Ch 10 *Nurse Anesthesia* (5th ed.). St. Louis, MO: Elsevier.

64. Which of the following factors has the greatest effect on the level of spinal anesthesia?

    (A) Age
    (B) Patient height
    (C) Position of patient during injection
    (D) Drug volume

    Rationale: The most important factors affecting the level of spinal anesthesia are solution baricity, drug dose, injection site, and patient position both during and directly after injection. In general, higher levels are obtained with higher doses, higher sites of injection, and hypobaric solutions (when in head up position).

    Ref: Butterworth, J.F., Mackey, D.C., & Wasnick, J.D. (2013). Ch 45 *Morgan & Mikhail's Clinical Anesthesiology* (5th ed.). New York, NY: McGraw-Hill.
    Hadzic, A. (2007). Ch 13 *Textbook of Regional Anesthesia and Acute Pain Management*. New York, NY: McGraw-Hill.

65. How much blood could a 90-kg adult female patient lose and still maintain a hematocrit of 30%, provided the preoperative hematocrit was 42%?

    (A) 702 mL
    (B) 2,106 mL
    (C) 2,457 mL
    (D) 5,850 mL

    Rationale: Calculation
    Correct answer: B.

    Step 1: Calculate EBV for a female: 90 kg × 65 mL/kg = 5850 mL (D is incorrect).

    Step 2: Calculate $RBCV_{42}$: 5850 × 42% = 2,457 mL (C is incorrect).

    Step 3: Calculate $RBCS_{30}$: 5850 × 30% = 1,755 mL.

    Step 4: Calculate red cell loss at 30%: 2,457-1,755 = 702 mL (A is incorrect).

    Step 5: Calculate ABL: 702 mL × 2 = 2,106 mL (B is correct).

    Ref: Butterworth, J.F., Mackey, D.C., & Wasnick, J.D. (2013). Ch 51 *Morgan & Mikhail's Clinical Anesthesiology* (5th ed.). New York, NY: McGraw-Hill.

66. Interruption of pain impulses can be accomplished through the administration of intrathecal opioids. These opioids act by binding to which of the following sites?

    (A) Periaqueductal gray
    (B) Dorsal root ganglia
    (C) Anterior horn
    (D) Dorsal horn

    Rationale: Small quantities of opioids injected within the intrathecal or epidural space produce analgesia segmentally, confined to the sensory nerves entering the dorsal horn of the spinal cord in the vicinity of the area of injection. Presynaptic opioid receptors inhibit primary afferent release of substance P and other neurotransmitters. Postsynaptic opoid receptors decrease spinothalamic tract activity in the dorsal horn.

Ref: Butterworth, J.F., Mackey, D.C., & Wasnick, J.D. (2013). Ch 47 *Morgan & Mikhail's Clinical Anesthesiology* (5th ed.). New York, NY: McGraw-Hill.

Hadzic, A. (2007). Ch 68 *Textbook of Regional Anesthesia and Acute Pain Management*. New York, NY: McGraw-Hill.

67. Epidural morphine was administered for postoperative pain control. What is the duration of action?

    (A) 12-24 hours

    (B) 4-6 hours

    (C) 24-48 hours

    (D) 2-6 hours

    Rationale: The duration of action for sufentanil 4-6 hours; and fentanyl 2-6 hours.

    Ref: Butterworth, J.F., Mackey, D.C., & Wasnick, J.D. (2013). Ch 45 *Morgan & Mikhail's Clinical Anesthesiology* (5th ed.). New York, NY: McGraw-Hill.

    Nagelhout, J.J., & Plaus, K.L. (2014). Ch 44 *Nurse Anesthesia* (5th ed.). St. Louis, MO: Elsevier.

68. A 20-kg child is scheduled for a urology procedure. What is the appropriate dose for a caudal anesthetic?

    (A) 10 mL

    (B) 5 mL

    (C) 3 mL

    (D) 25 mL

    Rationale: The local anesthetic dose for a caudal block is 0.5-1 mL/kg in children.

    Ref: Butterworth, J.F., Mackey, D.C., & Wasnick, J.D. (2013). Ch 45 *Morgan & Mikhail's Clinical Anesthesiology* (5th ed.). New York, NY: McGraw-Hill.

    Nagelhout, J.J., & Plaus, K.L. (2014). Ch 44 *Nurse Anesthesia* (5th ed.). St. Louis, MO: Elsevier.

69. Which of the following peripheral nerve block(s) would provide the most effective analgesia for a total knee arthroplasty?

    (A) Femoral nerve block

    (B) Femoral nerve block and obturator nerve block

    (C) Sciatic nerve block and psoas block

    (D) Sciatic and popliteal block

    Rationale: Patients undergoing total knee arthroplasty experience significant postoperative pain. Surgical anesthesia for knee procedures utilizing a tourniquet can be provided through blockade of the femoral, lateral femoral cutaneous, obturator, and sciatic nerves.

In order to provide exclusively regional anesthesia for this procedure, of the listed options, only the sciatic nerve block and the psoas block, also known as the lumbar plexus block (which covers the lateral femoral cutaneous, femoral, and obturator nerves) covers the nerves involved.

Ref: Butterworth, J.F., Mackey, D.C., & Wasnick, J.D. (2013). Ch 46 *Morgan & Mikhail's Clinical Anesthesiology* (5th ed.). New York, NY: McGraw-Hill.

Hadzic, A. (2007). Ch 37 *Textbook of Regional Anesthesia and Acute Pain Management*. New York, NY: McGraw-Hill.

70. Which mechanisms of action are common among nonsteroidal anti-inflammatory drugs?

    Select (2) two

    (A) Inhibition of cyclooxygenase

    (B) Inhibition of prostaglandin synthesis

    (C) Inhibition of lipoxygenase

    (D) Inhibition of leukotriene synthesis

    Rationale: Nonsteroidal anti-inflammatory drugs inhibit cyclooxygenase and subsequent prostaglandin synthesis.

    Ref: Butterworth, J.F., Mackey, D.C., & Wasnick, J.D. (2013). Ch 10 *Morgan & Mikhail's Clinical Anesthesiology* (5th ed.). New York, NY: McGraw-Hill.

    Harvey, R., & Ferrier, D. (Eds.) (2011). Ch 17 *Lippincott's illustrated reviews: Biochemistry* (5th ed.). Philadelphia, PA: Lippincott Williams & Wilkins.

71. What factor is not associated with postoperative pulmonary complications?

    (A) ASA III

    (B) Cigarette smoking

    (C) Aortic aneurysm repair

    (D) Surgery lasting 3 hours

    Rationale: Factors that lead to postoperative pulmonary complications include each of the items except surgery lasting 3 hours. Surgery lasting 4 or more hours is linked to postoperative pulmonary complications.

    Ref: Butterworth, J.F., Mackey, D.C., & Wasnick, J.D. (2013). Ch 18 *Morgan & Mikhail's Clinical Anesthesiology* (5th ed.). New York, NY: McGraw-Hill.

72. Which muscle is likely to be unaffected by an axillary brachial plexus block?

    (A) Abductor pollicis brevis

    (B) Interosseous

(C) Brachialis

(D) Pronator teres

Rationale: The axillary block is one of the most common nerve blocks and potential for serious complication is low; however, the block is often incomplete. Blockade is at the level of terminal nerves after separation of the musculocutaneous nerve, which requires an additional injection for a complete block. The musculocutaneous nerve enters the coracobrachialis muscle, which it innervates, and goes on to supply the biceps brachii and the brachialis. Sensory innervation is provided to the skin on the radial side of the forearm to the radiocarpal joint.

Ref: Butterworth, J.F., Mackey, D.C., & Wasnick, J.D. (2013). Ch 46 *Morgan & Mikhail's Clinical Anesthesiology* (5th ed.). New York, NY: McGraw-Hill.

Hadzic, A. (2007). Ch 28 *Textbook of Regional Anesthesia and Acute Pain Management*. New York, NY: McGraw-Hill.

73. Which of the following does not define somatic nociceptive pain?

(A) Transduction

(B) Transmission

(C) Thermal

(D) Modulation

Rationale: Transduction, transmission, modulation, and perception are the processes involved with somatic nociceptive pain. Thermal, mechanical, or chemical stimuli result in an action potential via transduction.

Ref: Butterworth, J.F., Mackey, D.C., & Wasnick, J.D. (2013). Ch 47 *Morgan & Mikhail's Clinical Anesthesiology* (5th ed.). New York, NY: McGraw-Hill.

Nagelhout, J.J., & Plaus, K.L. (2014). Ch 51 *Nurse Anesthesia* (5th ed.). St. Louis, MO: Elsevier Saunders.

74. During an unremarkable spinal anesthetic a bilateral T2 level in a healthy parturient results in a cardiac arrest. Which of the following is most likely responsible?

(A) Decreased preload

(B) Effect of local anesthetic on the medulla

(C) Blockade of the carotid sinus

(D) Cardiogenic hypertensive chemoreflex

Rationale: Cardiac arrest occurs in approximately 0.07-0.15% of spinal anesthetics. Most of these episodes of cardiac arrests are due directly or indirectly to sympathetic blockade. Inhibiting sympathetic efferents decreases venous return with reduction in right atrial pressure by 36% with low spinals and 53% with high spinals. Volume depletion can increase this to 66% on average. Dramatic reduction in preload initiate three reflexes which can result in bradycardia or sinus arrest: (1) The pacemaker stretch reflex is a result of myocardial pacemaker cells firing in proportion to the degree of stretch. Decreased venous return results in decreased stretch and thus decreased firing. (2) Low pressure baroreceptors are stimulated in the right atrium and vena cava which causes bradycardia. (3) The Bezold–Jarisch reflex occurs when intracardiac mechanoreceptors in the left ventricle are stimulated producing bradycardia.

Ref: Butterworth, J.F., Mackey, D.C., & Wasnick, J.D. (2013). Ch 54 *Morgan & Mikhail's Clinical Anesthesiology* (5th ed.). New York, NY: McGraw-Hill.

Hadzic, A. (2007). Ch 13, 69 *Textbook of Regional Anesthesia and Acute Pain Management*. New York, NY: McGraw-Hill.

75. Which medications should be held on the day of surgery?

Select (2) two

(A) Oral hypoglycemic agents

(B) Tricyclic antidepressants

(C) Selective serotonin reuptake inhibitors

(D) Beta-adrenergic blockers

(E) Angiotensin-converting enzyme (ACE) inhibitors

Rationale: Stopping tricyclic antidepressants may lead to cholinergic symptoms, cardiac disturbances, and neurological symptoms. Stopping ACE inhibitors may result in atrial fibrillation and/or congestive heart failure. If beta-adrenergic blockers are held, cardiac disturbances, and withdrawal symptoms may occur.

Ref: Butterworth, J.F., Mackey, D.C., & Wasnick, J.D. (2013). Ch 18 *Morgan & Mikhail's Clinical Anesthesiology* (5th ed.). New York, NY: McGraw-Hill.

Miller, R.D., & Pardo, M.C. (2011). Ch 13 in *Basics of Anesthesia* (6th ed.). Philadelphia, PA: Elsevier.

Nagelhout, J.J., & Plaus, K.L. (2014). Ch 19 *Nurse Anesthesia* (5th ed.). St. Louis, MO: Elsevier.

76. What nerve injury results most often with the lithotomy position?

(A) Common peroneal

(B) Sciatic

(C) Obturator

(D) Saphenous

Rationale: Each of the nerves may be affected by the lithotomy position. The nerve most likely to be injured in the lithotomy position is the common peroneal.

Ref: Butterworth, J.F., Mackey, D.C., & Wasnick, J.D. (2013). Ch 54 *Morgan & Mikhail's Clinical Anesthesiology* (5th ed.). New York, NY: McGraw-Hill.

Miller, R.D., & Pardo, M.C. (2011). Ch 19 *Basics of Anesthesia* (6th ed.). Philadelphia, PA: Elsevier.

Nagelhout, J.J., & Plaus, K.L. (2014). Ch 20 *Nurse Anesthesia* (5th ed.). St. Louis, MO: Elsevier.

77. Which of the following explains the rapid onset of 2-chloroprocaine when used for epidural anesthesia?

(A) It is activated by ester hydrolysis.

(B) It is administered in high concentrations.

(C) It has high potency and lipid solubility.

(D) It has relatively low pKa.

Rationale: 2-chloroprocaine is a rapidly acting local anesthetic despite its slow onset in isolated nerves. Its high pKa of 9 and large charge would normally result in a slow onset of action. It, however, has a low toxicity and, therefore, can be administered in high concentrations of 3%. The resultant large number of molecules results in mass diffusion and therefore quick onset.

The onset of local anesthetic in isolated nerves (in vitro) is determined to a large extent by the concentration of lipid soluble (nonionized) agent administered to the nerve to be anesthetized. The relative concentration of nonionized to ionized form present in a particular agent is expressed by its pKa, the pH at which these amounts are equal. Agents which have a pKa closer to physiological pH exist in a nonionized state in larger concentrations, resulting in a faster onset. Reducing the pH of the agent by mixing it with an alkaline solution (sodium bicarbonate) increases the amount of nonionized free base available and thus increases speed of onset. Other characteristics such as ease of diffusion and concentration affect the clinical onset of action.

Ref: Butterworth, J.F., Mackey, D.C., & Wasnick, J.D. (2013). Ch 14 *Morgan & Mikhail's Clinical Anesthesiology* (5th ed.). New York, NY: McGraw-Hill.

Hadzic, A. (2007). Ch 15 *Textbook of Regional Anesthesia and Acute Pain Management.* New York, NY: McGraw-Hill.

78. A patient taking furosemide is scheduled for a total knee arthroscopy. What statement is true?

(A) Continue in patients with chronic renal failure.

(B) Discontinue.

(C) Continue in patients with diabetes.

(D) Discontinue in the elderly.

Rationale: Diuretics may be held without concern except for patients with chronic renal failure or congestive heart failure.

Ref: Butterworth, J.F., Mackey, D.C., & Wasnick, J.D. (2013). Ch 18 *Morgan & Mikhail's Clinical Anesthesiology* (5th ed.). New York, NY: McGraw-Hill.

Miller, R.D., & Pardo, MC. (2011). Ch 13 in *Basics of Anesthesia* (6th ed.). Philadelphia, PA: Elsevier.

Nagelhout, J.J., & Plaus, K.L. (2014). Ch 19 *Nurse Anesthesia* (5th ed.). St. Louis, MO: Elsevier.

79. What discontinuation issues may result for patients who take angiotensin converting enzyme (ACE) inhibitors?

(A) Potential clotting abnormalities

(B) Cholinergic symptoms

(C) Psychosis and agitation

(D) Atrial fibrillation

Rationale: Discontinuing preoperative medications may result in potential clotting abnormalities with nonsterioidal anti-inflammatories or antiplatelet drugs; cholinergic symptoms with tricyclic antidepressants; psychosis or agitation with selective serotonin reuptake inhibitors (SSRIs); and rebound hypertension and/or atrial fibrillation with ACE inhibitors.

Ref: Butterworth, J.F., Mackey, D.C., & Wasnick, J.D. (2013). Ch 18 & 27 *Morgan & Mikhail's Clinical Anesthesiology* (5th ed.). New York, NY: Lange Medical Books McGraw-Hill.

Miller, R.D., & Pardo, MC. (2011). Ch 13 in *Basics of Anesthesia* (6th ed.). Philadelphia, PA: Elsevier.

Nagelhout, J.J., & Plaus, K.L. (2014). Ch 19 *Nurse Anesthesia* (5th ed.). St. Louis, MO: Elsevier.

80. What is the fluid deficit for a 13-kg patient fasting for 6 hours?

    (A) 46 mL/hr
    (B) 53 mL/hr
    (C) 138 mL/hr
    (D) 276 mL/hr

    Rationale: Calculating the preexisting fluid for this patient is as follows:

    Step 1: Using the 4-2-1 rule for a 13-kg patient,

    $$4 \text{ mL/kg/hr} \times 10 \text{ kg} = 40 \text{ mL/hr}$$
    $$2 \text{ mL/kg/hr} \times 3 \text{kg} = 6 \text{ mL/hr}$$

    Total maintenance rate: 46 mL/hr.

    Step 2: To calculate the preexisting deficit, 46 mL/hr × 6 hr = 276 mL.

    Ref: Butterworth, J.F., Mackey, D.C., & Wasnick, J.D. (2013). Ch 51 *Morgan & Mikhail's Clinical Anesthesiology* (5th ed.). New York, NY: McGraw-Hill.
    Barash, P.G., Cullen, B.F., Stoelting, R.K., Calahan, M.K., & Stock, M.C. (2009). Ch 14 & 45 *Clinical Anesthesia* (6th ed.). Philadelphia, PA: Lippincott Williams & Wilkins.

81. Which of the following elements in the postoperative note are not required by the Center for Medicare and Medicaid Services (CMS)?

    (A) Mental status
    (B) Temperature
    (C) Pain
    (D) Urine output

    Rationale: In addition to A, B, and C, respiratory and cardiovascular parameters, nausea, vomiting, and hydration are required documentation per CMS.
    Ref: Butterworth, J.F., Mackey, D.C., & Wasnick, J.D. (2013). Ch 18 *Morgan & Mikhail's Clinical Anesthesiology* (5th ed.). New York, NY: McGraw-Hill.

82. Which nerve is blocked by injection through the thyrohyoid membrane to anesthetize the area between the vocal cords and the epiglottis?

    (A) Hypoglossal
    (B) Recurrent laryngeal
    (C) Superior laryngeal
    (D) Glossopharyngeal

    Rationale: Sensory innervation of the airway below the epiglottis is supplied by the vagus nerve. The internal branch of the superior laryngeal nerve provides sensation from the epiglottis to the vocal cords.

    Ref: Butterworth, J.F., Mackey, D.C., & Wasnick, J.D. (2013). Ch 19 *Morgan & Mikhail's Clinical Anesthesiology* (5th ed.). New York, NY: McGraw-Hill.
    Hadzic, A. (2007). Ch 19 *Textbook of Regional Anesthesia and Acute Pain Management*. New York, NY: McGraw-Hill.

83. Tachycardia, euphoria, delirium, and excitement are noted when conducting the preoperative evaluation in the emergency department. Which of the following is probably not related to the symptoms?

    (A) Narcotics
    (B) Cocaine
    (C) Hallucinogens
    (D) Marijuana

    Rationale: Opioids produce respiratory depression, hypotension, and bradycardia. Euphoria may occur as well as pinpoint pupils linked to overdose.
    Ref: Butterworth, J.F., Mackey, D.C., & Wasnick, J.D. (2013). Ch 18 *Morgan & Mikhail's Clinical Anesthesiology* (5th ed.). New York, NY: McGraw-Hill.
    Nagelhout, J.J., & Plaus, K.L. (2014). Ch 19 *Nurse Anesthesia* (5th ed.). St. Louis, MO: Elsevier.

84. Which of the following may cause prolonged sedation?

    Select (2) two
    (A) Echinacea
    (B) Ephedra
    (C) Garlic
    (D) Kava-kava
    (E) Valerian

    Rationale: Anesthetic implications for patients taking echinacea include allergic reactions, liver enzyme induction, and immune system dysfunction. The sympathomimetic effects of ephedra predispose to myocardial infarction and stroke. Garlic increases the possibility of bleeding.
    Ref: Butterworth, J.F., Mackey, D.C., & Wasnick J.D. (2013). Ch 18 *Morgan & Mikhail's Clinical Anesthesiology* (5th ed.). New York, NY: McGraw-Hill.
    Nagelhout, J.J., & Plaus, K.L. (2014). Ch 19 *Nurse Anesthesia* (5th ed.). St. Louis, MO: Elsevier.

85. Calculate the ideal body weight (BW) for a 6 feet, 90-kg male.

(A) 80 kg

(B) 177 kg

(C) 72 kg

(D) 145 kg

Rationale: The IBW for males is calculated by the following equation: 105 lb + 6 lb for every inch over 5 feet. For females, add 5 lb for every inch over 5 feet.
Ref: Nagelhout, J.J., & Plaus, K.L. (2014). Ch 19 *Nurse Anesthesia* (5th ed.). St. Louis, MO: Elsevier.

86. A morbidly obese male patient is scheduled for a bariatric surgery. Which of the following diagnostic tests should be ordered?

Select (3) three

(A) Chest X-ray

(B) 12-lead EKG

(C) Coagulation studies

(D) HCG

(E) Glucose tolerance test

Rationale: Diagnostic testing for bariatric surgery includes a CBC, complete chemistry, fasting blood glucose, lipid profile, iron, vitamin, and mineral levels. Chest X-ray, 12-lead EKG, and coagulation testing is indicated. The pregnancy test is not indicated.
Ref: Nagelhout, J.J., & Plaus, K.L. (2014). Ch 19 *Nurse Anesthesia* (5th ed.). St. Louis, MO: Elsevier.

87. A patient with two peripheral intravenous (PIV) lines is undergoing general endotracheal anesthesia (GETA) for an orthopedic procedure. A recent lab value reveals a serum potassium level of 2.9 mEq/L. Which intervention is appropriate for this patient?

(A) Administer IV replacement K^+ in dextrose solutions.

(B) Maintain $ETCO_2$ levels between 25-30 mmHg.

(C) Reduce the rocuronium re-dose by 25-50%.

(D) Administer IV replacement K^+ 20 mEq IV in 0.9% NS over 1 hour.

Rationale: Increased sensitivity to neuromuscular blockers is common in patients with hypokalemia, and, therefore, dosages should be reduced by 25-50%. A is incorrect because dextrose containing solutions will result in hyperglycemia and secondary insulin secretion, thus worsening hypokalemia. B is incorrect because hyperventilation will

cause further decreases in plasma K^+. D is incorrect because peripheral replacement of K^+ should not exceed 8 mEq/h. Rapid replacement (i.e., 10-20 mEq/L) requires central venous administration.
Ref: Butterworth, J.F., Mackey, D.C., & Wasnick, J.D. (2013). Ch 49 *Morgan & Mikhail's Clinical Anesthesiology* (5th ed.). New York, NY: McGraw-Hill.
Nagelhout, J.J., & Plaus, K.L. (2014). Ch 20 *Nurse Anesthesia* (5th ed.). St. Louis, MO: Elsevier.

88. What is the primary innervation of the lumbar facet joint?

(A) The spinal nerve at the level of the joint

(B) The spinal nerve superior to the joint

(C) Both the nerve at the joint level and the nerve immediately superior

(D) Neither the superior nor inferior spinal nerve

Rationale: Facet joints are innervated by the spinal nerve at the level of the joint and the immediately superior spinal nerve.
Ref: Butterworth, J.F., Mackey, D.C., & Wasnick, J.D. (2013). Ch 47 *Morgan & Mikhail's Clinical Anesthesiology* (5th ed.). New York, NY: McGraw-Hill.
Moore, K.L., Dalley, A. F., & Agur, A. M. R. (2010). Ch 4 *Clinically oriented anatomy*. Philadelphia, PA: Lippincott Williams & Wilkins.

89. What is the gold standard diagnostic test for obstructive sleep apnea?

(A) Polysomnography

(B) STOP–Bang questionnaire

(C) STOP questionnaire

(D) Bang questionnaire

Rationale: The STOP–Bang questionnaire is an obstructive sleep apnea screening tool.
Ref: Nagelhout, J.J., & Plaus, K.L. (2014). Ch 19 *Nurse Anesthesia* (5th ed.). St. Louis, MO: Elsevier.

90. A patient with rheumatoid arthritis is undergoing a total knee replacement. What is the recommended glucocorticoid dosing regimen?

(A) Usual corticosteroid dose + hydrocortisone 25 mg

(B) Usual corticosteroid dose + hydrocortisone 100 mg

(C) Usual corticosteroid dose + hydrocortisone 150 mg

(D) Usual corticosteroid dose + hydrocortisone 50 mg

Rationale: Steroid coverage is based on the degree of surgical stress. Total join replacements are considered moderate surgical stress. For minor procedures, 25 mg of hydrocortisone is recommended, whereas major stress procedures including cardiac and large vascular procedures require 100-150 mg every 8 hours for 2-3 days.

Ref: Nagelhout, J.J., & Plaus, K.L. (2014). Ch 19 *Nurse Anesthesia* (5th ed.). St. Louis, MO: Elsevier.

91. Which diagnostic finding is consistent with intracranial hypertension?

    (A) MRI with a 0.5 cm midline brain shift
    (B) CT with a 0.5 cm midline brain shift
    (C) CT with contrast with a 0.4 cm midline brain shift
    (D) MRI with a 0.4 cm midline brain shift

    Rationale: A cat scan (CT) that evidences a 0.5 midline brain shift represents a finding consistent with intracranial hypertension.

    Ref: Nagelhout, J.J., & Plaus, K.L. (2014). Ch 19 *Nurse Anesthesia* (5th ed.). St. Louis, MO: Elsevier.

92. Which surgical procedures pose the lowest risk for myocardial infarction within 30 days of surgery?

    Select (3) three
    (A) Liver transplant
    (B) Breast reduction
    (C) Hysterectomy

TABLE 3-3. Cardiac risk[1] stratification for noncardiac surgical procedures.

Risk Stratification	Procedure Examples
Vascular (reported cardiac risk often > 5%)	Aortic and other major vascular surgery Peripheral vascular surgery
Intermediate (reported cardiac risk generally 1-5%)	Intraperitoneal and intrathoracic surgery Carotid endarterectomy Head and neck surgery Orthopedic surgery Prostate surgery
Low[2] (reported cardiac risk generally < 1%)	Endoscopic procedures Superficial procedure Cataract surgery Breast surgery Ambulatory surgery

[1]Combined incidence of cardiac death and nonfatal myocardial infarction.
[2]These procedures do not generally require further preoperative cardiac testing.
Fleisher L, Beckman J, Brown K, et al: ACC/AHA 2007 guidelines on perioperative cardiovascular evaluation and care for noncardiac surgery. Circulation 2007;116:1971-1996.

    (D) Cataract
    (E) Prostatectomy

    Rationale: Liver transplant and prostatectomy are considered intermediate risk carrying a 1-5% likelihood of myocardial infarction following surgery. Vascular and aortic procedures carry the highest risk of infarct (>5%).

    Ref: Nagelhout, J.J., & Plaus, K.L. (2014). Ch 19 *Nurse Anesthesia* (5th ed.). St. Louis, MO: Elsevier.

93. What is the most common cause of nonsurgical bleeding following massive blood transfusion?

    (A) Dilutional thrombocytopenia
    (B) Citrate toxicity
    (C) Dilution of factors V and X
    (D) Dilution of factors II and VIII

    Rationale: Dilutional thrombocytopenia is the most common cause of nonsurgical bleeding following massive blood transfusion. Dilutional coagulopathy is also associated with massive transfusion, specifically dilution of factors V and VIII.

    Ref: Butterworth, J.F., Mackey, D.C., & Wasnick, J.D. (2013). Ch 51 *Morgan & Mikhail's Clinical Anesthesiology* (5th ed.). New York, NY: McGraw-Hill.

    Miller, R., Fleisher, L., Wiener-Krunish, J., Young, W., & Eriksson, L. Ch 55 *Miller's Anesthesia* (7th ed). Philadelphia, PA: Elsevier.

94. The patient weighs 120 kg. The Ideal Body Weight is 60 kg. What is the patient's classification?

    (A) Obese
    (B) Morbidly obese
    (C) Overweight
    (D) Moderate obesity

    Rationale: Morbid obesity is twice the ideal body weight. Obesity reflects 20% over the ideal body weight.

    Ref: Nagelhout, J.J., & Plaus, K.L. (2014). Ch 19 *Nurse Anesthesia* (5th ed.). St. Louis, MO: Elsevier.

95. An adult patient's platelet count is 25,000/μL. After transfusing the patient with 2 units of apheresis platelets, what would you expect the platelet count to be?

    (A) 30,000-35,000/μL
    (B) 55,000-85,000/μL
    (C) 85,000-145,000/μL
    (D) 145,000-165,000/μL

Rationale: One unit of apheresis platelets will increase the platelet count by 30,000-60,000/μL. Two units of apheresis platelets will increase the platelet count by 60,000-120,000/μL. A single unit of platelets will increase the platelet count by 5,000-10,000/μL.

Ref: Butterworth, J.F., Mackey, D.C., & Wasnick, J.D. (2013). Ch 51 *Morgan & Mikhail's Clinical Anesthesiology* (5th ed.). New York, NY: McGraw-Hill.

Barash, P.G., Cullen, B.F., Stoelting, R.K., Calahan, M.K., & Stock, M.C. (2009). Ch 16 *Clinical Anesthesia* (6th ed.). Philadelphia, PA: Lippincott Williams & Wilkins.

96. During the preoperative interview the patient shares that he/she perform, light housework, plays golf once a week, and walks to the grocery store to get the newspaper. What is his/her metabolic equivalent (METs)?

    (A) 1 MET
    (B) 2 METs
    (C) 3 METs
    (D) 4 METs

    Rationale: Good functional capacity (4 METs) includes those listed as well as heavy housework, short distance running, and climbing a flight of stairs without stopping. Poor functional capacity (1 MET) includes basic activities of daily living and walking one to two blocks (<4 mph).

    Ref: Nagelhout, J.J., & Plaus, K.L. (2014). Ch 21 *Nurse Anesthesia* (5th ed.). St. Louis, MO: Elsevier.

97. What AANA Standard guides the practice of providing postanesthesia report?

    (A) Standard I
    (B) Standard III
    (C) Standard V
    (D) Standard VII

    Rationale: Standard VII speaks to the need to "transfer responsibility" for continuity of care.

    Ref: American Association of Nurse Anesthetists (AANA): *AANA Scope and Standards of Nurse Anesthesia* Practice: Standard VII.

    Nagelhout, J.J., & Plaus, K.L. (2014). Ch 50 *Nurse Anesthesia* (5th ed.). St. Louis, MO: Elsevier.

98. Which statement about fresh frozen plasma (FFP) administration is correct?

    Select (2) two

    (A) Each unit of FFP will increase the level of each clotting factor by 2-3% in adults.
    (B) The initial therapeutic dose is 10-15 mL/kg.
    (C) It should be ABO-compatible.
    (D) It must be Rh-compatible.
    (E) The therapeutic goal is to achieve 80% of the normal coagulation factor concentration

    Rationale: A unit of FFP will increase the level of each clotting factor by 2-3% in adults. The initial therapeutic dose is generally 10-15 mL/kg and should be ABO-compatible. Rh compatibility is not

TABLE 3-4. Estimated energy requirements for various activities.

	Can you…		Can you…
1 MET	Take care of yourself?	4 METs	Climb a flight of stairs or walk up a hill?
	Eat, dress, or use the toilet?		Walk on level ground at 4 mph (6.4 kph)?
	Walk indoors around the house?		Run a short distance?
	Walk a block or 2 on level ground at 2-3 mph (3.2-4.8 kph)?		Do heavy work around the house like scrubbing floors or lifting or moving heavy furniture?
4 METs	Do light work around the house like dusting or washing dishes?		Participate in moderate recreational activities like golf, bowling, dancing, doubles tennis, or throwing a baseball or football?
		Greater than 10 METs	Participate in strenuous sports like swimming, singles tennis, football, basketball, or skiing?

kph indicates kilometers per hour; MET, metabolic equivalent; and mph, miles per hour.

Modified and reproduced, with permission, from Hlatky MA, Boineau RE, Higginbotham MB, et al. A brief self-administered questionnaire to determine functional capacity (the Duke Activity Status Index). Am J Cardiol. 1989;64:651-654.

mandatory. The therapeutic goal is to achieve 30% of the normal coagulation factor concentration.

Ref: Butterworth, J.F., Mackey, D.C., & Wasnick, J.D. (2013). Ch 51 *Morgan & Mikhail's Clinical Anesthesiology* (5th ed.). New York, NY: McGraw-Hill.

Barash, P.G., Cullen, B.F., Stoelting, R.K., Calahan, M.K., & Stock, M.C. (2009). Ch 16 *Clinical Anesthesia* (6th ed.). Philadelphia, PA: Lippincott Williams & Wilkins.

99. Which of the following are risk factors for postoperative nausea and vomiting?

Select (3) three

(A) Male
(B) History of motion sickness
(C) Opioids
(D) Strabismus surgery
(E) Cataract surgery
(F) Hypertension

Rationale: Females are more likely to experience PONV than males. General anesthesia and commonly used opioids, volatile agents, and nitrous oxide contribute to PONV. Patients who are hypotensive postoperatively are at risk for PONV. Certain surgeries are linked to PONV including gynecological and urinary procedures, breast and

TABLE 3-5. Risk factors for postoperative nausea and vomiting.

Patient factors
Young age
Female gender, particularly if menstruating on day of surgery or in first trimester of pregnancy
Large body habitus
History of prior postoperative emesis
History of motion sickness

Anesthetic techniques
General anesthesia
Drugs
  Opioids
  Volatile agents
  Nitrous oxide

Surgical procedures
Strabismus surgery
Ear surgery
Laparoscopy
Orchiopexy
Ovum retrieval
Tonsillectomy
Breast surgery

Postoperative factors
Postoperative pain
Hypotension

ear, nose, and throat surgery, as well as strabismus surgery.

Ref: Butterworth, J.F., Mackey, D.C., & Wasnick, J.D. (2013). Ch 56 *Morgan & Mikhail's Clinical Anesthesiology* (5th ed.). New York, NY: McGraw-Hill.

Nagelhout, J.J., & Plaus, K.L. (2014). Ch 50 *Nurse Anesthesia* (5th ed.). St. Louis, MO: Elsevier.

100. Which of the following statements is true regarding airway blocks?

(A) Topical lidocaine may produce methemoglobinemia.
(B) 4% lidocaine is injected into the trachea upon inspiration.
(C) Nerve blocks of the airway pose risk for aspiration.
(D) Local anesthesia to the mouth and pharynx blocks nerve transmission from the superior laryngeal nerve.

Rationale: Benzocaine is linked to methemoglobinemia. For transtracheal blocks, local anesthetic is injected into the trachea during end expiration. The trigeminal and glossopharyngeal nerves innervate the airway including the anterior 2/3 of the tongue.

Ref: Butterworth, J.F., Mackey, D.C., & Wasnick, J.D. (2013). Ch 19 *Morgan & Mikhail's Clinical Anesthesiology* (5th ed.). New York, NY: McGraw-Hill.

Nagelhout, J.J., & Plaus, K.L. (2014). Ch 22 *Nurse Anesthesia* (5th ed.). St. Louis, MO: Elsevier.

101. A patient is admitted to the Post Anesthesia Care Unit with shallow, rapid respirations, diaphoresis, and tachycardia. What is the most likely cause?

(A) Delayed awakening
(B) Hypothermia
(C) Emergence delirium
(D) Inadequate oxygenation

Rationale: Common causes of delayed awakening reflect metabolic, neurological, and prolonged action of anesthetic drugs. The patient's presentation is not consistent with delayed awakening. Signs and symptoms of hypothermia reflect depressed metabolism, central nervous system depression, bradyarrhythmias, and ventricular arrhythmias. Emergence delirium refers to patients with dysfunctional cognitive signs including agitation, restlessness, fear, lack of orientation, and similar symptoms.

Ref: Butterworth, J.F., Mackey, D.C., & Wasnick, J.D. (2013). Ch 56 *Morgan & Mikhail's Clinical Anesthesiology* (5th ed.). New York, NY: McGraw-Hill.
Nagelhout, J.J., & Plaus, K.L. (2014). Ch 50 *Nurse Anesthesia* (5th ed.). St. Louis, MO: Elsevier.

102. The anesthesia plan includes using topical cocaine for nasal surgery. What is the maximum dose?

(A) 50 mg
(B) 200 mg
(C) 400 mg
(D) 40 mg

Rationale: To avoid symptoms associated with overdose (arrhythmia, convulsions, respiratory, and cardiac arrest) use no > 200 mg (5 mL of 4% solution).
Ref: Butterworth, J.F., Mackey, D.C., & Wasnick, J.D. (2013). Ch 16 *Morgan & Mikhail's Clinical Anesthesiology* (5th ed.). New York, NY: McGraw-Hill.
Nagelhout, J.J., & Plaus, K.L. (2014). Ch 10 *Nurse Anesthesia* (5th ed.). St. Louis, MO: Elsevier.

103. What factors are associated with hypotension in the Post Anesthesia Care Unit?

Select (2) two
(A) Hypervolemia
(B) Nausea
(C) Arrhythmias
(D) Pain
(E) Shivering

Rationale: The main cause of hypotension the PACU is hypovolemia. Hypertension in the PACU reflects painful stimulation (surgical, intubation, bladder distention) and shivering.
Ref: Butterworth, J.F., Mackey, D.C., & Wasnick, J.D. (2013). Ch 56 *Morgan & Mikhail's Clinical Anesthesiology* (5th ed.). New York, NY: McGraw-Hill.

104. What constitutes the eutectic mixture of local anesthetic?

(A) Benzocaine and prilocaine
(B) Prilocaine and tetracaine
(C) Lidocaine and prilocaine
(D) Prilocaine and nesicaine

Rationale: EMLA cream is 5% lidocaine and 5% prilocaine (1:1 mixture).

105. During post anesthesia recovery the patient is snoring and use of the accessory muscle for ventilation are noted. What is the most likely cause?

(A) Airway obstruction
(B) Hypoventilation
(C) Hypoxemia
(D) Bronchospasm

Rationale: Airway obstruction may contribute to hypoventilation. Other signs and symptoms of hypoventilation include: decreased respiratory rate or tachypnea with shallow respirations. In the PACU, hypoventilation is the primary cause of hypoxemia resulting in varied signs and symptoms. Airway symptoms including wheezing, secretions, tachypnea, and accessory muscle use are prominent signs.
Ref: Butterworth, J.F., Mackey, D.C., & Wasnick, J.D. (2013). Ch 56 *Morgan & Mikhail's Clinical Anesthesiology* (5th ed.). New York, NY: McGraw-Hill.
Nagelhout, J.J., & Plaus, K.L. (2014). Ch 50 *Nurse Anesthesia* (5th ed.). St. Louis, MO: Elsevier.

106. Gabapentin is most helpful in treating which type of pain?

(A) Acute somatic pain
(B) Deep visceral pain
(C) Neuropathic pain
(D) Chronic arthritic joint pain

Rationale: Gabapentin and other anticonvulsants are most helpful when used in the treatment neuropathic pain
Ref: Butterworth, J.F., Mackey, D.C., & Wasnick, J.D. (2013). Ch 47 *Morgan & Mikhail's Clinical Anesthesiology* (5th ed.). New York, NY: McGraw-Hill.
Miller, R.D., Eriksson, L.I., Fleisher, L.A., Weiner-Kronish, J.P., & Young, W.L. (Eds.) (2010). Ch 58 *Miller's Anesthesia* (7th ed.). Philadelphia, PA: Elsevier.

107. When using EMLA cream, what is the maximum total dose for children >20 kg?

(A) 20 g
(B) 10 g
(C) 2 g
(D) 1 g

Rationale: The maximum total dose for adults differs from children. Children <3 months and 5 kg (1g); children 3 months to 12 years and > 5 kg (2 g) and children 1-6 years and < 10 kg (10 g). 20 g is allowed for 2-12 years (>20 kg).

Ref: Butterworth, J.F., Mackey, D.C., & Wasnick, J.D. (2013). Ch 16 *Morgan & Mikhail's Clinical Anesthesiology* (5th ed.). New York, NY: McGraw-Hill.

Nagelhout, J.J., & Plaus, K.L. (2014). Ch 10 *Nurse Anesthesia* (5th ed.). St. Louis, MO: Elsevier.

108. Which peripheral nerve block provides complete anesthesia for ankle surgery?

    (A) Femoral
    (B) Sciatic
    (C) Obturator
    (D) Popliteal

    Rationale: The femoral block is useful for analgesia but not total anesthesia for ankle procedures. For surgical procedures below the knee, the popliteal approach to sciatic nerve block provides complete anesthesia. Surgery above and below the knee and including the knee are anesthetized using other approaches to the sciatic nerve block. The obturator block is useful for knee procedures.

    Ref: Butterworth, J.F., Mackey, D.C., & Wasnick, J.D. (2013). Ch 46 *Morgan & Mikhail's Clinical Anesthesiology* (5th ed.). New York, NY: McGraw-Hill.

    Nagelhout, J.J., & Plaus, K.L. (2014). Ch 45 *Nurse Anesthesia* (5th ed.). St. Louis, MO: Elsevier.

109. Which nerve block results in the highest blood level of local anesthetic?

    (A) Sciatic
    (B) Intercostal
    (C) Paravertebral
    (D) Cervical plexus

    Rationale: Along with the highest complication rate of nerve blocks, the intercostal block results in the highest blood level of local anesthetic. The anatomy is a vessel-rich area.

    Ref: Butterworth, J.F., Mackey, D.C., & Wasnick, J.D. (2013). Ch 46 *Morgan & Mikhail's Clinical Anesthesiology* (5th ed.). New York, NY: McGraw-Hill.

    Nagelhout, J.J., & Plaus, K.L. (2014). Ch 45 *Nurse Anesthesia* (5th ed.). St. Louis, MO: Elsevier.

110. What are the fluid requirements for redistribution and evaporative surgical fluid losses during a bowl resection?

    (A) 0-2 mL/kg
    (B) 2-4 mL/kg
    (C) 4-8 mL/kg
    (D) 10-14 mL/kg

    Rationale: Redistribution and evaporative loss are replaced according to the degree of tissue trauma sustained during surgery: minimal tissue trauma (e.g., herniorrhaphy/short superficial procedure) requires 0-2 mL/kg; moderate tissue trauma (e.g., cholecystectomy) requires 2-4 mL/kg; and severe tissue trauma (e.g., bowel resection) requires 4-8 mL/kg.

    Ref: Butterworth, J.F., Mackey, D.C., & Wasnick, J.D. (2013). Ch 51 *Morgan & Mikhail's Clinical Anesthesiology* (5th ed.). New York, NY: McGraw-Hill.

    Nagelhout, J.J., & Plaus, K.L. (2014). Ch 20 *Nurse Anesthesia* (5th ed.). St. Louis, MO: Elsevier.

111. Which airway block provides anesthesia below the vocal cords?

    Select (2) two

    (A) Superior laryngeal nerve block
    (B) Transtracheal block
    (C) Glossopharyngeal block
    (D) Instilling local anesthetic onto the vocal cords

    Rationale: A glossopharyngeal nerve block anesthetizes the posterior third of the tongue. Instilling local anesthetic (lidocaine droplet spread) onto the vocal cords provides local anesthesia to the immediate area only.

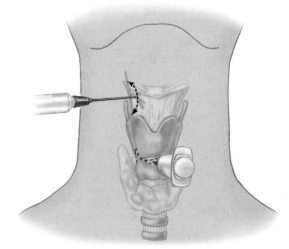

FIG. 3-4. Superior laryngeal nerve block and transtracheal block.

Ref: Butterworth, J.F., Mackey, D.C., & Wasnick, J.D. (2013). Ch 19 *Morgan & Mikhail's Clinical Anesthesiology* (5th ed.). New York, NY: McGraw-Hill.
Nagelhout, J.J., & Plaus, K.L. (2014). Ch 22 *Nurse Anesthesia* (5th ed.). St. Louis, MO: Elsevier.

112. Which of the following form the lumbar plexus?

    (A) L1–3 and T10
    (B) L1–4 and T10
    (C) L1–4 and T12
    (D) L1–3 and T12

    Rationale: L1–4 and T12 ventral rami form the lumbosacral plexus.
    Ref: Butterworth, J.F., Mackey, D.C., & Wasnick, J.D. (2013). Ch 46 *Morgan & Mikhail's Clinical Anesthesiology* (5th ed.). New York, NY: McGraw-Hill.
    Nagelhout, J.J., & Plaus, K.L. (2014). Ch 45 *Nurse Anesthesia* (5th ed.). St. Louis, MO: Elsevier.

113. What results when placing a femoral block with nerve stimulation?

    (A) Thigh adduction
    (B) Quadriceps twitch
    (C) Sciatic nerve block posterior approach
    (D) Sciatic nerve block anterior approach

    Rationale: Thigh adduction occurs with an obturator block. The posterior approach to sciatic nerve block results in a gluteal muscle twitch and plantar flexion or dorsiflexion. Foot inversion or plantar flexion is elicited when the anterior approach is used.
    Ref: Butterworth, J.F., Mackey, D.C., & Wasnick, J.D. (2013). Ch 46 *Morgan & Mikhail's Clinical Anesthesiology* (5th ed.). New York, NY: McGraw-Hill.
    Nagelhout, J.J., & Plaus, K.L. (2014). Ch 45 *Nurse Anesthesia* (5th ed.). St. Louis, MO: Elsevier Saunders.

114. Which phrase describes radiculopathy?

    (A) Abnormal sensation with or without a stimulus
    (B) Pain linked to noxious stimulation
    (C) Nerve distribution pain
    (D) Abnormal function of nerve roots

TABLE 3-6. Terms used in pain management.

Term	Description
Allodynia	Perception of an ordinarily nonnoxious stimulus as pain
Analgesia	Absence of pain perception
Anesthesia	Absence of all sensation
Anesthesia dolorosa	Pain in an area that lacks sensation
Dysesthesia	Unpleasant or abnormal sensation with or without a stimulus
Hypalgesia (hypoalgesia)	Diminished response to noxious stimulation (eg, pinprick)
Hyperalgesia	Increased response to noxious stimulation
Hyperesthesia	Increased response to mild stimulation
Hyperpathia	Presence of hyperesthesia, allodynia, and hyperalgesia usually associated with overreaction, and persistence of the sensation after the stimulus
Hypesthesia (hypoesthesia)	Reduced cutaneous sensation (eg, light touch, pressure, or temperature)
Neuralgia	Pain in the distribution of a nerve or a group of nerves
Paresthesia	Abnormal sensation perceived without an apparent stimulus
Radiculopathy	Functional abnormality of one or more nerve roots

Rationale: The unpleasant or abnormal sensation with or without a stimulus is dysesthesia. Hyperalgesia is the increased response to noxious stimulation. Neuralgia describes pain associated with nerve distribution.
Ref: Butterworth, J.F., Mackey, D.C., & Wasnick, J.D. (2013). Ch 47 *Morgan & Mikhail's Clinical Anesthesiology* (5th ed.). New York, NY: McGraw-Hill.
Nagelhout, J.J., & Plaus, K.L. (2014). Ch 51 *Nurse Anesthesia* (5th ed.). St. Louis, MO: Elsevier.

115. Which of the following are pain modulating excitatory neurotransmitters?

    Select (2) two
    (A) Substance P
    (B) Glycine
    (C) GABA
    (D) Glutamate
    (E) Serotonin

TABLE 3-7. Major neurotransmitters mediating or modulating pain.

Neurotransmitter	Receptor[1]	Effect on Nociception
Substance P	Neurokinin–1	Excitatory
Calcitonin gene-related peptide		Excitatory
Glutamate	NMDA, AMPA, kainate, quisqualate	Excitatory
Aspartate	NMDA, AMPA, kainate, quisqualate	Excitatory
Adenosine triphosphate (ATP)	P_1, P_2	Excitatory
Somatostatin		Inhibitory
Acetylcholine	Muscarinic	Inhibitory
Enkephalins	μ, δ, κ	Inhibitory
β-Endorphin	μ, δ, κ	Inhibitory
Norepinephrine	α_2	Inhibitory
Adenosine	A_1	Inhibitory
Serotonin	5-HT$_1$ (5-HT$_3$)	Inhibitory
γ-Aminobutyric acid (GABA)	A, B	Inhibitory
Glycine		Inhibitory

[1]NMDA, *N*-methyl-D-aspartate; AMPA, 2-(aminomethyl)phenylacetic acid; 5-HT, 5-hydroxytryptamine.

Rationale: Glycine, enkephalin, norepeinephrine, GABA, and serotonin are inhibitory neurotransmitters. Other excitatory substances include calcitonin, aspartate, and adenosine triphosphate.

Ref: Butterworth, J.F., Mackey, D.C., & Wasnick, J.D. (2013). Ch 47 *Morgan & Mikhail's Clinical Anesthesiology* (5th ed.). New York, NY: McGraw-Hill.

Nagelhout, J.J., & Plaus, K.L. (2014). Ch 51 *Nurse Anesthesia* (5th ed.). St. Louis, MO: Elsevier.

116. Which of the following physiological effects result from acute pain stimulation?

Select (3) three

(A) Increased myocardial workload

(B) Decreased vital capacity

(C) Decreased gastric emptying

(D) Decreased platelet aggregation

(E) Increased intestinal motility

Rationale: The physiological effects of pain include increased platelet aggregation leading to thrombosis as well as decreased intestinal motility with the potential for paralytic ileus.

Ref: Butterworth, J.F., Mackey, D.C., & Wasnick, J.D. (2013). Ch 47 *Morgan & Mikhail's Clinical Anesthesiology* (5th ed.). New York, NY: McGraw-Hill.

Nagelhout, J.J., & Plaus, K.L. (2014). Ch 51 *Nurse Anesthesia* (5th ed.). St. Louis, MO: Elsevier.

117. Vocal cord paralysis occurred following intubation. What is the most likely cause?

(A) Recurrent laryngeal nerve damage

(B) Epiglottic damage

(C) Esophageal damage

(D) Superior laryngeal nerve

Rationale: Stridor and respiratory distress result from injury to the superior laryngeal nerve. Unilateral damage to the recurrent laryngeal nerve results in vocal cord paralysis exhibited by hoarseness.

TABLE 3-8. The effects of laryngeal nerve injury on the voice.

Nerve	Effect of Nerve Injury
Superior laryngeal nerve	
Unilateral	Minimal effects
Bilateral	Hoarseness, tiring of voice
Recurrent laryngeal nerve	
Unilateral	Hoarseness
Bilateral	
Acute	Stridor, respiratory distress
Chronic	Aphonia
Vagus nerve	
Unilateral	Hoarseness
Bilateral	Aphonia

Ref: Butterworth, J.F., Mackey, D.C., & Wasnick, J.D. (2013). Ch 19 *Morgan & Mikhail's Clinical Anesthesiology* (5th ed.). New York, NY: Lange Medical Books McGraw-Hill.

Nagelhout, J.J., & Plaus, K.L. (2014). Ch 22 *Nurse Anesthesia* (5th ed.). St. Louis, MO: Elsevier.

118. A patient with a history of reflux and diabetes mellitus is scheduled for a bowel obstruction. Which of the following fasting guidelines apply?

(A) NPO for 8 hours

(B) Clear fluids up to 2 hours

(C) Light meal up to 6 hours

(D) NPO for 4 hours

Rationale: The patient's comorbidities and surgery are associated with increased risk for delayed gastric emptying and aspiration. Fasting guidelines remain conservative for patients at increased risk for aspiration. Relaxed fasting guidelines including a light meal or clear liquids apply only to patients not at risk for delayed gastric emptying.

Ref: Butterworth, J.F., Mackey, D.C., & Wasnick, J.D. (2013). Ch 18 *Morgan & Mikhail's Clinical Anesthesiology* (5th ed.). New York, NY: McGraw-Hill.

Miller, R.D., & Pardo, M.C. (2011). Ch 13 in *Basics of Anesthesia* (6th ed.). Philadelphia, PA: Elsevier.

119. A 40-year-old male with a history of well-controlled hypertension is scheduled for a carpal tunnel release. How will you classify the patient?

(A) ASA IV

(B) ASA III

(C) ASA II

(D) ASA I

Rationale: The American Society of Anesthesiologists (ASA) Physical Status Classification is used to assign patients a physical status prior to anesthesia and surgery. The patient's history of well-controlled hypertension is considered a mild systemic disease.

Ref: Butterworth, J.F., Mackey, D.C., & Wasnick, J.D. (2013). Ch 18 *Morgan & Mikhail's Clinical Anesthesiology* (5th ed.). New York, NY: McGraw-Hill.

Miller, R.D., & Pardo, M.C. (2011). Ch 13 in *Basics of Anesthesia* (6th ed.). Philadelphia, PA: Elsevier.

TABLE 3-9. American Society of Anesthesiologists' physical status classification of patients.[1]

Class	Definition
1	Normal healthy patient
2	Patient with mild systemic disease (no functional limitations)
3	Patient with severe systemic disease (some functional limitations)
4	Patient with severe systemic disease that is a constant threat to life (functionality incapacitated)
5	Moribund patient who is not expected to survive without the operation
6	Brain-dead patient whose organs are being removed for donor purposes
E	If the procedure is an emergency, the physical status is followed by "E" (e.g., "2E")

[1]Data from Committee on Standards and practice Parameters, Apfelbaum JL, Connis RT, et al: Practice advisory for preanesthesia evaluation: An updated report by the American Society of Anesthesiologists Task Force on Preanesthesia Evaluation. Anesthesiology 2012;116:522.

120. During the preoperative airway exam, you visualize the soft palate, faces, and uvula. How would you classify the patient's airway?

(A) Mallampati I

(B) Mallampati III

(C) Mallampati II

(D) Mallampati IV

Rationale: The Mallampati (MP) score correlates the ease of laryngoscopy and tracheal intubation with the ability to visualize oropharyngeal structures. Visualization of the soft palate, faces, uvula, and tonsillar pillars identifies the airway as a MP I. Visualization of the soft palate and base of the uvula is a MP III. No visualization of the soft palate identifies the airway as a MP IV.

Ref: Butterworth, J.F., Mackey, D.C., & Wasnick, J.D. (2013). Ch 19 *Morgan & Mikhail's Clinical Anesthesiology* (5th ed.). New York, NY: McGraw-Hill.

Miller, R.D., & Pardo, M.C. (2011). Ch 16 in *Basics of Anesthesia* (6th ed.). Philadelphia, PA: Elsevier.

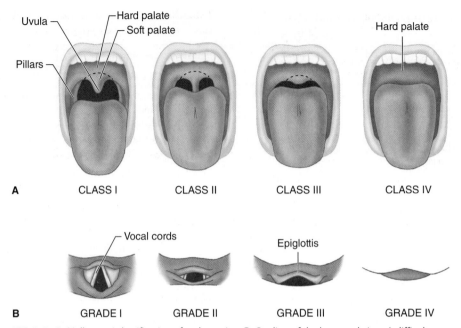

FIG. 3-5. **A**: Mallampati classification of oral opening. **B**: Grading of the laryngeal view. A difficult orotracheal intubation (grade III or IV) may be predicted by the inability to visualize certain pharyngeal structures (class III or IV) during the preoperative examination of a seated patient. (Reproduced, with permission, from Mallampati SR: Clinical signs to predict difficult tracheal intubation [hypothesis]. Can Anaesth Soc J 1983;30:316.)

121. A patient's lab values reveal digoxin toxicity and hyperkalemia. Which option for treating for hyperkalemia will you need to avoid in this patient?

    (A) 10 units regular insulin with 30-50 g dextrose 50% IV

    (B) 3-5 mL of 10% calcium chloride IV

    (C) 45 mEq sodium bicarbonate IV

    (D) 30 g sodium polystyrene PR

    Rationale: Administering calcium to patients who take digoxin potentiates digoxin toxicity. This patient is digoxin toxic so administering calcium will only cause further deterioration.

    Ref: Butterworth, J.F., Mackey, D.C., & Wasnick, J.D. (2013). Ch 49 *Morgan & Mikhail's Clinical Anesthesiology* (5th ed.). New York, NY: McGraw-Hill.

    Barash, P.G., Cullen, B.F., Stoelting, R.K., Calahan, M.K., & Stock, M.C. (2009). Ch 14 *Clinical Anesthesia* (6th ed.). Philadelphia, PA: Lippincott Williams & Wilkins.

122. A patient is scheduled for knee arthroscopy. The blood glucose is elevated along with the A_{1c}. What will you do first?

    (A) Notify the surgeon that the surgery will be delayed.

    (B) Proceed with the surgery.

    (C) Cancel the surgery.

    (D) Call the endocrinologist.

    Rationale: The elective case may be rescheduled or placed on the schedule later in the day. An insulin infusion may be needed to lower the blood sugar closer to normal limits. An endocrine consult is in order following surgery.

    Ref: Butterworth, J.F., Mackey, D.C., & Wasnick, J.D. (2013). Ch 18 *Morgan & Mikhail's Clinical Anesthesiology* (5th ed.). New York, NY: McGraw-Hill.

    Nagelhout, J.J., & Plaus, K.L. (2014). Ch 20 *Nurse Anesthesia* (5th ed.). St. Louis, MO: Elsevier.

123. What is the primary intracellular cation?

    (A) Potassium

    (B) Sodium

    (C) Calcium

    (D) Chloride

    Rationale: Sodium is the primary extracellular cation. Calcium and chloride are minimally concentrated in the intracellular fluid.

TABLE 3-10. The composition of fluid compartments.

| | Gram-Molecular Weight | Intracellular (mEq/L) | Extracellular | |
			Intravascular (mEq/L)	Interstitial (mEq/L)
Sodium	23.0	10	145	142
Potassium	39.1	140	4	4
Calcium	40.1	<1	3	3
Magnesium	24.3	50	2	2
Chloride	35.5	4	105	110
Bicarbonate	61.0	10	24	28
Phosphorus	31.0[1]	75	2	2
Protein (g/dL)		16	7	2

[1]PO_4^{3-} is 95 g.

Ref: Butterworth, J.F., Mackey, D.C., & Wasnick, J.D. (2013). Ch 49 *Morgan & Mikhail's Clinical Anesthesiology* (5th ed.). New York, NY: McGraw-Hill.

Nagelhout, J.J., & Plaus, K.L. (2014). Ch 20 *Nurse Anesthesia* (5th ed.). St. Louis, MO: Elsevier.

124. What mechanism results in the greatest amount of heat loss in the operating room?

   (A) Convection
   (B) Evaporation
   (C) Radiation
   (D) Conduction

   Rationale: Radiation (60%) results in the most heat lost in the operating room. Evaporation, convection, and conduction follow.

   Ref: Longnecker, D.E., Brown, D.L., Newman, M.F., & Zapol, W.M. (2012). Ch 88 *Anesthesiology* (2nd ed.). New York, NY: McGraw-Hill.

125. What is the average blood volume of an 80-kg male?

   (A) 5 L
   (B) 6 L
   (C) 5.2 L
   (D) 6.4 L

   Rationale: The average blood volume for a male is 75 mL/kg; 65 mL/kg for a female; and 80 mL/kg for an infant.

   Ref: Butterworth, J.F., Mackey, D.C., & Wasnick, J.D. (2013). Ch 51 *Morgan & Mikhail's Clinical Anesthesiology* (5th ed.). New York, NY: McGraw-Hill.

126. How much additional fluid will you administer to a patient undergoing a herniorrhaphy?

   (A) 4-8 mL/kg
   (B) 0-2 mL/kg
   (C) 2-4 mL/kg
   (D) 10 mL/kg

   Rationale: Surgical procedures with minimal trauma require the least amount of additional fluid replacement. A herniorrhaphy is an example of a minimally invasive procedure with little tissue trauma. Moderate tissue trauma requires 2-4 mL/kg and large tissue trauma surgeries required 4-8 mL/kg.

TABLE 3-11. Redistribution and evaporative surgical fluid losses.

Degree of Tissue Trauma	Additional Fluid Requirement
Minimal (eg, herniorrhaphy)	0-2 mL/kg
Moderate (eg, cholecystectomy)	2-4 mL/kg
Severe (eg, bowel resection)	4-8 mL/kg

Ref: Butterworth, J.F., Mackey, D.C., & Wasnick, J.D. (2013). Ch 51 *Morgan & Mikhail's Clinical Anesthesiology* (5th ed.). New York, NY: McGraw-Hill.

Nagelhout, J.J., & Plaus, K.L. (2014). Ch 20 *Nurse Anesthesia* (5th ed.). St. Louis, MO: Elsevier.

127. What statement is true regarding colloids?

   (A) Inexpensive
   (B) Increase plasma volume
   (C) Used for initial resuscitation
   (D) Used primarily for extracellular expansion

   Rationale: As compared to crystalloids, colloids are expensive and are useful in increasing the plasma volume. Crystalloids are typically used for initial resuscitation and extracellular fluid replacement.

   Ref: Butterworth, J.F., Mackey, D.C., & Wasnick, J.D. (2013). Ch 51 *Morgan & Mikhail's Clinical Anesthesiology* (5th ed.). New York, NY: McGraw-Hill.

Nagelhout, J.J., & Plaus, K.L. (2014). Ch 20 *Nurse Anesthesia* (5th ed.). St. Louis, MO: Elsevier.

128. While receiving a blood transfusion during general anesthesia tachycardia and hypotension develop. What is the most likely cause?

(A) Delayed hemolytic reaction

(B) Anaphylactic reaction

(C) Urticarial reaction

(D) Acute hemolytic reaction

Rationale: When a patient receives incompatible ABO blood, hemolytic reactions result. When patients are awake symptoms include chills, flank pain, nausea, and fever. Patients undergoing general anesthesia exhibit tachycardia hypotension, hemoglobinuria, and oozing. Delayed hemolytic reactions develop 2-21 days after the transfusion and are mild compared to the acute hemolytic reaction. Anaphylactic reactions occur in patients with IgA deficiency. Urticarial reactions are linked to plasma proteins.

Ref: Butterworth, J.F., Mackey, D.C., & Wasnick, J.D. (2013). Ch 51 *Morgan & Mikhail's Clinical Anesthesiology* (5th ed.). New York, NY: McGraw-Hill.

Nagelhout, J.J., & Plaus, K.L. (2014). Ch 20 *Nurse Anesthesia* (5th ed.). St. Louis, MO: Elsevier.

129. What statement is true regarding a patient who is awake in the supine position?

(A) The blood pressure decreases due to autoregulation.

(B) Venous return decreases.

(C) Blood pressure remains relatively constant.

(D) Sympathetic outflow increases.

Rationale: When a patient goes from standing to the supine position, venous return increases. Sympathetic outflow decreases while parasympathetic activity increases due to activation of afferent baroreceptors. Activated atrial and ventricular receptors also decrease sympathetic outflow. These processes along with activation of atrial reflexes results in maintenance of arterial blood pressure.

Ref: Butterworth, J.F., Mackey, D.C., & Wasnick, J.D. (2013). Ch 51 *Morgan & Mikhail's Clinical Anesthesiology* (5th ed.). New York, NY: McGraw-Hill.

Miller, R.D., & Pardo, M.C. (2011). Ch 19 *Basics of Anesthesia* (6th ed.). Philadelphia, PA: Elsevier.

130. What effect does the lithotomy position have on arterial pressure?

(A) Lower than supine position

(B) Higher than supine position

(C) Lower than Trendelenburg

(D) Lower than sitting position

Rationale: The blood pressure in the lithotomy position remains the same as or higher than the supine position. Auto transfusion from the lower extremities occurs in the lithotomy position. Trendelenberg position typically increases blood pressure whereas the sitting position often results in a lower blood pressure.

Ref: Butterworth, J.F., Mackey, D.C., & Wasnick, J.D. (2013). Ch 54 *Morgan & Mikhail's Clinical Anesthesiology* (5th ed.). New York, NY: McGraw-Hill.

Miller, R.D., & Pardo, M.C. (2011). Ch 19 *Basics of Anesthesia* (6th ed.). Philadelphia, PA: Elsevier.

Nagelhout, J.J., & Plaus, K.L. (2014). Ch 20 *Nurse Anesthesia* (5th ed.). St. Louis, MO: Elsevier.

131. A patient experiences low vision following a lumbar laminectomy in the prone position. What is the etiology?

(A) Decreased intracranial pressure

(B) Decreased venous pressure

(C) Increased cerebral blood flow

(D) Decreased ocular perfusion pressure

Rationale: Physiological changes in the prone position include increased intracranial pressure; increased venous pressure and decreased cerebral blood flow. Postoperative vision loss is due to increased ocular venous pressure as well as decreased ocular perfusion pressure.

Ref: Butterworth, J.F., Mackey, D.C., & Wasnick, J.D. (2013). Ch 54 *Morgan & Mikhail's Clinical Anesthesiology* (5th ed.). New York, NY: McGraw-Hill.

Miller, R.D., & Pardo, M.C. (2011). Ch 19 *Basics of Anesthesia* (6th ed.). Philadelphia, PA: Elsevier.

Nagelhout, J.J., & Plaus, K.L. (2014). Ch 20 *Nurse Anesthesia* (5th ed.). St. Louis, MO: Elsevier.

132. Where will you measure the blood pressure for patients undergoing surgery in the lateral decubitus position?

(A) Nondependent arm

(B) Both arms

(C) Dependent arm

(D) Right thigh

Rationale: Avoiding compression of the neurovascular bundle in the dependent arm is necessary. To determine perfusion to the extremity, monitor the blood pressure in the dependent arm intermittently. Checking a radial pulse is another safety measure.

Ref: Butterworth, J.F., Mackey, D.C., & Wasnick, J.D. (2013). Ch 54 *Morgan & Mikhail's Clinical Anesthesiology* (5th ed.). New York, NY: McGraw-Hill.

Miller, R.D., & Pardo, M.C. (2011). Ch 19 *Basics of Anesthesia* (6th ed.). Philadelphia, PA: Elsevier.

Nagelhout, J.J., & Plaus, K.L. (2014). Ch 20 *Nurse Anesthesia* (5th ed.). St. Louis, MO: Elsevier.

133. A sudden decreased SpO_2, blood pressure, and $ETCO_2$ occur during general anesthesia. A mill-wheel murmur exists. What is the most likely cause?

    (A) Venous air embolism
    (B) Pneumocephalus
    (C) Fat embolism
    (D) Cardiovascular accident

    Rationale: Classic signs of a venous air embolism include marked hemodynamic changes, falling end-tidal carbon dioxide, increased nitrogen, arrhythmias and a mill-wheel murmur.

    Ref: Butterworth, J.F., Mackey, D.C., & Wasnick, J.D. (2013). Ch 27 *Morgan & Mikhail's Clinical Anesthesiology* (5th ed.). New York, NY: Lange Medical Books McGraw-Hill.

    Miller, R.D., & Pardo, M.C. (2011). Ch 19 *Basics of Anesthesia* (6th ed.). Philadelphia, PA: Elsevier.

    Nagelhout, J.J., & Plaus, K.L. (2014). Ch 21 *Nurse Anesthesia* (5th ed.). St. Louis, MO: Elsevier.

134. What nerve injury is most likely to occur when the arm is pronated?

    (A) Brachial plexus
    (B) Ulnar nerve
    (C) Radial nerve
    (D) Suprascapular nerve

    Rationale: To avoid injury to the ulnar nerve, the forearm is supinated. An additional measure to avoid injury include the use of elbow padding and flexing elbows <90 degrees.

    Ref: Butterworth, J.F., Mackey, D.C., & Wasnick, J.D. (2013). Ch 27 *Morgan & Mikhail's Clinical Anesthesiology* (5th ed.). New York, NY: McGraw-Hill.

    Miller, R.D., & Pardo, M.C. (2011). Ch 19 *Basics of Anesthesia* (6th ed.). Philadelphia, PA: Elsevier.

    Nagelhout, J.J., & Plaus, K.L. (2014). Ch 21 *Nurse Anesthesia* (5th ed.). St. Louis, MO: Elsevier.

135. In the supine position, what nerve injury is associated with arm abduction >90 degrees and lateral rotation of the head?

    (A) Ulnar nerve
    (B) Brachial plexus
    (C) Radial nerve
    (D) Suprascapular nerve

    Rationale: Ulnar nerve symptoms may result from injury to the brachial plexus. Keeping the arms abducted <90 degrees as well as proper head alignment minimizes stretching of the brachial plexus.

    Ref: Butterworth, J.F., Mackey, D.C., & Wasnick, J.D. (2013). Ch 54 *Morgan & Mikhail's Clinical Anesthesiology* (5th ed.). New York, NY: McGraw-Hill.

    Miller, R.D., & Pardo, M.C. (2011). Ch 19 *Basics of Anesthesia* (6th ed.). Philadelphia, PA: Elsevier.

    Nagelhout, J.J., & Plaus, K.L. (2014). Ch 21 *Nurse Anesthesia* (5th ed.). St. Louis, MO: Elsevier.

136. Following surgery in the lithotomy position the patient exhibits foot drop and the inability to extend the toes. What nerves are most likely injured?

    (A) Sciatic and common peroneal
    (B) Femoral and sciatic
    (C) Common peroneal and femoral
    (D) Obturator and sciatic

    Rationale: Foot drop and the inability to extend the toes are seen with sciatic and common peroneal nerve injury. These nerves are the most commonly injured when placed in the lithotomy position. Injury to the obturator and femoral nerves results in a femoral neuropathy demonstrated by decreased hip flexion, inability to extend the knee, and/or sensory loss (superior thigh and anteromedial or medial leg).

    Ref: Butterworth, J.F., Mackey, D.C., & Wasnick, J.D. (2013). Ch 54 *Morgan & Mikhail's Clinical Anesthesiology* (5th ed.). New York, NY: McGraw-Hill.

    Miller, R.D., & Pardo, M.C. (2011). Ch 19 *Basics of Anesthesia* (6th ed.). Philadelphia, PA: Elsevier.

    Nagelhout, J.J., & Plaus, K.L. (2014). Ch 21 *Nurse Anesthesia* (5th ed.). St. Louis, MO: Elsevier.

137. Which patient requires a preoperative chest X-ray?

    (A) 55-year-old smoker undergoing a laparoscopic cholecystectomy
    (B) 65-year-old chronic stable bronchitic undergoing a carpal tunnel release

(C) 60-year-old undergoing a transurethral resection of the prostate

(D) 50-year-old undergoing a mitral valve replacement

Rationale: Preoperative chest X-rays are indicated for patients with acute or chronic symptomatic pulmonary dysfunction, cardiac conditions, or malignancies of the chest.

Ref: Nagelhout, J.J., & Plaus, K.L. (2014). Ch 19 *Nurse Anesthesia* (5th ed.). St. Louis, MO: Elsevier.

138. What is the average distance from the skin to the epidural space?

(A) 1 cm

(B) 1.5 cm

(C) 5 cm

(D) 7.5 cm

Rationale: The distance from the skin to the epidural space ranges from 2.5-8 cm.

Ref: Butterworth, J.F., Mackey, D.C., & Wasnick, J.D. (2013). Ch 45 *Morgan & Mikhail's Clinical Anesthesiology* (5th ed.). New York, NY: McGraw-Hill.

Miller, R.D., & Pardo, M.C. (2011). Ch 17 *Basics of Anesthesia* (6th ed.). Philadelphia, PA: Elsevier.

Nagelhout, J.J., & Plaus, K.L. (2014). Ch 44 *Nurse Anesthesia* (5th ed.). St. Louis, MO: Elsevier.

139. What statement is false regarding the lateral decubitus position?

(A) Rhabdomyolysis may occur.

(B) Flex the dependent arm <90 degrees.

(C) Pad the lateral aspect of the dependent leg.

(D) Pulmonary blood flow to the dependent lung decreases.

Rationale: In the lateral decubitus position, blood flow to the dependent lung is increased.

Ref: Butterworth, J.F., Mackey, D.C., & Wasnick, J.D. (2013). Ch 54 *Morgan & Mikhail's Clinical Anesthesiology* (5th ed.). New York, NY: McGraw-Hill.

Miller, R.D., & Pardo, M.C. (2011). Ch 19 *Basics of Anesthesia* (6th ed.). Philadelphia, PA: Elsevier.

Nagelhout, J.J., & Plaus, K.L. (2014). Ch 20 *Nurse Anesthesia* (5th ed.). St. Louis, MO: Elsevier.

140. In what position is a venous air embolism (VAE) most likely to occur?

(A) Lateral decubitus

(B) Sitting

(C) Prone

(D) Trendelenburg

Rationale: In surgeries above the level of the heart, the risk of VAE exists. Any position where the surgery is above the level of the heart predisposes the patient to VAE. Open sinuses allow for the entrainment of air.

Ref: Butterworth, J.F., Mackey, D.C., & Wasnick, J.D. (2013). Ch 27 *Morgan & Mikhail's Clinical Anesthesiology* (5th ed.). New York, NY: McGraw-Hill.

Miller, R.D., & Pardo, M.C. (2011). Ch 19 *Basics of Anesthesia* (6th ed.). Philadelphia, PA: Elsevier.

141. A T6 sensory level is identified following administration of a spinal anesthetic. At what level is the sympathetic block?

(A) T4

(B) T10

(C) T6

(D) T8

Rationale: Differential blockade exists following administration of a spinal anesthetic. The sympathetic block is two or more segments higher than the sensory block, which is two segments higher than a motor block.

Ref: Butterworth, J.F., Mackey, D.C., & Wasnick, J.D. (2013). Ch 45 *Morgan & Mikhail's Clinical Anesthesiology* (5th ed.). New York, NY: McGraw-Hill.

Miller, R.D., & Pardo, M.C. (2011). Ch 17 *Basics of Anesthesia* (6th ed.). Philadelphia, PA: Elsevier.

Nagelhout, J.J., & Plaus, K.L. (2014). Ch 44 *Nurse Anesthesia* (5th ed.). St. Louis, MO: Elsevier.

142. In which patient is spinal anesthesia contraindicated?

(A) 30-year-old who takes daily garlic

(B) 50-year-old taking subcutaneous heparin injections

(C) 25-year-old taking NSAIDs

(D) 40-year-old who received thrombolytic therapy

Rationale: Herbal remedies including garlic, ginkgo and ginseng increase the risk of bleeding, but are not contraindicated for regional anesthesia. No contraindication exists for patients taking aspirin, NSAIDs, or subcutaneous heparin. Thrombolytic therapy is an absolute contraindication for regional anesthesia.

Ref: Butterworth, J.F., Mackey, D.C., & Wasnick, J.D. (2013). Ch 45 *Morgan & Mikhail's Clinical Anesthesiology* (5th ed.). New York, NY: McGraw-Hill.

Miller, R.D., & Pardo, M.C. (2011). Ch 17 *Basics of Anesthesia* (6th ed.). Philadelphia, PA: Elsevier.

Nagelhout, J.J., & Plaus, K.L. (2014). Ch 44 *Nurse Anesthesia* (5th ed.). St. Louis, MO: Elsevier.

143. What factor least affects the spread of spinal local anesthetic?

(A) Baricity

(B) Drug dosage

(C) Site of injection

(D) Drug volume

Rationale: While each of the factors affects the spread of local anesthetic in the CSF, drug volume least affects the spread. Other factors influencing the spread of spinal local anesthetic include age, curvature of the spine, intraabdominal pressure, needle direction, patient height, and pregnancy.

TABLE 3-12. Factors affecting the dermatomal spread of spinal anesthesia.

Most important factors
Baricity of anesthetic solution
Position of the patient
    During injection
    Immediately after injection
Drug dosage
Site of injection

Other factors
Age
Cerebrospinal fluid
Curvature of the spine
Drug volume
Intraabdominal pressure
Needle direction
Patient height
Pregnancy

Ref: Butterworth, J.F., Mackey, D.C., & Wasnick, J.D. (2013). Ch 45 *Morgan & Mikhail's Clinical Anesthesiology* (5th ed.). New York, NY: McGraw-Hill.

Miller, R.D., & Pardo, M.C. (2011). Ch 17 *Basics of Anesthesia* (6th ed.). Philadelphia, PA: Elsevier.

Nagelhout, J.J., & Plaus, K.L. (2014). Ch 44 *Nurse Anesthesia* (5th ed.). St. Louis, MO: Elsevier.

144. How do transient neurologic symptoms (TNS) differ from cauda equina syndrome?

(A) TNS persists for several weeks following surgery.

(B) Cauda equina syndrome disappears within 10 days following surgery.

(C) TNS symptoms spontaneously disappear.

(D) Cauda equina syndrome symptoms include severe radicular back pain.

Rationale: Cauda equine syndrome is a persistent condition that results in lower extremity weakness, bowel and bladder dysfunction. TNS occurs within 24 hours of surgery. Mild to severe radicular back pain results, but symptoms spontaneously disappear.

Ref: Butterworth, J.F., Mackey, D.C., & Wasnick, J.D. (2013). Ch 45 *Morgan & Mikhail's Clinical Anesthesiology* (5th ed.). New York, NY: McGraw-Hill.

Miller, R.D., & Pardo, M.C. (2011). Ch 17 *Basics of Anesthesia* (6th ed.). Philadelphia, PA: Elsevier.

145. What local anesthetic is linked to cauda equnia syndrome?

(A) Ropivacaine

(B) Bupivacaine

(C) Tetracaine

(D) Lidocaine

Rationale: Administration of spinal lidocaine and epidural 2-chloroprocaine (inadvertent dural puncture) has been implicated in cauda equina syndrome as well as transient neurological symptoms.

Ref: Butterworth, J.F., Mackey, D.C., & Wasnick, J.D. (2013). Ch 45 *Morgan & Mikhail's Clinical Anesthesiology* (5th ed.). New York, NY: McGraw-Hill.

Miller, R.D., & Pardo, M.C. (2011). Ch 17 *Basics of Anesthesia* (6th ed.). Philadelphia, PA: Elsevier.

Nagelhout, J.J., & Plaus, K.L. (2014). Ch 44 *Nurse Anesthesia* (5th ed.). St. Louis, MO: Elsevier Saunders.

146. Spinal anesthesia using tetracaine 12 mg is given for a patient undergoing a transurethral resection of the prostate. If you add epinephrine what is the longest anticipated duration?

(A) 0.5 hour

(B) 1 hour

(C) 2 hours

(D) 3 hours

Rationale: Addition of epinephrine to tetracaine extends the duration of action from 2-4 hours.

TABLE 3-13. Dosages and actions of commonly used spinal anesthetic agents.

Drug	Preparation	Doses (mg)			Duration (min)	
		Perineum, Lower Limbs	Lower Abdomen	Upper Abdomen	Plain	Epinephrine
Procaine	10% solution	75	125	200	45	60
Bupivacaine	0.75% in 8.25% dextrose	4-10	12-14	12-18	90-120	100-150
Tetracaine	1% solution in 10% glucose	4-8	10-12	10-16	90-120	120-240
Lidocaine[1]	5% in 7.5% glucose	25-50	50-75	75-100	60-75	60-90

[1]No longer widely used for outpatients, particularly those undergoing surgery in the lithotomy position.

Ref: Butterworth, J.F., Mackey, D.C., & Wasnick, J.D. (2013). Ch 45 *Morgan & Mikhail's Clinical Anesthesiology* (5th ed.). New York, NY: McGraw-Hill.

Miller, R.D., & Pardo, M.C. (2011). Ch 17 *Basics of Anesthesia* (6th ed.). Philadelphia, PA: Elsevier.

Nagelhout, J.J., & Plaus, K.L. (2014). Ch 44 *Nurse Anesthesia* (5th ed.). St. Louis, MO: Elsevier.

147. Which clotting factor is the first to become inactivated shortly after a patient has begun warfarin therapy?

    (A) IV
    (B) V
    (C) VII
    (D) IX

    Rationale: Because factor VII has the shortest half-life (4-6 hours), it is the first factor to become inactivated after a patient begins treatment with warfarin.

    Ref: Butterworth, J.F., Mackey, D.C., & Wasnick, J.D. (2013). Ch 32 *Morgan & Mikhail's Clinical Anesthesiology* (5th ed.). New York, NY: McGraw-Hill.

    Barash, P.G., Cullen, B.F., Stoelting, R.K., Calahan, M.K., & Stock, M.C. (2009). Ch 16 *Clinical Anesthesia* (6th ed.). Philadelphia, PA: Lippincott Williams & Wilkins.

148. Following administration of 15 mg spinal bupivacaine, the patient's heart rate and blood pressure fall precipitously. What is the cause?

    (A) Sympathetic blockade
    (B) Motor blockade
    (C) Sensory blockade
    (D) Sensory and motor blockade

    Rationale: Administration of a spinal anesthetic may cause blocking the cardiac accelerators (T1–T4) and decreasing venous return with resultant bradycardia. Venous return, cardiac output and systemic vascular resistance decrease in response to sympathetic nervous system blockade.

    Ref: Butterworth, J.F., Mackey, D.C., & Wasnick, J.D. (2013). Ch 45 *Morgan & Mikhail's Clinical Anesthesiology* (5th ed.). New York, NY: McGraw-Hill.

149. A patient states that their feet are numb following administration of an epidural test dose. What is the most likely cause?

    (A) Intravascular injection
    (B) Local anesthetic toxicity
    (C) Intrathecal injection
    (D) Normal response to a test dose

    Rationale: The test dose determines correct epidural needle placement. Inadvertent injection of an epidural test dose into the intrathecal space results in signs and symptoms consistent with a spinal anesthetic. Intravascular injection is demonstrated by tachycardia.

    Ref: Butterworth, J.F., Mackey, D.C., & Wasnick, J.D. (2013). Ch 45 *Morgan & Mikhail's Clinical Anesthesiology* (5th ed.). New York, NY: McGraw-Hill.

    Miller, R.D., & Pardo, M.C. (2011). Ch 17 *Basics of Anesthesia* (6th ed.). Philadelphia, PA: Elsevier.

    Nagelhout, J.J., & Plaus, K.L. (2014). Ch 44 *Nurse Anesthesia* (5th ed.). St. Louis, MO: Elsevier.

150. Twenty-four hours following an epidural anesthetic the patient complains of occipital headache, nausea, vomiting, and double vision. What is the most likely cause?

(A) Neurologic injury

(B) Spinal hematoma

(C) Epidural hematoma

(D) Postdural puncture headache

Rationale: Signs and symptoms are consistent with a postdural puncture headache. Specifically, a headache associated with changes in position (i.e., sitting or standing worsens the pain). Sharp back and leg pain with accompanying motor weakness are symptoms of spinal or epidural hematoma.

Ref: Butterworth, J.F., Mackey, D.C., & Wasnick, J.D. (2013). Ch 45 *Morgan & Mikhail's Clinical Anesthesiology* (5th ed.). New York, NY: McGraw-Hill.

Nagelhout, J.J., & Plaus, K.L. (2014). Ch 44 *Nurse Anesthesia* (5th ed.). St. Louis, MO: Elsevier.

151. What factor does not influence the spread of local anesthetic placed in the epidural space?

(A) Concentration

(B) Dose

(C) Site of injection

(D) Age

Rationale: The dose and site of injection influence the spread of local anesthetic. The density of the block is influenced by the concentration of local anesthetic. With advanced age, the dose of local anesthetic decreases due to anatomical changes. Additional factors that influence the spread of local anesthetic in the epidural space are pregnancy, weight, height, rate of injection, and patient position.

Ref: Butterworth, J.F., Mackey, D.C., & Wasnick, J.D. (2013). Ch 45 *Morgan & Mikhail's Clinical Anesthesiology* (5th ed.). New York, NY: McGraw-Hill.

Miller, R.D., & Pardo, M.C. (2011). Ch 17 *Basics of Anesthesia* (6th ed.). Philadelphia, PA: Elsevier.

Nagelhout, J.J., & Plaus, K.L. (2014). Ch 44 *Nurse Anesthesia* (5th ed.). St. Louis, MO: Elsevier.

152. A patient is scheduled for a thoracotomy. A thoracic epidural is placed. What volume of local anesthetic will you use?

(A) 15 mL

(B) 10 mL

(C) 18 mL

(D) 20 mL

Rationale: Cervical and thoracic epidural volume is calculated based upon 0.7-1.0 mL/segment. For lumbar epidural anesthesia, 1-2 mL/segment volume is administered.

Ref: Butterworth, J.F., Mackey, D.C., & Wasnick, J.D. (2013). Ch 45 *Morgan & Mikhail's Clinical Anesthesiology* (5th ed.). New York, NY: McGraw-Hill.

Miller, R.D., & Pardo, M.C. (2011). Ch 17 *Basics of Anesthesia* (6th ed.). Philadelphia, PA: Elsevier.

Nagelhout, J.J., & Plaus, K.L. (2014). Ch 44 *Nurse Anesthesia* (5th ed.). St. Louis, MO: Elsevier.

153. What is the best approach to avoiding cardiac arrest during spinal anesthesia?

(A) Decrease preload

(B) Give prophylactic ephedrine

(C) Increase preload

(D) Give prophylactic atropine

Rationale: Preload is essential when administering spinal and epidural anesthesia. Giving a fluid bolus improves preload in light of a sympathetic blockade. When significant bradycardia occurs following administration of local anesthetic, give ephedrine and atropine in sequence. These measures will help avoid cardiac arrest.

Ref: Butterworth, J.F., Mackey, D.C., & Wasnick, J.D. (2013). Ch 45 *Morgan & Mikhail's Clinical Anesthesiology* (5th ed.). New York, NY: McGraw-Hill.

Miller, R.D., & Pardo, M.C. (2011). Ch 17 *Basics of Anesthesia* (6th ed.). Philadelphia, PA: Elsevier.

Nagelhout, J.J., & Plaus, K.L. (2014). Ch 44 *Nurse Anesthesia* (5th ed.). St. Louis, MO: Elsevier.

154. What patient is least likely to experience a postdural puncture headache?

(A) 70-year-old male

(B) 40-year-old male

(C) 20-year-old female

(D) 60-year-old female

Rationale: Risk factors linked to post dural puncture headache include age, gender, needle size, and pregnancy. Young females represent the highest risk population. The incidence of PDPH in females is greater than males. The incidence of PDPH is greater in younger versus older populations.

Ref: Butterworth, J.F., Mackey, D.C., & Wasnick, J.D. (2013). Ch 45 *Morgan & Mikhail's Clinical Anesthesiology* (5th ed.). New York, NY: McGraw-Hill.

Miller, R.D., & Pardo, M.C. (2011). Ch 17 *Basics of Anesthesia* (6th ed.). Philadelphia, PA: Elsevier.

Nagelhout, J.J., & Plaus, K.L. (2014). Ch 44 *Nurse Anesthesia* (5th ed.). St. Louis, MO: Elsevier.

155. What ultrasound frequency is used when placing an epidural or spinal?

    (A) 2-5 MHz
    (B) 5-10 MHz
    (C) 10-15 MHz
    (D) 20-25 MHz

    Rationale: The ultrasound probe for peripheral nerve blocks utilizes high frequency. Lower frequency ultrasound probes are used for spinal and epidural placement.

    Ref: Nagelhout, J.J., & K.L., Plaus (2014). Ch 44 *Nurse Anesthesia* (5th ed.). St. Louis, MO: Elsevier.

156. Which statement is true regarding ultrasound for peripheral nerve blocks?

    (A) Structures that appear white on the ultrasound screen are hypoechoic.
    (B) Low frequencies are used for peripheral nerve blocks.
    (C) Structures that appear white on the ultrasound screen are hyperechoic.
    (D) High-frequency transducers offer a low resolution picture.

    Rationale: Hypoechoic refers to dark structures on the ultrasound screen. Higher frequencies are used for peripheral nerve blocks, whereas lower frequencies are used for spinal and epidural anesthesia when ultrasound technology is employed. High-frequency transducers provide high resolution pictures but poor tissue penetration. Low-frequency transducers allow for deeper tissue penetration.

    Ref: Butterworth, J.F., Mackey, D.C., & Wasnick, J.D. (2013). Ch 46 *Morgan & Mikhail's Clinical Anesthesiology* (5th ed.). New York, NY: McGraw-Hill.

    Miller, R.D., & Pardo, M.C. (2011). Ch 18 *Basics of Anesthesia* (6th ed.). Philadelphia, PA: Elsevier.

    Nagelhout, J.J., & Plaus, K.L. (2014). Ch 45 *Nurse Anesthesia* (5th ed.). St. Louis, MO: Elsevier.

157. What is the innervation of the brachial plexus?

    (A) C5–C8 and T1
    (B) C4–C8
    (C) C4–C8 and T1
    (D) C5–C7 and T1–T2

    Rationale: The C4 and T2 innervation is minimal or absent.

    Ref: Butterworth, J.F., Mackey, D.C., & Wasnick, J.D. (2013). Ch 46 *Morgan & Mikhail's Clinical Anesthesiology* (5th ed.). New York, NY: McGraw-Hill.

    Miller, R.D., & Pardo, M.C. (2011). Ch 18 *Basics of Anesthesia* (6th ed.). Philadelphia, PA: Elsevier.

    Nagelhout, J.J., & Plaus, K.L. (2014). Ch 45 *Nurse Anesthesia* (5th ed.). St. Louis, MO: Elsevier.

158. What brachial plexus approach is indicated for a patient undergoing a shoulder surgery?

    (A) Supraclavicular
    (B) Infraclavicular
    (C) Interscalene
    (D) Axillary

    Rationale: Surgeries distal to the mid-humerus employ supraclavicular, infraclavicular, and axillary blocks. The interscalene block is used for surgeries proximal to the humerus including the shoulder.

    Ref: Butterworth, J.F., Mackey, D.C., & Wasnick, J.D. (2013). Ch 46 *Morgan & Mikhail's Clinical Anesthesiology* (5th ed.). New York, NY: McGraw-Hill.

    Miller, R.D., & Pardo, M.C. (2011). Ch 18 *Basics of Anesthesia* (6th ed.). Philadelphia, PA: Elsevier.

    Nagelhout, J.J., & Plaus, K.L. (2014). Ch 45 *Nurse Anesthesia* (5th ed.). St. Louis, MO: Elsevier.

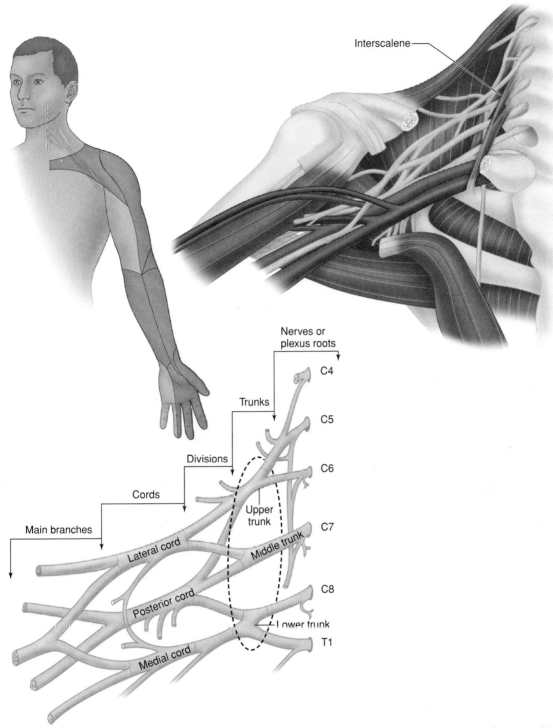

FIG. 3-6. An interscalene block is appropriate for shoulder and proximal humerus procedures. The ventral rami of C5–C8 and T1 form the brachial plexus.

159. Which would result from excessive pressure on the sciatic nerve by the piriformis muscle?

(A) Chronic pain in the perineum with voiding difficulty

(B) Anterior thigh pain and weakness upon standing

(C) Gluteal pain with paresthesia in the posterior thigh

(D) Lumbar vertebral pain exacerbated by flexion of the lower back

Rationale: The sciatic nerve emerges from the greater sciatic foramen immediately approximate to the piriformis muscle. Nerve compression by this muscle results in gluteal pain and posterior paresthesia.

Ref: Butterworth, J.F., Mackey, D.C., & Wasnick, J.D. (2013). Ch 47 *Morgan & Mikhail's Clinical Anesthesiology* (5th ed.). New York, NY: McGraw-Hill.

Moore, K.L., Dalley, A. F., & Agur, A. M. R. (2010). Ch 5 *Clinically oriented anatomy.* Philadelphia, PA: Lippincott Williams & Wilkins.

160. Which of the following is appropriate to use for intravenous regional anesthesia?

(A) 0.5% lidocaine with epinephrine 50 mL

(B) 5.0% lidocaine with epinephrine 40 mL

(C) 0.5% lidocaine 50 mL

(D) 0.5% bupivacaine 50 mL

Rationale: Vasoconstrictors are contraindicated in regional blocks involving extremities. Low versus high local anesthetic concentration is used. In addition, preservatives are contraindicated. Bupivacaine should not be used in light of potential systemic toxicity.

Ref: Butterworth, J.F., Mackey, D.C., & Wasnick, J.D. (2013). Ch 46 *Morgan & Mikhail's Clinical Anesthesiology* (5th ed.). New York, NY: McGraw-Hill.

Miller, R.D., & Pardo, M.C. (2011). Ch 18 *Basics of Anesthesia* (6th ed.). Philadelphia, PA: Elsevier.

Nagelhout, J.J., & Plaus, K.L. (2014). Ch 45 *Nurse Anesthesia* (5th ed.). St. Louis, MO: Elsevier.

161. For which medication is regional anesthesia an absolute contraindication?

(A) Clopidogrel

(B) Unfractionated heparin

(C) Low-molecular-weight heparin

(D) Thrombolytics

Rationale: Regional anesthesia may be performed safely when the waiting period is adhered to for each of the medications except thrombolytics.

Ref: Butterworth, J.F., Mackey, D.C., & Wasnick, J.D. (2013). Ch 45 *Morgan & Mikhail's Clinical Anesthesiology* (5th ed.). New York, NY: McGraw-Hill.

Nagelhout, J.J., & Plaus, K.L. (2014). Ch 44 *Nurse Anesthesia* (5th ed.). St. Louis, MO: Elsevier.

162. The patient received a Bier Block for hand surgery. The case was completed in 10 minutes. When will you deflate the tourniquet?

(A) 10 minutes after the local anesthetic is injected.

(B) 20 minutes after the local anesthetic is injected.

(C) 30 minutes after the local anesthetic is injected.

(D) 40 minutes after the local anesthetic is injected.

Rationale: The tourniquet should remain inflated for a minimum of 20 minutes after the local anesthetic is injected to avoid local anesthetic toxicity.

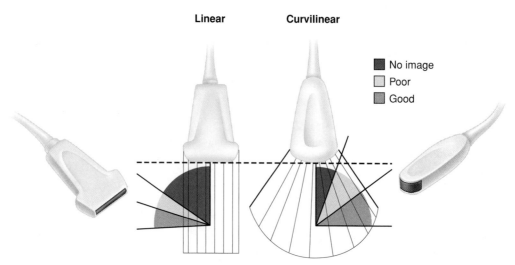

FIG. 3-7. A linear probe offers higher resolution with less penetration. A curvilinear probe provides better penetration with lower resolution.

Ref: Butterworth, J.F., Mackey, D.C., & Wasnick, J.D. (2013). Ch 46 *Morgan & Mikhail's Clinical Anesthesiology* (5th ed.). New York, NY: McGraw-Hill.

Miller, R.D., & Pardo, M.C. (2011). Ch 18 *Basics of Anesthesia* (6th ed.). Philadelphia, PA: Elsevier.

Nagelhout, J.J., & Plaus, K.L. (2014). Ch 45 *Nurse Anesthesia* (5th ed.). St. Louis, MO: Elsevier.

163. What statement is true regarding digital nerve blocks?

    (A) A small gauge needle is inserted at the distal aspect of the selected digit.

    (B) 2-3 mL of lidocaine with epinephrine is used.

    (C) A small gauge needle is inserted at the medial and lateral borders of the base of the selected digit.

    (D) 2-3 mL of lidocaine is used.

    Rationale: The digital block is performed by injecting 2-3 mL of a nonepinephrine containing local anesthetic solution at the base of the selected digit.

    Ref: Butterworth, J.F., Mackey, D.C., & Wasnick, J.D. (2013). Ch 46 *Morgan & Mikhail's Clinical Anesthesiology* (5th ed.). New York, NY: McGraw-Hill.

164. What is the definition of persistent postsurgical pain?

    (A) Pain resulting from outpatient surgery sufficient to require inpatient care

    (B) Pain for > 1-2 weeks following surgery

    (C) Pain for > 1-2 months following surgery

    (D) Pain for > 1 year following surgery

    Rationale: Chronic pain persisting beyond 4-8 weeks following surgery defines persistent postsurgical pain.

    Ref: Butterworth, J.F., Mackey, D.C., & Wasnick, J.D. (2013). Ch 48 *Morgan & Mikhail's Clinical Anesthesiology* (5th ed.). New York, NY: Lange Medical Books McGraw Hill.

    Hemmings, H.C., & T. D. Egan, T.D. (Eds.) (2013). Ch 14 *Pharmacology and physiology for anesthesia: Foundations and clinical application.* Philadelphia, PA: Elsevier.

165. Where is local anesthetic injected in a radial block at the wrist?

    (A) Medial to the ulnar artery at the wrist

    (B) Lateral to the radial artery at the wrist

    (C) Medial to the radial artery at the wrist

    (D) Lateral to the ulnar artery at the wrist

Rationale: The radial nerve block at the wrist requires injecting 3-5 mL of local anesthetic lateral to the radial artery. The ulnar nerve block requires injecting local anesthetic medial to the ulnar artery at the wrist.

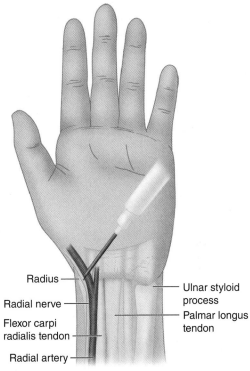

FIG. 3-8. Radial nerve block at the wrist.

Ref: Butterworth, J.F., Mackey, D.C., & Wasnick, J.D. (2013). Ch 46 *Morgan & Mikhail's Clinical Anesthesiology* (5th ed.). New York, NY: McGraw-Hill.

166. Which nerve provides sensation to the anteromedial foot and medial lower leg?

    (A) Deep peroneal

    (B) Sural

    (C) Superficial peroneal

    (D) Saphenous

Rationale: The deep peroneal nerve provides sensation to webbing between the first and second digits. The superficial personal nerve supplies sensation to the dorsum of the foot and toes. The sural nerve provides sensation to the lateral foot.

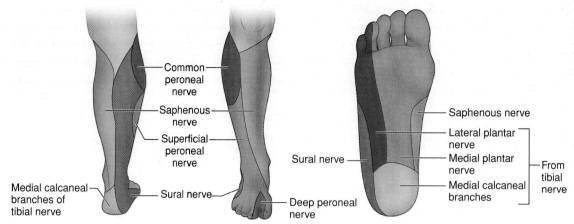

FIG. 3-9. Cutaneous innervation of the foot.

Ref: Butterworth, J.F., Mackey, D.C., & Wasnick, J.D. (2013). Ch 46 *Morgan & Mikhail's Clinical Anesthesiology* (5th ed.). New York, NY: Lange Medical Books McGraw-Hill.
Nagelhout, J.J., & Plaus, K.L. (2014). Ch 45 *Nurse Anesthesia* (5th ed.). St. Louis, MO: Elsevier.

167. Calculate the Aldrete Score for a patient with the following criteria:

SpO_2 >92% (room air); shallow breathing; blood pressure +/−20 mmHg of normal; arousable on calling, and moves all extremities.

Answer: 8

Rationale: The Aldrete Score provides discharge criteria. Each criterion (Oxygenation, respiration, circulation, consciousness, and activity earn 2 points maximum. Full deep breathing and coughing receive 2 points as compared to shallow or limited breathing (1 point). A fully awake patient receives 2 points as compared to a patient who arouses on calling (1 point).

Ref: Butterworth, J.F., Mackey, D.C., & Wasnick, J.D. (2013). Ch 56 *Morgan & Mikhail's Clinical Anesthiology* (5th ed.). New York, NY: McGraw-Hill.
Nagelhout, J.J., & Plaus, K.L. (2014). Ch 50 *Nurse Anesthesia* (5th ed.). St. Louis, MO: Elsevier.

TABLE 3-14. Postanesthetic Aldrete recovery score.[1,2]

Original Criteria	Modified Criteria	Point Value
Color	**Oxygenation**	
Pink	SpO_2 > 92% on room air	2
Pale or dusky	SpO_2 > 90% on oxygen	1
Cyanotic	SpO_2 < 90% on oxygen	0
Respiration		
Can breathe deeply and cough	Breathes deeply and coughs freely	2
Shallow but adequate exchange	Dyspneic, shallow or limited breathing	1
Apnea or obstruction	Apnea	0
Circulation		
Blood pressure within 20% of normal	Blood pressure ± 20 mm Hg of normal	2
Blood pressure within 20-50% of normal	Blood pressure ± 20-50 mm Hg of normal	1
Blood pressure deviating >50% from normal	Blood pressure > ± 50 mm Hg of normal	0
Consciousness		
Awake, alert, and oriented	Fully awake	2
Arousable but readily drifts back to sleep	Arousable on calling	1
No response	Not responsive	0
Activity		
Moves all extremities	Same	2
Moves two extremities	Same	1
No movement	Same	0

[1]Data from Aldrete JA, Kronlik D: A postanesthetic recovery score. Anesth Analg 1970;49:924 and Aldrete JA: The postanesthesia recovery score revisited. J Clin Anesth 1995;7:89.

[2]Ideally, the patient should be discharged when the total score is 10, but a minimum of 9 is required.

168. What artery provides the majority of the blood supply to the anterior, lower 2/3 of the spinal cord?

(A) Posterior spinal artery

(B) Artery of Adamkiewicz

(C) Posterior inferior cerebellar artery

(D) Intercostal arteries

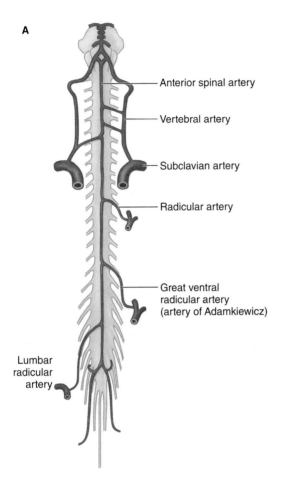

A

— Anterior spinal artery

— Vertebral artery

— Subclavian artery

— Radicular artery

— Great ventral radicular artery (artery of Adamkiewicz)

Lumbar radicular artery

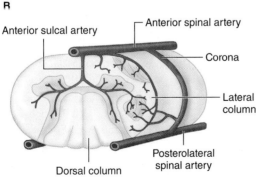

R

Anterior sulcal artery

— Anterior spinal artery

— Corona

— Lateral column

Dorsal column

Posterolateral spinal artery

FIG. 3-10. Arterial supply to the spinal cord. **A:** Anterior view showing principal sources of blood supply. **B:** Cross-sectional view through the spinal cord showing paired posterior spinal arteries and a single anterior spinal artery. (Adapted and reproduced, with permission, from Waxman SG: *Correlative Neuroanatomy*, 24th ed. McGraw-Hill, 2000.)

Rationale: Blood flow to the posterior 1/3 of the spinal cord is provided by the posterior spinal artery. The posterior inferior cerebellar artery feeds the posterior spinal arteries. The intercostal arteries provide blood flow to the anterior and posterior spinal arteries. The largest of the arteries supplying the spinal cord is the arteria radicularis magna (Artery of Adamkiewicz).

Ref: Butterworth, J.F., Mackey, D.C., & Wasnick, J.D. (2013). Ch 45 *Morgan & Mikhail's Clinical Anesthesiology* (5th ed.). New York, NY: McGraw-Hill.
Miller, R.D., & Pardo, M.C. (2011). Ch 17 *Basics of Anesthesia* (6th ed.). Philadelphia, PA: Elsevier.

169. After placing a spinal anesthetic the sensory block is assessed at T8. Where is the most likely level of the motor block?

(A) T4

(B) T6

(C) T10

(D) T2

Rationale: A motor block typically is typically two or more segments below the sensory block.

Ref: Butterworth, J.F., Mackey, D.C., & Wasnick, J.D. (2013). Ch 45 *Morgan & Mikhail's Clinical Anesthesiology* (5th ed.). New York, NY: McGraw-Hill.
Miller, R.D., & Pardo, M.C. (2011). Ch 17 *Basics of Anesthesia* (6th ed.). Philadelphia, PA: Elsevier.
Nagelhout, J.J., & Plaus, K.L. (2014). Ch 44 *Nurse Anesthesia* (5th ed.). St. Louis, MO: Elsevier.

170. Which of the following characterize A-*a* nerve fibers?

Select (3) three

(A) Diameter 0.5-1 μm

(B) Heavy myelination

(C) Diameter 15-20 μm

(D) Motor function

E) Light myelination

F) Pain and temperature

Rationale: B fibers are lightly myelinated, 1-4 μm in diameter possessing preganglionic and autonomic function. C fibers are not myelinated, 0.5-1 μm in diameter and are responsible for touch and temperature sensation.

Ref: Nagelhout, J.J., & Plaus, K.L. (2014). Ch 44 *Nurse Anesthesia* (5th ed.). St. Louis, MO: Elsevier.

171. Following administration of spinal anesthesia the patient becomes hypotensive and bradycardic. What nerve fibers are affected?

(A) T1–T4
(B) T5–T6
(C) T7–T8
(D) T10–T12

Rationale: Blocking the cardiac accelerator fibers results in bradycardia and hypotension.

Ref: Butterworth, J.F., Mackey, D.C., & Wasnick, J.D. (2013). Ch 45 *Morgan & Mikhail's Clinical Anesthesiology* (5ᵗʰ ed.). New York, NY: McGraw-Hill.

Miller, R.D., & Pardo, M.C. (2011). Ch 17 *Basics of Anesthesia* (6ᵗʰ ed.). Philadelphia, PA: Elsevier.

Nagelhout, J.J., & Plaus, K.L. (2014). Ch 44 *Nurse Anesthesia* (5ᵗʰ ed.). St. Louis, MO: Elsevier.

172. Which clotting factor is not synthesized in the liver?

(A) II
(B) IV
(C) VII
(D) VIII

Rationale: Most clotting factors are synthesized in the liver except factor VIII, that is, von Willebrand factor, which is synthesized by vascular endothelial cells.

Ref: Butterworth, J.F., Mackey, D.C., & Wasnick, J.D. (2013). Ch 32 *Morgan & Mikhail's Clinical Anesthesiology* (5ᵗʰ ed.). New York, NY: McGraw-Hill.

Barash, P.G., Cullen, B.F., Stoelting, R.K., Calahan, M.K., & Stock, M.C. (2009). Ch 16 *Clinical Anesthesia* (6ᵗʰ ed.). Philadelphia, PA: Lippincott Williams & Wilkins.

173. A 70-year-old patient with emphysema is undergoing an open cholecystectomy. What is the best anesthetic choice for this patient?

(A) Spinal
(B) Epidural
(C) General
(D) MAC

Rationale: Regional anesthesia is used with caution for patients with pulmonary disease, specifically for surgical procedures above the umbilicus. The patient would benefit, however, from epidural analgesia.

Ref: Butterworth, J.F., Mackey, D.C., & Wasnick, J.D. (2013). Ch 45 *Morgan & Mikhail's Clinical Anesthesiology* (5ᵗʰ ed.). New York, NY: McGraw-Hill.

174. Which of the following are relative contraindications for regional anesthesia?

Select (3) three

(A) Uncooperative patient
(B) Preexisting neurological deficits
(C) Severe aortic stenosis
(D) Patient refusal
(E) Stenotic valvular disease

Rationale: Absolute contraindications for regional anesthesia include severe aortic, mitral stenosis, or hypovolemia; increased intracranial pressure, injection at the site of injection, patient refusal, and bleeding diathesis. Extreme caution is used when considering regional anesthesia for patients with coagulopathies. The risks and benefits must be weighed.

TABLE 3-15. Contraindications to neuraxial blockade.

Absolute
Infection at the site of injection
Patient refusal
Coagulopathy or other bleeding diathesis
Severe hypovolemia
Increased intracranial pressure
Severe aortic stenosis
Severe mitral stenosis

Relative
Sepsis
Uncooperative patient
Preexisting neurological deficits
Demyelinating lesions
Stenotic valvular heart lesions
Left ventricular outflow obstruction (hypertrophic obstructive cardiomyopathy)
Severe spinal deformity

Controversial
Prior back surgery at the site of injection
Complicated surgery
Prolonged operation
Major blood loss
Maneuvers that compromise respiration

Ref: Butterworth, J.F., Mackey, D.C., & Wasnick, J.D. (2013). Ch 45 *Morgan & Mikhail's Clinical Anesthesiology* (5ᵗʰ ed.). New York, NY: McGraw-Hill.

Miller, R.D., & Pardo, M.C. (2011). Ch 17 *Basics of Anesthesia* (6ᵗʰ ed.). Philadelphia, PA: Elsevier.

Nagelhout, J.J., & Plaus, K.L. (2014). Ch 44 *Nurse Anesthesia* (5ᵗʰ ed.). St. Louis, MO: Elsevier.

175. A patient who takes ticlopidine requests a spinal anesthetic for a total knee replacement. What is the waiting period for ticlopidine?

(A) 7 days
(B) 14 days

(C) 48 hour

(D) 8 hour

Rationale: The waiting period to provide regional anesthesia for patients taking antiplatelet drugs varies. The waiting period for clopidogrel is 7 days; abciximab is 48 hours; and eptifibatide is 8 hours.

Ref: Butterworth, J.F., Mackey, D.C., & Wasnick, J.D. (2013). Ch 45 *Morgan & Mikhail's Clinical Anesthesiology* (5th ed.). New York, NY: McGraw-Hill.

Nagelhout, J.J., & Plaus, K.L. (2014). Ch 44 *Nurse Anesthesia* (5th ed.). St. Louis, MO: Elsevier.

176. Where is Tuffier's line located?

    (A) L4

    (B) L2

    (C) L1

    (D) L3

Rationale: Tuffier's line is located just above the iliac crests crossing the L4–5 vertebrae.

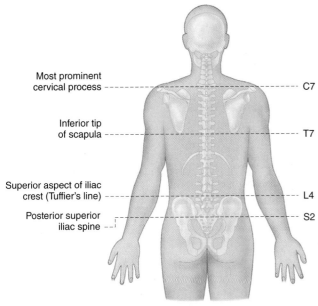

FIG. 3-11. Surface landmarks for identifying spinal levels.

    Ref: Butterworth, J.F., Mackey, D.C., & Wasnick, J.D. (2013). Ch 45 *Morgan & Mikhail's Clinical Anesthesiology* (5th ed.). New York, NY: McGraw-Hill.

Miller, R.D., & Pardo, M.C. (2011). Ch 17 *Basics of Anesthesia* (6th ed.). Philadelphia, PA: Elsevier.

177. What is the correct order of anatomical structure used when placing an epidural needle?

    (A) Skin, subcutaneous tissue, supraspinous ligament, interspinous ligament, ligamentum flavum, epidural space

    (B) Skin, subcutaneous tissue, interspinous ligament, supraspinous ligament, ligamentum flavum, epidural space

    (C) Skin, subcutaneous tissue, interspinous ligament, supraspinous ligament, ligamentum flavum, dura, subarachnoid space

    (D) Skin, subcutaneous tissue, interspinous ligament, supraspinous ligament, ligamentum flavum, dura, epidural space

Rationale: Once the needle reaches the epidural space, further advancement penetrates the dura reaching the subarachnoid space and presence of cerebral spinal fluid.

    Ref: Butterworth, J.F., Mackey, D.C., & Wasnick, J.D. (2013). Ch 45 *Morgan & Mikhail's Clinical Anesthesiology* (5th ed.). New York, NY: McGraw-Hill.

Miller, R.D., & Pardo, M.C. (2011). Ch 17 *Basics of Anesthesia* (6th ed.). Philadelphia, PA: Elsevier.

Nagelhout, J.J., & Plaus, K.L. (2014). Ch 44 *Nurse Anesthesia* (5th ed.). St. Louis, MO: Elsevier.

178. Which statement is true of Aδ fibers?

    (A) Aδ fibers are myelinated, synapse in Rexed laminae I and V, and transmit primarily mechanical or thermal pain.

    (B) Aδ fibers are unmyelinated, synapse in Rexed laminae II and VII, and transmit primarily mechanical or thermal pain.

    (C) Aδ fibers are myelinated, synapse in Rexed laminae III and X, and transmit primarily mechanical or thermal pain.

    (D) Aδ fibers are unmyelinated, synapse in Rexed laminae IV and VI, and transmit primarily mechanical or thermal pain.

Rationale: Aδ fibers are myelinated, terminate in laminae I and V, and respond to mechanical and thermal stimuli.

    Ref: Butterworth, J.F., Mackey, D.C., & Wasnick, J.D. (2013). Ch 47 *Morgan & Mikhail's Clinical Anesthesiology* (5th ed.). New York, NY: McGraw-Hill.

Hall, J.E. (2011). Ch 48 Guyton and Hall *Textbook of Medical Physiology* (12th ed.). Philadelphia, PA: Elsevier.

179. Which laminae receive input from C fibers?

    (A) III, IV, VI

    (B) I, VI, X

    (C) II, VII, IX

    (D) I, II, V

Rationale: Signals from C fibers travel to laminae I, II, V.

Ref: Butterworth, J.F., Mackey, D.C., & Wasnick, J.D. (2013). Ch 47 *Morgan & Mikhail's Clinical Anesthesiology* (5th ed.). New York, NY: McGraw-Hill.

Nagelhout, J.J., & Plaus, K.L. (2014). Ch 51 *Nurse Anesthesia* (5th ed.). St. Louis, MO: Elsevier.

180. How would postoperative pain localized to the site of skin incision be classified?

(A) Visceral pain

(B) Deep somatic pain

(C) Superficial somatic pain

(D) Referred pain

Rationale: This is an example of acute superficial somatic pain.

Ref: Butterworth, J.F., Mackey, D.C., & Wasnick, J.D. (2013). Ch 47 *Morgan & Mikhail's Clinical Anesthesiology* (5th ed.). New York, NY: McGraw-Hill.

Hall, J.E. (2011). Ch 47 *Guyton and Hall Textbook of Medical Physiology* (12th ed.). Philadelphia, PA: Saunders.

181. Referred pain from the diaphragm can be expected in which dermatome?

(A) C4

(B) C7

(C) T4

(D) T7

Rationale: Diaphragmatic innervation originates in cervical levels 3, 4, and 5.

TABLE 3-16. Patterns of referred pain.

Location	Cutaneous Dermatome
Central diaphragm	C4
Lungs	T2–T6
Aorta	T1–L2
Heart	T1–T4
Esophagus	T3–T8
Pancreas and spleen	T5–T10
Stomach, liver, and gallbladder	T6–T9
Adrenals	T8–L1
Small intestine	T9–T11
Colon	T10–L1
Kidney, ovaries, and testes	T10–L1
Ureters	T10–T12
Uterus	T11–L2
Bladder and prostate	S2–S4
Urethra and rectum	S2–S4

Ref: Butterworth, J.F., Mackey, D.C., & Wasnick, J.D. (2013). Ch 47 *Morgan & Mikhail's Clinical Anesthesiology* (5th ed.). New York, NY: McGraw-Hill.

Moore, K.L., Dalley, A.F., & Agur, A.M.R. (2010). Ch 2 *Clinically Oriented Anatomy*. Philadelphia, PA: Lippincott Williams & Wilkins.

182. What is the surface landmark of the fourth cervical cutaneous dermatome?

(A) Anterior neck

(B) Shoulder

(C) Biceps

(D) Xiphoid

Rationale: Referred diaphragm pain occurs in the shoulder due to innervation at C3–C5.

Ref: Butterworth, J.F., Mackey, D.C., & Wasnick, J.D. (2013). Ch 47 *Morgan & Mikhail's Clinical Anesthesiology* (5th ed.). New York, NY: McGraw-Hill.

Moore, K.L., Dalley, A.F., & Agur, A.M.R. (2010). Ch 1 *Clinically Oriented Anatomy*. Philadelphia, PA: Lippincott Williams & Wilkins.

183. Which act to diminish pain signals?

Select (2) two

(A) Glutamate

(B) Enkephalin

(C) Substance P

(D) ß-Endorphin

Rationale: Endogenous opioids modulate pain by decreasing severity.

TABLE 3-17. Major neurotransmitters mediating or modulating pain.

Neurotransmitter	Receptor[1]	Effect on Nociception
Substance P	Neurokinin–1	Excitatory
Calcitonin gene-related peptide		Excitatory
Glutamate	NMDA, AMPA, kainate, quisqualate	Excitatory
Aspartate	NMDA, AMPA, kainate, quisqualate	Excitatory
Adenosine triphosphate (ATP)	P_1, P_2	Excitatory
Somatostatin		Inhibitory
Acetylcholine	Muscarinic	Inhibitory
Enkephalins	μ, δ, κ	Inhibitory
β-Endorphin	μ, δ, κ	Inhibitory
Norepinephrine	α_2	Inhibitory

TABLE 3-17. Major neurotransmitters mediating or modulating pain. (Continued)

Neurotransmitter	Receptor[1]	Effect on Nociception
Adenosine	A₁	Inhibitory
Serotonin	5-HT₁ (5-HT₃)	Inhibitory
γ-Aminobutyric acid (GABA)	A, B	Inhibitory
Glycine		Inhibitory

[1]NMDA, N-methyl-D-aspartate; AMPA, 2-(aminomethyl)phenylacetic acid; 5-HT, 5-hydroxytryptamine.

Ref: Butterworth, J.F., Mackey, D.C., & Wasnick, J.D. (2013). Ch 47 *Morgan & Mikhail's Clinical Anesthesiology* (5th ed.). New York, NY: McGraw-Hill.

Hall, J.E. (2011). Ch 48 *Guyton and Hall textbook of medical physiology* (12th ed.). Philadelphia, PA: Saunders.

184. What complication is associated with using 6% hetastarch in volumes > 20 mL/kg?

   (A) Interference with blood typing

   (B) Coagulopathy

   (C) Kidney failure

   (D) Anaphylaxis

   Rationale: Hetastarch in doses > 20 mL/kg has been known to produce coagulopathy. Dextran I doses > 20 mL/kg is associated with interference with blood typing and kidney failure. Unlike dextran, which is antigenic and known to cause anaphylaxis, hetastarch is nonantigenic.

   Ref: Butterworth, J.F., Mackey, D.C., & Wasnick, J.D. (2013). Ch 51 *Morgan & Mikhail's Clinical Anesthesiology* (5th ed.). New York, NY: McGraw-Hill.

   Barash, P.G., Cullen, B.F., Stoelting, R.K., Calahan, M.K., & Stock, M.C. (2009). Ch 16 *Clinical Anesthesia* (6th ed.). Philadelphia, PA: Lippincott Williams & Wilkins.

185. Which portion of the spinal cord is most associated with transmission of pain signals?

   (A) Dorsal horn

   (B) Central canal

   (C) Ventral horn

   (D) Pia mater

   Rationale: The proximal portion of pain receptors terminate in the dorsal horn.

Ref: Butterworth, J.F., Mackey, D.C., & Wasnick, J.D. (2013). Ch 47 *Morgan & Mikhail's Clinical Anesthesiology* (5th ed.). New York, NY: McGraw-Hill.

Hemmings, H.C., & T. D. Egan, T.D. (Eds.) (2013). Ch 14 *Pharmacology and Physiology for Anesthesia: Foundations and Clinical Application*. Philadelphia, PA: Elsevier.

186. Which of the following does not relieve pain by decreasing inflammation?

   (A) Acetaminophen

   (B) Ketorolac

   (C) Ibuprofen

   (D) Celecoxib

   Rationale: Acetaminophen does not exert an anti-inflammatory effect.

   Ref: Butterworth, J.F., Mackey, D.C., & Wasnick, J.D. (2013). Ch 10 *Morgan & Mikhail's Clinical Anesthesiology* (5th ed.). New York, NY: McGraw-Hill.

   Hemmings, H.C., & Egan, T.D. (Eds.) (2013). Ch 16 *Pharmacology and Physiology for Anesthesia: Foundations and Clinical Application*. Philadelphia, PA: Elsevier.

187. Which are mechanisms of action for gabapentin?

   Select (2) two

   (A) GABA agonist effect

   (B) Calcium channel blockade

   (C) Excitatory neurotransmitter inhibition

   (D) Inhibition of prostaglandin synthesis

   Rationale: Possible mechanisms include calcium or sodium channel blockade and inhibition of excitatory neurotransmitters in the central nervous system.

   Ref: Butterworth, J.F., Mackey, D.C., & Wasnick, J.D. (2013). Ch 47 *Morgan & Mikhail's Clinical Anesthesiology* (5th ed.). New York, NY: McGraw-Hill.

   Hemmings, H.C., & Egan, T.D. (Eds.) (2013). Ch 16 *Pharmacology and Physiology for Anesthesia: Foundations and Clinical Application*. Philadelphia, PA: Elsevier.

188. Which of these analgesic agents is a GABA agonist?

   (A) Baclofen

   (B) Pregabalin

   (C) Dexmedetomidine

   (D) Celecoxib

Rationale: Baclofen is a GABA agonist.

Ref: Butterworth, J.F., Mackey, D.C., & Wasnick, J.D. (2013). Ch 47 *Morgan & Mikhail's Clinical Anesthesiology* (5th ed.). New York, NY: McGraw-Hill.

Miller, R.D., Eriksson, L.I., Fleisher, L.A., Weiner-Kronish, J.P., & Young, W.L. (Eds.) (2010). Ch 58 *Miller's Anesthesia* (7th ed.). Philadelphia, PA: Elsevier.

189. What is the most common level of approach to perform a stellate ganglion block?

    (A) C3

    (B) C4

    (C) C5

    (D) C6

Rationale: An anterior approach is made toward Chassaignac's tubercle, which is the transverse process of C6.

Ref: Butterworth, J.F., Mackey, D.C., & Wasnick, J.D. (2013). Ch 47 *Morgan & Mikhail's Clinical Anesthesiology* (5th ed.). New York, NY: McGraw-Hill.

Brown, D.L. (2006). Ch 26 *Atlas of Regional Anesthesia* (4th ed.). Philadelphia, PA: Elsevier.

190. What are mechanisms of action for duloxetine?

Select (2) two

    (A) Monoamine oxidase inhibition

    (B) Serotonin reuptake inhibition

    (C) α_2 receptor agonist effect

    (D) Norepinephrine reuptake inhibition

Rationale: This drug inhibits serotonin and norepinephrine reuptake.

Ref: Butterworth, J.F., Mackey, D.C., & Wasnick, J.D. (2013). Ch 47 *Morgan & Mikhail's Clinical Anesthesiology* (5th ed.). New York, NY: McGraw-Hill.

Nagelhout, J.J., & Plaus, K.L. (2014). Ch 51 *Nurse Anesthesia* (5th ed.). St. Louis, MO: Elsevier.

191. Which is an α_2 agonist?

    (A) Carbamazepine

    (B) Tapentadol

    (C) Phenytoin

    (D) Tizanidine

Rationale: Tizanidine is an α_2 agonist sometimes useful in spastic pain.

Ref: Butterworth, J.F., Mackey, D.C., & Wasnick, J.D. (2013). Ch 47 *Morgan & Mikhail's Clinical Anesthesiology* (5th ed.). New York, NY: McGraw-Hill.

Brunton, C. Chabner, & B. Knollman (Eds.) (2011). Ch 12 *Goodman & Gilman's The Pharmacological Basis of Therapeutics* (12th ed.). New York, NY: McGraw-Hill.

192. Which route of administration of fentanyl is subject to the hepatic first-pass effect?

    (A) Transdermal patch

    (B) Intravenous injection

    (C) Sublingual spray

    (D) Oral tablet

Rationale: Gastrointestinal absorption is subject to hepatic first-pass effect.

Ref: Butterworth, J.F., Mackey, D.C., & Wasnick, J.D. (2013). Ch 47 *Morgan & Mikhail's Clinical Anesthesiology* (5th ed.). New York, NY: McGraw-Hill.

Stoelting, R.K., & Hillier, S.C. (Eds.) (2006). Ch 1 *Pharmacology & Physiology in Anesthetic Practice* (4th ed.). Philadelphia, PA: Lippincott Williams & Wilkins.

193. What would be the correct classification of hyperalgesia with sympathetic dysfunction following a traumatic injury that included direct nerve damage persisting beyond the standard healing period in the absence of other conditions that may be responsible for the pain?

    (A) Complex regional pain syndrome type I

    (B) Reflex sympathetic dystrophy

    (C) Complex regional pain syndrome type II

    (D) Persistent allodynia

Rationale: Precipitating injury to the nerve itself identifies complex regional pain syndrome type II. Type I does not include distinct injury to the nerve. Reflex sympathetic dystrophy is a synonym for type I.

Ref: Butterworth, J.F., Mackey, D.C., & Wasnick, J.D. (2013). Ch 47 *Morgan & Mikhail's Clinical Anesthesiology* (5th ed.). New York, NY: McGraw-Hill.

Miller, R., & Pardo, M. Jr. (Eds.) (2011). Ch 43 *Basics of anesthesia* (6th ed.). Philadelphia, PA: Elsevier.

194. Following placement of a stellate ganglion block the patient becomes hoarse. What has occurred?

    (A) Phrenic nerve block

    (B) Recurrent laryngeal nerve block

    (C) Subdural injection

    (D) Pneumothorax

Rationale: Unilateral recurrent laryngeal nerve block results in hoarseness.

Ref: Butterworth, J.F., Mackey, D.C., & Wasnick, J.D. (2013). Ch 47 *Morgan & Mikhail's Clinical Anesthesiology* (5th ed.). New York, NY: McGraw-Hill.

Brown, D.L. (2010). Ch 28 *Atlas of regional anesthesia* (4th ed.). Philadelphia, PA: Elsevier.

195. Which are appropriate for inclusion in an epidural steroid injection?

Select (3) three

(A) Saline

(B) Methylprednisolone acetate

(C) Triamcinolone diacetate

(D) Fentanyl

Rationale: Opioids are not indicated.

Ref: Butterworth, J.F., Mackey, D.C., & Wasnick, J.D. (2013). Ch 47 *Morgan & Mikhail's Clinical Anesthesiology* (5th ed.). New York, NY: McGraw-Hill.

Longnecker, D., Brown, D., Newman, M., & Zapol, W. (Eds.) (2012). Ch 92 *Anesthesiology* (2nd ed.), New York, NY: McGraw-Hill.

196. Which steroid has the smallest particulate size?

(A) Methylprednisolone acetate

(B) Triamcinolone diacetate

(C) Dexamethasone sodium phosphate

(D) Betamethasone

Rationale: Dexamethasone has the smallest particulate size, which minimizes the risk of vasoocclusive complications if inadvertently injected into a vessel during an epidural steroid injection.

Ref: Butterworth, J.F., Mackey, D.C., & Wasnick, J.D. (2013). Ch 47 *Morgan & Mikhail's Clinical Anesthesiology* (5th ed.). New York, NY: McGraw-Hill.

Longnecker, D., Brown, D., Newman, M., & Zapol, W. (Eds.) (2012). Ch 92 *Anesthesiology* (2nd ed.), New York, NY: McGraw-Hlll.

197. What is the maximal volume of solution that can be safely injected into the lumbar facet joint?

(A) 1 mL

(B) 2 mL

(C) 3 mL

(D) 4 mL

Rationale: Intra-articular facet injection should be limited to 1-1.5 mL total volume to avoid damage to the capsule.

Ref: Butterworth, J.F., Mackey, D.C., & Wasnick, J.D. (2013). Ch 47 *Morgan & Mikhail's Clinical Anesthesiology* (5th ed.). New York, NY: McGraw-Hill.

Longnecker, D., Brown, D., Newman, M., & Zapol, W. (Eds.) (2012). Ch 92, *Anesthesiology* (2nd ed.), New York, NY: McGraw-Hill.

198. Which is an indication for a celiac plexus block?

(A) Post-traumatic hypoperfusion of the arm

(B) Lower extremity vascular insufficiency

(C) Intractable lumbar pain

(D) Pain resulting from pancreatic malignancy

Rationale: Pain associated with an intra-abdominal malignancy is a primary indication for this intervention.

Ref: Butterworth, J.F., Mackey, D.C., & Wasnick, J.D. (2013). Ch 47 *Morgan & Mikhail's Clinical Anesthesiology* (5th ed.). New York, NY: McGraw-Hill.

Miller, R.D., Eriksson, L.I., Fleisher, L.A., Weiner-Kronish, J.P., & Young, W.L. (Eds.) (2010). Ch 58 *Miller's Anesthesia* (7th ed.). Philadelphia, PA: Elsevier.

Longnecker, D., Brown, D., Newman, M., & Zapol, W. (Eds.) (2012). Ch 91 *Anesthesiology* (2nd ed.). New York, NY: McGraw-Hill.

199. Which class of nerve fiber will be the site of therapeutic stimulation for a transcutaneous electrical nerve stimulation (TENS) unit?

(A) Aδ fibers

(B) C fibers

(C) Aß fibers

(D) B fibers

Rationale: TENS units are effective through activation of large diameter afferent fibers such as Aß fibers. Aδ, B, and C fibers all have comparably smaller diameters.

Ref: Butterworth, J.F., Mackey, D.C., & Wasnick, J.D. (2013). Ch 47 *Morgan & Mikhail's Clinical Anesthesiology* (5th ed.). New York, NY: McGraw-Hill.

Longnecker, D., Brown, D., Newman, M., & Zapol, W. (Eds.) (2012). Ch 91 *Anesthesiology* (2nd ed.). New York, NY: McGraw-Hill.

200. When selecting a needle for spinal anesthesia, which type is most likely to cause a post dural puncture headache?

(A) 20-g Quincke

(B) 22-g Whitacre

(C) 22-g Sprotte

(D) 22-g Quincke

Rationale: Cutting needles (Quincke) are more likely to cause postdural puncture headaches as compared to pencil point needles. Larger gauge needles are also more likely to cause postdural puncture headaches.

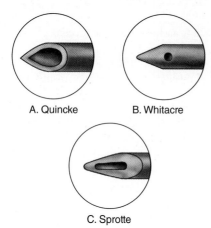

A. Quincke   B. Whitacre

C. Sprotte

FIG. 3-12. Spinal needles.

Ref: Butterworth, J.F., Mackey, D.C., & Wasnick, J.D. (2013). Ch 45 *Morgan & Mikhail's Clinical Anesthesiology* (5th ed.). New York, NY: McGraw-Hill.

Miller, R.D., & Pardo, M.C. (2011). Ch 17 *Basics of Anesthesia* (6th ed.). Philadelphia, PA: Elsevier.

Nagelhout, J.J., & Plaus, K.L. (2014). Ch 44 *Nurse Anesthesia* (5th ed.). St. Louis, MO: Elsevier.

201. An adult patient with moderate aortic regurgitation receives a spinal anesthetic. A blood pressure drop to 68/42 is treated with 100 μg of phenylephrine. How will this dose impact the patient's underlying disease state?

    (A) It will improve the regurgitation.
    (B) It will exacerbate the regurgitation.
    (C) It will have no impact on the regurgitation.
    (D) Phenylephrine is contraindicated in this patient.

    Rationale: Phenylephrine can be used to treat anesthetic-induced hypotension in a patient with aortic regurgitation but the doses should be small and incremental, that is, 25-50 μg. Larger doses such as 100 μg will increase the systemic vascular resistance and exacerbate the regurgitation.
    Ref: Butterworth, J.F., Mackey, D.C., & Wasnick, J.D. (2013). Ch 21 *Morgan & Mikhail's Clinical Anesthesiology* (5th ed.). New York, NY: McGraw-Hill.

    Nagelhout, J.J., & Plaus, K.L. (2014). Ch 23 *Nurse Anesthesia* (5th ed.). St. Louis, MO: Elsevier.

202. Which estimated blood volume is correctly paired with its age group?

    (A) Preterm neonate: 85 mL/kg
    (B) 6-month old: 90 mL/kg
    (C) Adult male: 80 mL/kg
    (D) Adult female: 65 mL/kg

    Rationale: The estimated blood volume for an adult female is 65 mL/kg. The estimated blood volume for a preterm neonate ranges from 95-100 mL/kg; for an infant, 80 mL/kg; and for an adult male, 80 mL/kg.
    Ref: Butterworth, J.F., Mackey, D.C., & Wasnick, J.D. (2013). Ch 51 *Morgan & Mikhail's Clinical Anesthesiology* (5th ed.). New York, NY: Lange Medical Books McGraw-Hill.

    Barash, P.G., Cullen, B.F., Stoelting, R.K., Calahan, M.K., & Stock, M.C. (2009). Ch 45 *Clinical Anesthesia* (6th ed.). Philadelphia, PA: Lippincott Williams & Wilkins.

203. How will the symptoms of an acute hemolytic transfusion reaction manifest in a patient under general anesthesia?

    (A) Fever, unexplained tachycardia, hypotension and diffuse oozing in surgical field
    (B) Nausea, fever, flank pain, unexplained tachycardia, and hypotension
    (C) Hemoglobinuria, chest and flank pain, fever, and hypotension
    (D) Hypertension, unexplained tachycardia, fever, erythema, and hives

    Rationale: Unlike the symptoms of acute hemolytic reaction in awake patients (chills, nausea, fever, chest pain, and flank pain), in anesthetized patients, these symptoms are masked. Symptoms include fever, unexplained tachycardia, hypotension, hemoglobinuria, and diffuse oozing in the surgical field.
    Ref: Butterworth, J.F., Mackey, D.C., & Wasnick, J.D. (2013). Ch 51 *Morgan & Mikhail's Clinical Anesthesiology* (5th ed.). New York, NY: McGraw-Hill.

    Barash, P.G., Cullen, B.F., Stoelting, R.K., Calahan, M.K., & Stock, M.C. (2009). Ch 16 *Clinical Anesthesia* (6th ed.). Philadelphia, PA: Lippincott Williams & Wilkins.

204. An injection of 0.5% ropivacaine is placed into the brachial plexus via the interscalene approach. Which of the following is most likely to be spared?

    (A) Sensation of the radial side of the forearm
    (B) Sensation of the medial upper arm

(C) Sensation of half of the fourth and all of the fifth fingers

(D) Sensation of the palmar surface of the first three fingers

Rationale: The interscalene block of the brachial plexus is the most proximal approach to the brachial plexus and idea for shoulder surgery with advantages of clear landmarks and a low risk of pneumothorax because of the distance to the dome of the pleura.

This approach can be used for forearm and hand surgery; however, blockade of the inferior trunk is typically incomplete. The inferior trunk provides innervation to C8 and T1. Supplementation at the site of the ulnar nerve can assist with providing coverage for that distribution.

Ref: Butterworth, J.F., Mackey, D.C., & Wasnick, J.D. (2013). Ch 46 *Morgan & Mikhail's Clinical Anesthesiology* (5th ed.). New York, NY: McGraw-Hill.

Hadzic, A. (2007). Ch 25 *Textbook of Regional Anesthesia and Acute Pain Management.* New York, NY: McGraw-Hill.

205. How does an opioid inhibit postsynaptic nociceptive signal transmission?

Select (2) two

(A) Hyperpolarization

(B) Excitation

(C) Opening calcium channels

(D) Opening potassium channels

Rationale: Opioids impede postsynaptic signal transmission by opening potassium channels resulting in hyperpolarization.

Ref: Butterworth, J.F., Mackey, D.C., & Wasnick, J.D. (2013). Ch 10 *Morgan & Mikhail's Clinical Anesthesiology* (5th ed.). New York, NY: McGraw-Hill.

Miller, R.D., Eriksson, L.I., Fleisher, L.A., Weiner-Kronish, J.P., & Young, W.L. (Eds.) (2010). Ch 27 *Miller's Anesthesia* (7th ed.). Philadelphia, PA: Elsevier.

206. When administering a spinal anesthetic, which nerve roots are easily blocked?

(A) Smaller, unmyelinated

(B) Larger, myelinated

(C) Smaller, myelinated

(D) Larger, unmyelinated

Rationale: Smaller myelinated nerves are blocked easier than larger, unmyelinated nerve roots.

Ref: Butterworth, J.F., Mackey, D.C., & Wasnick, J.D. (2013). Ch 45 *Morgan & Mikhail's Clinical Anesthesiology* (5th ed.). New York, NY: Lange Medical Books McGraw-Hill.

Miller, R.D., & Pardo, M.C. (2011). Ch 17 *Basics of Anesthesia* (6th ed.). Philadelphia, PA: Elsevier Saunders.

207. Which corticosteroid has the most potent glucocorticoid activity?

(A) Hydrocortisone

(B) Prednisone

(C) Methylprednisolone

(D) Dexamethasone

Rationale: The relative glucocorticoid potency of dexamethasone is roughly 25 times that of hydrocortisone.

Ref: Butterworth, J.F., Mackey, D.C., & Wasnick, J.D. (2013). Ch 47 *Morgan & Mikhail's Clinical Anesthesiology* (5th ed.). New York, NY: McGraw-Hill.

Calvey, T.N. & Williams, N.E. (Eds.) (2008). Ch 17 *Pharmacology for Anaesthetists* (5th ed.). Malden, MA: Blackwell Publishing.

208. Where does the spinal cord end in a 5-year-old?

(A) L1

(B) L2

(C) L3

(D) L4

Rationale: The spinal cord ends at L1 in adults and L3 in children.

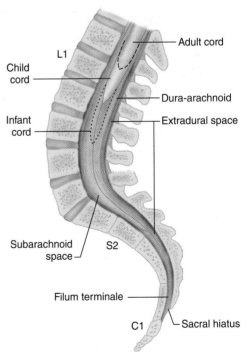

FIG. 3-13. Sagittal view through the lumbar vertebrae and sacrum. Note the end of the spinal cord rises with development from approximately L3-L1. The dural sac normally ends at S2.

Ref: Butterworth, J.F., Mackey, D.C., & Wasnick, J.D. (2013). Ch 45 *Morgan & Mikhail's Clinical Anesthesiology* (5th ed.). New York, NY: McGraw-Hill.

Miller, R.D., & Pardo, M.C. (2011). Ch 17 *Basics of Anesthesia* (6th ed.). Philadelphia, PA: Elsevier.

Nagelhout, J.J., & Plaus, K.L. (2014). Ch 44 *Nurse Anesthesia* (5th ed.). St. Louis, MO: Elsevier.

209. When is a type and screen preferable to a type and cross match?

(A)   The probability of transfusing blood is low.

(B)   The probability of transfusing blood is high.

(C)   The patient has high risk for alloimmunization.

(D)   The patient has a history of a positive antibody screen.

Rationale: A type and screen is preferable when the probability of transfusing blood is low. A type and cross is preferable when the probability of transfusing blood is high.

Ref: Butterworth, J.F., Mackey, D.C., & Wasnick, J.D. (2013). Ch 51 *Morgan & Mikhail's Clinical Anesthesiology* (5th ed.). New York, NY: McGraw-Hill.

Barash, P.G., Cullen, B.F., Stoelting, R.K., Calahan, M.K., & Stock, M.C. (2009). Ch 16 *Clinical Anesthesia* (6th ed.). Philadelphia, PA: Lippincott Williams & Wilkins.

CHAPTER 4

Advanced Principles
Questions

1. During induction of general anesthesia, the pregnant patient quickly desaturates. Which factors most likely caused the desaturation?

   (A) Increased functional residual capacity and increased oxygen consumption
   (B) Decreased residual volume and increased expiratory reserve volume
   (C) Decreased functional residual capacity and increased oxygen consumption
   (D) Increased residual volume and decreased expiratory reserve volume

2. Which cardiac variable leads to heart failure resulting from obesity?

   (A) Decreased preload
   (B) Left ventricular systolic dysfunction
   (C) Decreased afterload
   (D) Hypotension

3. What is the average weight of a 6-year-old?

   (A) 15 kg
   (B) 18 kg
   (C) 21 kg
   (D) 24 kg

4. Which of the following are considered symptomatic of fat embolism following a long bone fracture?

   Select (3) three
   (A) Dyspnea
   (B) Confusion
   (C) Petechiae
   (D) Decreased free fatty acids
   (E) One week post fracture

5. An 80-year-old female with moderate aortic stenosis is undergoing an emergent open reduction and internal fixation of her left hip. Preoperative vital signs include a blood pressure of 175/95 mmHg and a heart rate in sinus rhythm of 65 beats per minute. Shortly after induction with propofol and general anesthesia maintained with sevoflurane, the patient's heart rate increases to an irregular 133 beats per minute. The blood pressure decreases to 69/55 mmHg. What would be the most effective action to restore the patient to a stable hemodynamic profile?

   (A) Administer 100 μg of phenylephrine intravenously.
   (B) Request that the surgery begin immediately so that a painful stimulus may increase blood pressure.
   (C) Cardiovert the patient with a synchronized transthoracic shock of 170 joules.
   (D) Administer a 500 mL bolus of Lactated Ringer's.

6. What finding is most likely during preoperative examination of an awake and alert patient with a posterior cerebral artery aneurysm?

   (A) Brown Séquard syndrome
   (B) Abnormal gaze or pupil response
   (C) Decorticate posturing
   (D) Hypertensive crisis

7. What is the uterine blood flow at term?

   (A) 200-300 mL/min
   (B) 300-400 mL/min
   (C) 400-500 mL/min
   (D) 600-700 mL/min

8. What is resting cerebral oxygen consumption?

   (A) 3.5 mL/100g/min
   (B) 5 mL/100g/min
   (C) 100 mL/min
   (D) 250 mL/min

9. What dose of protamine sulfate would be appropriate to reverse 5,000 units of heparin?

   (A) 500 μg
   (B) 5 mg
   (C) 50 mg
   (D) 5 μg

10. Which of the following may be harmful when in proximity to the Magnetic Resonance Imaging (MRI) machine?

    Select (3) three
    (A) Implanted medication pumps
    (B) Pacing wires
    (C) Cardiac pacemakers
    (D) Pulse oximeter
    (E) Precordial stethoscope

11. A patient is scheduled for bariatric surgery. What is the recommended induction dose for propofol?

    (A) Dose based on lean body weight
    (B) Dose based on total body weight
    (C) Decrease dose by 30%
    (D) Decrease dose by 10%

12. What is an indication of significant venous air embolism during a seated craniotomy?

    (A) Increased end-tidal carbon dioxide
    (B) Unchanged end-tidal carbon dioxide
    (C) Decreased end-tidal carbon dioxide

13. For which heart rhythm is cardioversion not indicated?

    (A) Atrial flutter
    (B) Atrial fibrillation
    (C) Stable ventricular tachycardia
    (D) Pulseless ventricular tachycardia

14. A patient with dysmenorrhea is scheduled for dilation and curettage (D & C). What preoperative testing is required?

    (A) CBC
    (B) Electrolyte panel
    (C) Chest X-ray
    (D) HCG

15. The addition of an intravenous inotrope will tend to move the Frank–Starling curve in which direction?

    (A) Up
    (B) Down
    (C) Left
    (D) Right

16. During an uncomplicated vaginal delivery, what is the expected blood loss?

    (A) 250 mL
    (B) 400 mL
    (C) 750 mL
    (D) 800 mL

17. What should the activated clotting time be prior to initiation of cardiopulmonary bypass (CPB)?

    (A) <150 seconds
    (B) >200 seconds but <350 seconds
    (C) >350 seconds but <450 seconds
    (D) >400 seconds

18. What level of neural blockade is needed for analgesia during the first stage of labor?

    (A) T10–L1 motor level
    (B) T10–S4 sensory level
    (C) T10–L1 sensory level
    (D) T10–S4 motor level

19. How is cardiac index calculated?

    (A) $\dfrac{Cardiac\ Output}{Stroke\ Volume}$

    (B) $\dfrac{Cardiac\ Output}{Systemic\ Vascular\ Resistance}$

    (C) $\dfrac{Cardiac\ Output}{Body\ Surface\ Area}$

    (D) $\dfrac{Cardiac\ Output}{Heart\ Rate}$

20. What is the goal of hemodynamic management for the patient with mitral stenosis?

    (A) Avoiding bradycardia
    (B) Maintenance of sinus rhythm
    (C) Aggressive volume resuscitation
    (D) Inotropic support with phosphodiesterase inhibitors

21. A peribulbar block was performed. There was notable resistance during the injection. The patient becomes agitated and complains of pain. What do you suspect?

    (A) Retrobulbar hemorrhage
    (B) Globe puncture
    (C) Extraocular muscle palsy
    (D) Intravascular injection

22. Which sign is associated with placenta previa?

    (A) Painless vaginal bleeding
    (B) Uterine irritability
    (C) Painful vaginal bleeding
    (D) Coagulopathy

23. What sign is not an effect of hyperparathyroidism?

    (A) Hypertension
    (B) Ventricular arrhythmias
    (C) Muscle weakness
    (D) Hypochloremic metabolic acidosis

24. Which factors contribute to respiratory fatigue in neonates and infants?

    (A) Respiratory musculature composed of primarily type-one muscle fibers
    (B) Increased dead space

    (C) Respiratory musculature composed of primarily type-two muscle fibers
    (D) Decreased chest wall compliance

25. Which valvular disorder leads to the largest ventricular volume?

    (A) Mitral stenosis
    (B) Aortic stenosis
    (C) Mitral regurgitation
    (D) Aortic regurgitation

26. Which narcotic analgesic is not used for patient controlled analgesia (PCA)?

    (A) Meperidine
    (B) Morphine
    (C) Fentanyl
    (D) Hydromorphone

27. With which patient would the anesthetist most want to maintain spontaneous ventilation while under general anesthesia?

    (A) Severe aortic stenosis
    (B) Severe mitral regurgitation
    (C) Acute pulmonary edema
    (D) Mitral valve prolapse

28. The "a" wave on the central venous pressure tracing corresponds to which on the EKG tracing?

    (A) P wave
    (B) QRS wave
    (C) QT interval
    (D) T wave

29. What do you anticipate during laparoscopic cholecystectomy?

    (A) Increased functional residual capacity
    (B) Increased closing capacity
    (C) Decreased functional residual capacity
    (D) Decreased peak inspiratory pressure

30. Which of the following symptoms is consistent with cardiac tamponade?

    (A) Hypotension, tachycardia, tachypnea, muffled heart sounds, and pulsus paradoxus
    (B) Hypertension, tachycardia, tachypnea, and widened pulse pressure
    (C) Jugular venous distension, muffled heart sounds, and bradycardia
    (D) Hypotension, widened pulse pressure, and tachycardia

31. Which of the following are absolute contraindications for electroconvulsive therapy (ECT)?

    Select (3) three
    (A) Myocardial infarction <6 weeks
    (B) Pheochromocytoma
    (C) Glaucoma
    (D) Pregnancy
    (E) Cerebrovascular accident <3 months

32. What is the most common cause of acute epiglottitis?

    (A) *Streptococcus pneumoniae*
    (B) Allergic reaction
    (C) *Haemophilus influenzae B*
    (D) Viral infection

33. The patient is scheduled for a thyroidectomy. What are your primary anesthetic concerns?

    Select (3) three
    (A) Arrhythmias
    (B) Tachycardia
    (C) Body temperature
    (D) Hypotension
    (E) Corneal abrasion

34. What is the lowest recommended $PaCO_2$ if hyperventilation is used during intracranial tumor resection?

    (A) 35 mmHg
    (B) 30 mmHg
    (C) 25 mmHg
    (D) 20 mmHg

35. How is coronary perfusion pressure defined?

    (A) Difference between mean arterial pressure; central venous pressure
    (B) Difference between aortic diastolic pressure; left-ventricular end-diastolic pressure
    (C) Difference between aortic systolic pressure; left-ventricular end-diastolic pressure
    (D) Difference between systolic pressure; central venous pressure

36. What results when a limb tourniquet is released?

    Select (3) three
    (A) Temperature decrease
    (B) Metabolic acidosis
    (C) Metabolic alkalosis
    (D) Temperature increase
    (E) End-tidal CO_2 increase

37. Which patient faces the greatest risk of complete cardiovascular collapse?

    (A) 75-year-old female with bilateral carotid artery disease with an aortic valve area of 1.1 cm^2 undergoing left carotid endarterectomy
    (B) 82-year-old male with severe mitral regurgitation and severe tricuspid regurgitation with atrial fibrillation undergoing bowel resection for colon cancer
    (C) 67-year-old male with aortic valve area of 0.7 cm^2 undergoing left carotid endarterectomy
    (D) 59-year-old male with aortic valve area of 0.7 cm^2 undergoing colon resection for ischemic colon

38. While observing the fetal heart monitor during labor you note a decrease in the fetal heart rate. What is the probable cause?

    (A) Epidural opioids
    (B) Terbutaline
    (C) Ritodrine
    (D) Atropine

39. Estimate the total difference in cerebral blood flow if $PaCO_2$ is decreased from 40 mmHg to 34 mmHg. Assume total brain weight is 1,400 grams.

    (A) 0-50 mL/min
    (B) 30-60 mL/min
    (C) 60-120 mL/min
    (D) 90-180 mL/min

40. Which of the following rate control agents should be avoided in patients undergoing general anesthesia with acute onset wide-complex supraventricular tachycardia (SVT)?

    (A) Digitalis
    (B) Adenosine
    (C) Esmolol
    (D) Amiodarone

41. Which factors contribute to the rapid development of hypoxia during apnea in neonates?

    Select (2) two
    (A) Low functional residual capacity
    (B) Low basal metabolic rate
    (C) High oxygen reserve
    (D) High oxygen demand

42. A 100-kg patient is administered 40,000 units of heparin. Five minutes later the ACT was measured to be 182 seconds. What is the next step?

    (A) Proceed with cardiopulmonary bypass.
    (B) Wait 5 more minutes and recheck ACT.
    (C) Administer an additional 40,000 units of heparin.
    (D) Administer two units of fresh frozen plasma.

43. Because you are concerned with monitoring factors contributing to cerebral ischemia during mediastinoscopy, where will you place your monitors?

    (A) Blood pressure cuff on right arm; arterial line in left hand
    (B) Blood pressure cuff on right arm; pulse oximeter on right hand
    (C) Blood pressure cuff on left arm; arterial line in right hand
    (D) Blood pressure cuff on left arm; pulse oximeter on left hand

44. Which symptom is not present in advanced aortic stenosis?

    (A) Angina
    (B) Dyspnea on exertion
    (C) Orthostatic syncope
    (D) Dyspnea at rest

45. Which nerve is at greatest risk for injury during thyroid surgery?

    (A) Recurrent laryngeal nerve
    (B) Superior laryngeal nerve
    (C) Facial nerve
    (D) Glossopharyngeal nerve

46. Which statements are true regarding gastrointestinal changes during pregnancy?

    Select (3) three
    (A) Pregnant patients are considered a "full stomach".
    (B) Gastric acid increases.
    (C) Gastric volume increases.
    (D) Lower esophageal sphincter relaxation occurs due to progesterone and estrogen.
    (E) Stomach elevates and rotates during pregnancy.

47. What is the level of the larynx in a child?

    (A) C1–C3
    (B) C2–C4
    (C) C3–C5
    (D) C4–C7

48. How does obesity affect the functional residual capacity (FRC) during general anesthesia?

    (A) Increases FRC 50%
    (B) Decreases FRC 20%
    (C) Increases FRC 20%
    (D) Decreases FRC 50%

49. Which is least adaptive in an infant as compared to an adult?

    (A) Heart rate
    (B) Cardiac output
    (C) Stroke volume
    (D) Chest wall

50. A spinal anesthetic is planned for an obese patient. How will you adjust the dose of local anesthetic?

(A) Decrease 20%.
(B) Increase 20%.
(C) Decrease 10%.
(D) Increase 10%.

51. What is the primary determinant of cerebral perfusion?

(A) Position
(B) Mean arterial pressure
(C) Intracranial pressure
(D) Central venous pressure

52. What is the efferent limb of the oculocardiac reflex?

(A) Cranial nerve V
(B) Cranial nerve X
(C) Cranial nerve I
(D) Cranial nerve III

53. What factor is increased in a neonate as compared with an adult?

(A) Surface area to weight ratio
(B) Systolic blood pressure
(C) Plasma protein concentration
(D) Lung compliance

54. When dosing medications for obese patients, what is the best weight parameter to use?

(A) Total body weight
(B) Ideal body weight
(C) Lean body weight
(D) Total body mass index

55. Which is true regarding morbidity and mortality in pediatric anesthesia?

(A) Anesthetic risk is directly related to patient age.
(B) Anesthetic risk is greatest in patients younger than 1 year.
(C) Anesthetic risk is greater now than in the past.
(D) Anesthetic risk is similar throughout childhood.

56. With which of the following preoperative EKG findings will the anesthetist be particularly careful to avoid bradycardia?

(A) Sinus rhythm with prolonged QT interval
(B) Sinus rhythm with left bundle branch block
(C) Sinus rhythm with premature ventricular complexes
(D) Atrial fibrillation

57. The patient is scheduled for a total knee arthroscopy under general anesthesia. The patient's history includes retina surgery using sulfur hexafluoride 2 months ago. What will you avoid?

(A) Nitrous oxide
(B) Rocuronium
(C) Sevoflurane
(D) Fentanyl

58. What is the maintenance intravenous fluid replacement rate for a toddler weighing 12 kg?

(A) 48 mL/hr
(B) 44 mL/hr
(C) 40 mL/hr
(D) 36 mL/hr

59. How much intravenous replacement fluid should be given in the first hour of an anesthetic for a child weighing 16 kg? The child last ate at 0400. The current time is 0700.

(A) 52 mL
(B) 104 mL
(C) 208 mL
(D) 130 mL

60. Which feature of a pediatric endotracheal tube will have greatest influence on work of breathing?

(A) External diameter
(B) Length
(C) Internal diameter
(D) Curvature

61. During laparoscopic bariatric surgery, you apply positive end expiratory pressure (PEEP). What is the recommended upper limit?

(A) 5 cm H_2O
(B) 10 cm H_2O
(C) 15 cm H_2O
(D) 20 cm H_2O

62. Which of the following agents will cause the greatest decreased afterload?

(A) Verapamil
(B) Nicardipine
(C) Metoprolol
(D) Nitroglycerine

63. What is the correct internal diameter and depth for an endotracheal tube placed in a 4-year-old?

(A) Internal diameter 3.5 mm at a depth of 12 cm
(B) Internal diameter 5.0 cm at a depth of 10 cm
(C) Internal diameter of 4.5 mm at a depth of 13.5 cm
(D) Internal diameter of 5.0 mm at a depth of 15 cm

64. You are planning to add fentanyl to the epidural for labor. How much will you add to the local anesthetic solution?

(A) 5 mg
(B) 10 µg
(C) 50 µg
(D) 0.5 mg

65. A patient with ischemic cardiomyopathy, with a preoperative ejection fraction of 15%, presents for a general anesthetic. After induction of general anesthesia, the vital signs include a blood pressure of 79/61 mmHg and a heart rate of 54 beats per minute. What intravenous drip is best?

(A) Epinephrine
(B) Vasopressin
(C) Phenylephrine
(D) Milrinone

66. Which solution is appropriate for replacement of calculated fluid deficits, blood loss, or third-space loss in the pediatric patient?

(A) Lactated Ringer's solution
(B) 5% dextrose in water
(C) 5% dextrose in 0.45% normal saline
(D) 25% albumin

67. Which estimation of blood volume per kilogram is correct for a 2-week-old?

(A) 65 mL
(B) 75 mL
(C) 85 mL
(D) 95 mL

68. Which patient requires the highest minimum alveolar concentration (MAC)?

(A) Newborn of 35 weeks' gestation
(B) A 4-month-old
(C) An 18-month-old
(D) A 3-year-old

69. If intramuscular succinylcholine were indicated, what would be the correct dose for a child?

(A) 1 mg/kg
(B) 2 mg/kg
(C) 3 mg/kg
(D) 4 mg/kg

70. Why does an infant require an increased induction dose (mg/kg) of propofol than an adult?

(A) Enzyme induction
(B) Increased central volume of distribution
(C) Immature renal function
(D) Decreased adipose for redistribution

71. What is the best means to avoid lung overdistension for obese ventilated patients?

(A) Tidal volume 10-15 mL/kg
(B) Tidal volume 12-15 mL/kg
(C) Tidal volume 6-10 mL/kg
(D) Tidal volume 4-8 mL/kg

72. Which patient is at greatest risk of central apnea following anesthesia?

    (A) A 3-month-old born at 40 weeks' gestation
    (B) A 9-week-old born at 39 weeks' gestation
    (C) A 4-month-old born at 30 weeks' gestation
    (D) An 8-month-old born at 28 weeks' gestation

73. Following administration of intrathecal anesthesia for cesarean section, the patient is unable to speak, loses consciousness, and is hypotensive. What is the most likely cause?

    (A) High spinal
    (B) Use of ropivacaine
    (C) Spinal hematoma
    (D) Use of bupivacaine

74. What is the best position for optimizing airway patency during pediatric airway management?

    (A) Small pad placed under the shoulders
    (B) Small pad placed behind the head
    (C) The "sniffing position"
    (D) "Ramp" of towels behind the back

75. What is the best indication for a caudal block in a pediatric patient?

    (A) Anesthesia or analgesia for procedures below the xyphoid process
    (B) Analgesia for the first stage of labor
    (C) Anesthesia or analgesia for procedures below the umbilicus
    (D) Significant deformity of the sacral region

76. Which valve disorder most likely predisposes a patient to coronary ischemia with hypotension?

    (A) Mitral stenosis
    (B) Mitral regurgitation
    (C) Aortic stenosis
    (D) Aortic regurgitation

77. What is the hallmark laboratory finding associated with pyloric stenosis?

    (A) Hypokalemic hypochloremic metabolic acidosis
    (B) Hypokalemic hyperchloremic metabolic alkalosis
    (C) Hyperkalemic hypochloremic metabolic acidosis
    (D) Hypokalemic hypochloremic metabolic alkalosis

78. Which of the following is true regarding a patient with septal defects?

    (A) An increase in SVR relative to PVR will increase cyanosis.
    (B) An increase in PVR relative to SVR favors right to left shunting.
    (C) An increase in PVR relative to SVR will decrease risk of paradoxical air embolism.
    (D) Eisenmenger syndrome is most often due to left ventricular hypertrophy.

79. What is the most common site of herniation in congenital diaphragmatic hernia?

    (A) Right foramen of Bochdalek
    (B) Foramen of Morgagni
    (C) Left foramen of Bochdalek
    (D) Foramen of Luschka

80. Which is the most common type of tracheoesophageal fistula?

    (A) Type IIIb, esophageal atresia with a fistula between the distal esophagus and trachea
    (B) Type I, proximal tracheoesophageal fistula without distal fistula between stomach and trachea
    (C) Type IIIc, fistula between the trachea and both the upper and lower esophageal sections
    (D) Type II, esophageal atresia without communication with the trachea

81. Which statement is true regarding omphalocele and gastroschisis?

    (A) Gastroschisis is less common and presents with a peritoneal covering.
    (B) Omphalocele is less common and presents without peritoneal covering.
    (C) Gastroschisis is more common and presents without peritoneal covering.
    (D) Omphalocele is more common and presents with a peritoneal covering.

82. Which congenital cardiac malformation is most commonly associated with Down syndrome?

    (A) Transposition of the great vessels
    (B) Coarctation of the aorta
    (C) Endocardial cushion defect
    (D) Aortic stenosis

83. Which of the following is an anatomic characteristic of the pediatric airway that distinguishes it from the adult patient?

    (A) The rima glottis is the narrowest point of the airway until the age of 5.
    (B) The tongue is proportionately smaller.
    (C) The larynx is located at the level of C4.
    (D) The epiglottis is flat and flexible.

84. Which type of surgical procedure will result in the greatest increase in afterload accompanied by acute hypertension during aortic cross-clamping?

    (A) Stanford Type A dissection of the ascending aorta
    (B) Suprarenal descending aortic aneurysm
    (C) Infrarenal descending aortic aneurysm
    (D) Stanford Type B dissection

85. At what gestational age does surfactant production begin?

    (A) 30 weeks
    (B) 34 weeks
    (C) 26 weeks
    (D) 32 weeks

86. Which of the following correctly describes omphalocele?

    (A) It is due to occlusion of the omphalomesenteric artery.
    (B) 40-60% of patients have associated anomalies.
    (C) The defect is periumbilical.
    (D) Incidence is approximately 1 in 15,000 births.

87. During a repeat cesarean section a term infant is delivered. On assessment at 1 minute, the infant has a heart rate of 90, blue extremities, whimpering to stimulus, breathing regularly, and active with good muscle tone. What is the 1 minute Apgar score?

    (A) 5
    (B) 6
    (C) 7
    (D) 8

88. Which complications are most concerning following carotid endarterectomy?

    Select (2) two
    (A) Hypertension
    (B) Hypoxemia
    (C) Hypotension
    (D) Delayed emergence

89. Cleft palate, micrognathia, glossoptosis, and congenital heart disease are key characteristics of which syndromes?

    (A) Treacher Collins
    (B) VATER
    (C) Pierre–Robin
    (D) Prader–Willi

90. Which induction agent produces effects desirable for patients with Tetralogy of Fallot?

    (A) Etomidate
    (B) Ketamine
    (C) Midazolam
    (D) Propofol

91. Which of the following is true regarding a transplanted heart?

    (A) No response to atropine
    (B) No response to isoproterenol
    (C) No response to milrinone
    (D) No response to epinephrine

92. Which inhaled agent is most suitable for a pediatric inhalation induction?

    (A) Isoflurane
    (B) Desflurane
    (C) Sevoflurane
    (D) Enflurane

93. Which of the following variables is not associated with aging?

    (A) Increased volume of distribution for lipid soluble drugs
    (B) Reduced plasma volume
    (C) Decreased volume of distribution for lipid soluble drugs
    (D) Reduced plasma protein binding

94. An elderly patient with coronary artery disease is scheduled for an umbilical hernia repair. You note a decreased albumin level. What do you expect when administering an intravenous induction dose of propofol?

    (A) Higher free drug fraction
    (B) Decreased drug effect
    (C) Lower free drug fraction
    (D) Similar drug effect

95. What is the effect of aging on the minimum alveolar concentration (MAC)?

    (A) MAC of volatile anesthetics increases 50% after age 60.
    (B) MAC of volatile anesthetics decreases 10% after age 50.
    (C) MAC of volatile anesthetics decreases 4% per decade after 40 years of age.
    (D) MAC of volatile anesthetics increases 4% per decade after 40 years of age.

96. What is the best induction dose for an 80-year-old weighing 100 kg?

    (A) Propofol 100 mg
    (B) Sodium pentothal 250 mg
    (C) Etomidate 40 mg
    (D) Ketamine 100mg

97. What is the definition of premature birth?

    (A) Birth prior to 42 weeks' gestation
    (B) Birth prior to 37 weeks' gestation
    (C) Birth prior to 32 weeks' gestation
    (D) Birth prior to 35 weeks' gestation

98. Which body mass index (BMI) is categorized as obese Class I?

    (A) 18.5%
    (B) 24.9%
    (C) 29.9%
    (D) 32.1%

99. Total body water will be the largest percentage of body weight in which patient?

    (A) A neonate
    (B) An infant
    (C) A toddler
    (D) A school-age child

100. Which sign is associated with metabolic syndrome?

    (A) High levels of high-density lipoprotein cholesterol
    (B) Hypotension
    (C) High triglyceride levels
    (D) Small waist circumference

101. The patient is undergoing a latissimus dorsi myocutaneous flap for reconstruction of the breast. What is the desired mean arterial pressure?

    (A) MAP > 55 mmHg
    (B) MAP > 60 mmHg
    (C) MAP > 65 mmHg
    (D) MAP > 70 mmHg

102. Which patient appropriately fasted for an anesthetic to begin at 1000?

    (A) A child who had cereal at 0500
    (B) A child who had clear liquids at 0900
    (C) An infant who breast-fed at 0500
    (D) An infant who had formula at 0700

103. Which dose of morphine is appropriate for intrathecal post-cesarean section analgesia?

(A) 2.5 mg

(B) 50 μg

(C) 0.2 mg

(D) 100 μg

104. When is it best to avoid teratogenic drugs?

(A) 1-2 weeks' gestation

(B) 3-10 weeks' gestation

(C) 12-15 weeks' gestation

(D) 20-25 weeks' gestation

105. Which variable is not linked to postdural puncture headache following placement of a spinal anesthetic for cesarean section?

(A) 26-g needle

(B) Cutting needles

(C) 20-g needle

(D) Beveled needles

106. Which symptoms are associated with pregnant patients in the supine position?

(A) Hypotension, nausea

(B) Nausea, hypertension

(C) Normotension, nausea

(D) Hypertension, vomiting

107. Which of the following physiologic changes occurs during pregnancy?

(A) Hypocoagulation

(B) Plasma volume decreases

(C) Hypercoagulation

(D) Red cell mass decreases

108. The patient requests an epidural for abdominal hysterectomy. Which sensory level is needed for epidural anesthesia?

(A) T12

(B) T10

(C) T8

(D) T6

109. The patient is scheduled for a laparoscopic cholecystectomy. Which of the following is true?

(A) Central venous pressure decreases.

(B) Lung compliance increases.

(C) Intra-abdominal pressure decreases.

(D) Functional residual capacity decreases.

110. During a laparoscopic hernia repair, you notice a sudden drop in blood pressure and oxygen saturation and decreased end-tidal carbon dioxide. What is the most likely cause?

(A) CO_2 embolus

(B) Tension pneumothorax

(C) Hemorrhage

(D) Pneumomediastinum

111. Which of the following is true about the infant airway?

(A) The tongue is small in relation to the mandible.

(B) The larynx is located at the C2–C3 vertebrae.

(C) The epiglottis is stiff and flat.

(D) The larynx is located at C5–C6.

112. While reversing heparin, the anesthetist notes that the blood pressure has dropped precipitously to 42/23 mmHg. What will you do first?

(A) Administer 100 μg of epinephrine IV.

(B) Administer 10 μg of epinephrine IV.

(C) Administer 50 mg of Benadryl and 125 mg of methylprednisolone IV.

(D) Begin chest compressions.

113. By how much are neuraxial requirements for cesarean section decreased?

(A) 10%

(B) 20%

(C) 30%

(D) 50%

114. What are the normal physiological changes associated with pregnancy?

Select (3) three

(A) MAC decreases by 50%.

(B) Functional residual capacity decreases by 20%.

(C) Respiratory rate decreases by 15%.

(D) Plasma volume increases by 55%.

(E) Heart rate increases by 20%.

(F) Hemoglobin increases by 10%.

115. What is the best size endotracheal tube used for a patient undergoing general anesthesia for cesarean section?

(A) 5.5 mm

(B) 6.5 mm

(C) 7.5 mm

(D) 8.5 mm

116. How does propofol affect uterine blood flow (UBF)?

(A) Decreases UBF

(B) No change on UBF

(C) Dose-related increase in UBF

(D) Dose-related decrease in UBF

117. What statement is false regarding the use of metoclopramide in pregnant patients?

(A) Speeds gastric emptying

(B) Increases pH

(C) Decreases gastric volume

(D) Increases lower esophageal sphincter tone

118. A patient is scheduled for a radical neck dissection. History includes neck radiation. How will you manage this patient's airway?

(A) Standard IV induction

(B) Rapid sequence induction

(C) Laryngeal mask airway

(D) Awake fiberoptic intubation

119. Within 1 minute following the epidural test dose, the patient complains of heavy legs. What is the most likely cause?

(A) Intravascular injection

(B) Incomplete epidural analgesia

(C) Unintentional intrathecal block

(D) Local anesthetic toxicity

120. The patient is receiving echothiophate eye drops for glaucoma. You plan to use succinylcholine. What should you expect?

(A) Shortened onset of action

(B) Shortened duration of action

(C) Prolonged duration of action

(D) Prolonged onset of action

121. The patient has severe preeclampsia. When will you avoid regional anesthesia?

(A) Platelet count 100,000/µL

(B) Platelet count 150,000/µL

(C) Platelet count 125,000/µL

(D) Platelet count 75,000/µL

122. What fetal monitoring pattern is associated with umbilical cord compression?

(A) Variable decelerations

(B) Late decelerations

(C) Early decelerations

(D) Increased variability

123. During labor the patient experiences an abrupt onset of constant abdominal pain accompanied by hypotension. What is the most likely cause?

(A) Uterine rupture

(B) Placenta previa

(C) Placenta abruption

(D) Hemorrhage

124. Which of the following increases intraocular pressure?

Select (2) two

(A) Hypotension

(B) Hypoventilation

(C) Hypertension

(D) Hyperventilation

125. During radical neck dissection, you note new onset bradycardia, arrhythmias, and prolonged QT intervals. What is the probable cause of these symptoms?

    (A) Denervation of carotid sinus
    (B) Manipulation of the carotid sinus
    (C) Venous air embolism
    (D) Denervation of carotid bodies

126. The patient is scheduled for laser removal of vocal cord papilloma. What will you avoid?

    (A) Eye protection with colored glasses
    (B) Nitrous oxide
    (C) Eye protection with wet gauze
    (D) Oxygen and air mixture

127. Fifteen minutes ago you transported a patient to the postanesthesia care unit following tonsillectomy. The patient is bleeding. How will you induce this patient?

    (A) Rapid sequence induction
    (B) Standard induction
    (C) Awake intubation
    (D) Standard induction with a glidescope

128. Which of the following is associated with a peribulbar block?

    Select (3) three
    (A) Intraconal procedure
    (B) Patient gaze is supranasal.
    (C) Extraconal procedure
    (D) Patient gaze is straight ahead.
    (E) 5-8 mL local anesthetic is used.

129. Which statement is true regarding the use of inhalational agents during pregnancy?

    (A) Uterine blood flow is increased.
    (B) Uteroplacental blood flow is increased.
    (C) Uteroplacental blood flow is decreased.
    (D) Uterine blood flow is unchanged.

130. The patient is scheduled for an endoscopic sinus surgery. Which of the following will not minimize blood loss?

    (A) Head-up position
    (B) Cocaine 4%

    (C) Supine position
    (D) Hypotensive technique

131. A patient is scheduled for surgery involving a Le Fort II fracture. During the preoperative interview, periorbital edema and raccoon eyes hematoma are noted. What is your main anesthetic concern?

    (A) Securing the airway
    (B) Bleeding
    (C) Emergence with a wired jaw
    (D) Postoperative respiratory compromise

132. What are the clinical signs of hyperthyroidism?

    Select (3) three
    (A) Polyuria
    (B) Weight gain
    (C) Nervousness
    (D) Paresthesias
    (E) Hypertension

133. What is the hemodynamic priority for anesthetic management of an unrepaired aortic dissection?

    (A) Decrease blood pressure with arterial vasodilators to decrease risk of rupture or further dissection.
    (B) Increase blood pressure to ensure adequate perfusion distal to the aneurysm.
    (C) Decrease shear force on the aneurysm using beta-blockers to decrease risk of rupture of further dissection.
    (D) Decrease heart rate with medications in order to decrease myocardial oxygen demand.

134. The patient is scheduled for a laryngeal endoscopy. Jet ventilation is planned. What statement is false regarding jet ventilation?

    (A) High-pressure (30-60 psi) is used.
    (B) FiO_2 of 30% or less is used.
    (C) End-tidal CO_2 is accurate.
    (D) Expiration is passive.

135. A patient undergoing repair of a descending thoracic aortic aneurysm is found postoperatively to exhibit loss of lower extremity motor function bilaterally. What is the most likely cause?

(A) Blood flow to the motor cortex of the brain was decreased during cross-clamp.

(B) Blood flow to the anterior spinal cord was damaged during the surgery.

(C) Blood flow to the posterior spinal cord was damaged during the surgery.

(D) This is a normal occurrence when blood flow to the lower extremities has been restricted as in aortic cross clamping.

136. The patient is undergoing a mediastinoscopy. What will you consider for this patient?

Select (3) three

(A) Blood pressure in the left arm

(B) Large bore IV

(C) Blood pressure in the right arm

(D) Air embolism

(E) Superior laryngeal nerve damage

137. What statements are true regarding cardioversion?

Select (2) two

(A) 50-100 joules are used initially for atrial flutter.

(B) Electrical shock is synchronized with the "R" wave.

(C) 200-300 joules are used initially to convert atrial flutter.

(D) Electrical shock is asynchronous.

(E) Electrical shock is synchronized with the "Q" wave.

138. What do you anticipate with distention of the bowel during colonoscopy?

(A) Tachycardia

(B) Hypertension

(C) Bradycardia

(D) EKG changes

139. The patient is scheduled for Computed Tomography (CT) scan with intravenous contrast media (ICM). What is your main concern?

(A) Patient must not move during the CT

(B) Patient anxiety

(C) Hypothermia

(D) Allergic reaction

140. A patient is scheduled for electroconvulsive therapy. What is your main anesthetic concern when calculating dosages for induction agents?

(A) Anterograde amnesia

(B) Seizure quality

(C) Parasympathetic stimulation

(D) Sympathetic stimulation

141. A patient with an intestinal obstruction is scheduled for surgery. The patient's history includes pancreatitis and GERD. What is the best approach to airway management?

(A) Awake fiberoptic intubation

(B) Endotracheal intubation

(C) LMA

(D) Intubating LMA

142. When is cardiac output greatest?

(A) Immediately following delivery

(B) Third trimester

(C) Second trimester

(D) First trimester

143. Which of the following would be the most appropriate induction technique for a patient undergoing drainage of a severe cardiac tamponade via subxiphoid approach or pericardiocentesis?

(A) Propofol, high dose fentanyl, succinylcholine, and intubate. Maintain with light sevoflurane and positive pressure ventilation.

(B) Ketamine, high dose fentanyl, succinylcholine, and intubate. Maintain with light sevoflurane.

(C) Inhalational induction and LMA insertion. Maintain with light sevoflurane and ketamine supplementation.

(D) High dose fentanyl, midazolam, and mask ventilate patient.

144. A sedated patient experiences headache, nausea and vomiting during stereotactic Gamma Knife surgery. What is the most likely cause?

(A) Hemorrhage
(B) Perforated aneurysm
(C) Radiocontrast reaction
(D) Embolization

145. Which of the following medications shortens the duration of a seizure during electroconvulsive therapy (ECT)?

(A) Caffeine
(B) Etomidate
(C) Ketamine
(D) Propofol

146. The patient is undergoing a mastectomy. During surgery, isosulfan blue dye is injected. What do you expect?

(A) Tachycardia
(B) Increased oxygen saturation
(C) Bradycardia
(D) Decreased oxygen saturation

147. Following cystoscopy the patient's blood pressure falls. What is the most likely cause?

(A) Sympathectomy
(B) Blood loss
(C) Vasoconstriction due to spinal anesthesia
(D) Lowering legs from lithotomy position

148. Pain relief during the second stage of labor requires neural blockade at what sensory level?

(A) T10 to T12
(B) T12 to S1
(C) T10 to S1
(D) T10 to S4

149. Which condition benefits most from epidural steroid injections?

(A) Radiculopathy
(B) Intractable cancer pain
(C) Intra-abdominal neoplasms
(D) Phantom limb pain

150. Which of the following has mainly analgesic and anti-pyretic properties?

(A) Acetaminophen
(B) Ketorolac
(C) Fentanyl
(D) Codeine

151. Which statement regarding the use of epidural analgesia and anesthesia for preeclamptic patients is true?

(A) Circulating catecholamines are decreased.
(B) Decreases intervillous blood flow.
(C) Epidural block should be avoided.
(D) Epidural blocks are difficult to place.

152. The patient is taking duloxetine and fluoxetine for chronic neuropathic pain. The patient complains of fever, agitation, sweating, and anxiety. What is the most likely cause?

(A) Duloxetine overdose
(B) Fluoxetine sensitivity
(C) Combined use of fluoxetine and duloxetine
(D) Allergic reaction to duloxetine

153. A patient is receiving tocolytic therapy for preterm labor. Which of the following is most concerning for this patient?

(A) Hyperkalemia
(B) Hypoglycemia
(C) Pulmonary edema
(D) Increased systemic vascular resistance

154. Which of the following are systemic effects of hydrocortisone?

Select (3) three
(A) Adrenal-pituitary insufficiency
(B) Cushing syndrome
(C) Hypertension
(D) Sodium depletion
(E) Hypotension

155. How is the renal system affected by pregnancy?

     Select (2) two
     (A) Renal plasma flow increases.
     (B) Glomerular filtration rate increases.
     (C) Tubular absorption of glucose increases.
     (D) Renal blood flow decreases.

156. When giving epidural steroid injections what dose will you use to avoid systemic effects?

     (A) Methylprednisolone acetate 40 mg
     (B) Triamcinolone diacetate 100 mg
     (C) Methylprednisolone acetate 20 mg
     (D) Triamcinolone diacetate 120 mg

157. The patient is scheduled for in vitro fertilization (IVF). Which medications are considered safe for this patient?

     Select (3) three
     (A) Morphine
     (B) Fentanyl
     (C) Demerol
     (D) NSAIDs
     (E) Nitrous oxide

158. Which statement is false regarding open breast biopsy?

     (A) Postoperative nausea and vomiting is increased.
     (B) Smooth emergence minimizes hematoma formation.
     (C) Monitor the EKG for ST-segment changes when local anesthetic with epinephrine is used.
     (D) The blood pressure cuff is placed on the non-operative arm and IV placed on the operative side.

159. The patient is undergoing a modified radical mastectomy. When planning the general anesthetic, why would you check with the surgeon?

     (A) Determine the patient's risk for postoperative nausea and vomiting.
     (B) Type and cross-match preoperatively.
     (C) Determine what if any neuromuscular blockers will be used.
     (D) Determine when to give antiemetics.

160. What is your primary concern when caring for a patient undergoing hysteroscopy?

     (A) Vasovagal response to uterine traction
     (B) Postoperative pain
     (C) Lithotomy positioning
     (D) Absorption of glycine or saline solution

161. The patient is scheduled for a total abdominal hysterectomy. Why is the patient likely to become hypotensive following induction?

     (A) Bowel prep
     (B) Chronic bleeding
     (C) Anemia
     (D) Position changes

162. During a cystoscopy, the patient complains of upper abdominal pain and nausea. The patient is diaphoretic. What is the most likely cause?

     (A) Bladder perforation
     (B) Stent placement
     (C) Biopsy
     (D) Stone removal

163. What emergency medication is essential for penile surgery?

     (A) Midazolam
     (B) Propofol
     (C) Fentanyl
     (D) Glycopyrrolate

164. What is the primary anesthetic concern for patients undergoing rectal surgery?

     (A) Postoperative pain
     (B) Relaxation of the anal sphincter
     (C) Fluid and electrolyte balance
     (D) Postoperative nausea and vomiting

165. During a total knee arthroplasty with spinal anesthesia the patient develops hypotension, arrhythmias, and loses consciousness. What is the most likely cause?

     (A) Hemorrhage
     (B) Fluid imbalance
     (C) Tourniquet pain
     (D) Methyl methacrylate

166. Which is the preferred method of airway management in a child with acute epiglottitis?

(A) Rapid sequence induction followed by laryngoscopy

(B) Awake laryngoscopy

(C) Inhalation induction maintaining spontaneous respiration

(D) Urgent tracheostomy

167. Which factor does not contribute to decreased uterine blood flow?

(A) Systemic hypotension

(B) Uterine vasoconstriction

(C) Uterine contractions

(D) Uterine vasodilation

168. Which of the following physiologic changes occur with limb tourniquets?

(A) Cellular acidosis

(B) Metabolic alkalosis

(C) Cellular alkalosis

(D) Metabolic acidosis

169. While undergoing a shoulder arthroscopy with regional anesthesia the patient exhibits tachycardia, agitation, diaphoresis, hypotension, and jugular vein distention. What is the most likely cause?

(A) Tension pneumothorax

(B) Subcutaneous emphysema

(C) Pneumomediastinum

(D) Failed regional block

170. Which of the following risk factors are linked to post-operative vision loss (POVL)?

Select (3) three

(A) Female

(B) Thin

(C) Obese

(D) Male

(E) <18 years

(F) >18 years

171. The patient is scheduled for a total hip arthroplasty (THR). What are your anesthetic concerns?

Select (3) three

(A) Hemorrhage

(B) Thromboembolism

(C) Tourniquet pain

(D) Bone cement implantation syndrome

(E) Postoperative pain

172. How are hypotensive bradycardic episodes (HBEs) that occur during shoulder surgery defined?

Select (2) two

(A) Any heart rate <50 bpm

(B) Any systolic blood pressure <90 mmHg

(C) Heart rate decrease of 30 bpm in 3 minutes

(D) Heart rate decrease of 20 bpm in 5 minutes

173. Your patient is undergoing an elective coronary artery bypass graft (CABG). The patient was managed on heparin therapy for five days preoperatively. The patient is now on cardiopulmonary bypass and the perfusionist is having difficulty maintaining total heparinization. What is the most likely cause?

(A) Antithrombin deficiency

(B) Factor V deficiency

(C) Factor VIII deficiency

(D) Factor IV deficiency

174. Which condition is associated with carbamazepine taken during pregnancy?

(A) Spina bifida

(B) Pyloric stenosis

(C) Biliary atresia

(D) Hypospadias

175. A patient is undergoing an elective abdominal aortic aneurysm (AAA) repair. What drug are you most likely to administer after aortic clamping?

(A) Nitroglycerin

(B) Phenylephrine

(C) Milrinone

(D) Dopamine

176. A 5-year-old requires endotracheal intubation for an exploratory laparotomy. What size ETT will you select?

(A) 6
(B) 5
(C) 4
(D) 3

177. Which of the following is linked to late decelerations?

(A) Fetal head compression
(B) Begins 10-30 seconds following the peak of a contraction
(C) Begin with the contraction
(D) Umbilical cord compression

178. Which neurosurgical procedure places the patient at highest risk for postoperative diabetes insipidus?

(A) Resection of intracranial aneurysm in the anterior Circle of Willis
(B) Stereotactic biopsy of a lesion in the parietal lobe
(C) Tumor resection within the posterior fossa
(D) Transsphenoidal hypophysectomy

179. What is the correct placement of a precordial Doppler to monitor for venous air embolism?

(A) Midclavicular line at the first intercostal space
(B) Right sternal border at the third intercostal space
(C) Right midaxillary line at the fifth intercostal space
(D) Left sternal border at the fifth intercostal space

180. What is average total cerebral blood flow?

(A) 550 mL/min
(B) 650 mL/min
(C) 750 mL/min
(D) 850 mL/min

181. How is Minimum Alveolar Concentration (MAC) affected for inhaled anesthetics during pregnancy?

(A) MAC is increased 30%.
(B) MAC is decreased 15%.
(C) MAC is increased 25%.
(D) MAC is decreased 40%.

182. Calculate cerebral perfusion pressure (CPP) using the information provided and correctly interpret the result. Blood pressure is 130/90 mmHg, intracranial pressure is 12 mmHg, central venous pressure is 6 mmHg.

(A) CPP = 110 mmHg, high
(B) CPP = 97 mmHg, normal
(C) CPP = 105 mmHg, high
(D) CPP = 91 mmHg, normal

183. Inhalational anesthetic agents have what effects on the hearts conduction?

(A) Decrease AV node refractoriness
(B) Suppress SA node automaticity
(C) Increase pacing thresholds
(D) All of the above

184. For Frank–Starling's Law what does the x-axis and y-axis represent?

(A) Heart rate; cardiac output
(B) Ventricular end-diastolic volume; cardiac output
(C) Cardiac output; ventricular end-diastolic volume
(D) Afterload; systemic vascular resistance

185. The fetal scalp pH is 7.25. How would you interpret this value?

(A) Normal infant pH
(B) Abnormal infant pH
(C) Needs to be repeated to ensure accuracy
(D) Requires neonatal resuscitation

186. What does the formula,
$$\frac{\text{(end-diastolic volume)} - \text{(end-systolic volume)}}{\text{end-diastolic volume}}, \text{ represent?}$$

(A) Stroke volume
(B) Cardiac index
(C) Cardiac output
(D) Ejection fraction

187. A pacemaker is placed in a patient with symptomatic sinus bradycardia with a normally functioning atrioventricular node. What settings would be most appropriate?

    (A) AAI
    (B) AOO
    (C) DDD
    (D) DDI

188. Which of the following agents possesses combined alpha- and beta-adrenergic blocking affects?

    (A) Metoprolol
    (B) Esmolol
    (C) Propanolol
    (D) Labetalol

189. Which of the following would be appropriate anesthesia induction techniques for a severely hypertensive patient with coronary artery disease and moderate ventricular dysfunction?

    (A) Inhalational induction with sevoflurane
    (B) Inhalational induction with desflurane
    (C) Intravenous induction with ketamine
    (D) Intravenous induction with propofol

190. Which arrhythmia is best treated with magnesium sulfate?

    (A) Ventricular fibrillation
    (B) Polymorphic ventricular tachycardia in the presence of prolonged QT syndrome
    (C) Atrioventricular nodal reentrant tachycardia
    (D) Polymorphic ventricular tachycardia in the absence of prolonged QT syndrome

191. What is the goal of hemodynamic management for the patient with severe mitral valve regurgitation?

    (A) Aggressive volume resuscitation
    (B) Inotropic support
    (C) Afterload reduction
    (D) Maintenance of moderate bradycardia

192. Which patient is most at risk for catastrophic bleeding upon midline sternotomy?

    (A) Patient with ischemic cardiomyopathy on multiple vasopressor therapies undergoing aortic valve replacement
    (B) Patient with heparin induced thrombocytopenia to be treated with argatroban for cardiopulmonary bypass undergoing coronary artery bypass grafts
    (C) Patient with a previous coronary artery bypass grafting undergoing mitral valve repair
    (D) Obese patient with severe aortic stenosis undergoing aortic valve replacement

193. What is the approximate mean arterial blood pressure for the patient whose pressure is 115/70 mmHg?

    (A) 100 mmHg
    (B) 85 mmHg
    (C) 92.5 mmHg
    (D) 80 mmHg

194. In which valvular disorder is the left ventricular volume approximately normal, but left ventricular pressure higher than normal?

    (A) Mitral stenosis
    (B) Aortic stenosis
    (C) Mitral regurgitation
    (D) Aortic regurgitation

195. Measured systolic and pulse pressure will appear greatest when transduced and measured at which point?

    (A) Aortic root
    (B) Brachial artery
    (C) Radial artery
    (D) Dorsalis pedis

196. Which of the following is a relative contraindication to pulmonary artery catheter placement?

    (A) Atrial fibrillation
    (B) Left bundle branch block
    (C) Complete heart block
    (D) 1st-degree block

197. Which law explains the effect of post-intubation airway edema in children?

(A) Poiseuille's equation
(B) Dalton's law
(C) The Ideal Gas Law
(D) Avogadro's number

198. Which medication used for preeclampsia may extend the duration of rocuronium?

(A) Nitroglycerin
(B) Hydralazine
(C) Labetalol
(D) Magnesium

199. What is the normal fetal heart rate?

(A) 80-100 bpm
(B) 100-110 bpm
(C) 110-160 bpm
(D) >160 bpm

200. What is the best choice to improve hypotension resulting from aortocaval compression?

(A) Give oxygen via facemask.
(B) Turn the patient on his/her side.
(C) Give ephedrine.
(D) Give phenylephrine.

201. Which opioid causes the greatest respiration depression in newborns?

(A) Meperidine
(B) Morphine
(C) Fentanyl
(D) Remifentanil

202. The patient is scheduled for a parathyroidectomy. What is the anesthetic implication for hyperparathyroidism and neuromuscular blockade (NMB)?

(A) Decrease NMB dose.
(B) Titrate NMB carefully.
(C) No relationship exists.
(D) No change in the response to NMB.

203. A patient undergoes bronchoscopy for removal of a foreign body. What neuromuscular blocker (NMB) is the best choice for this procedure?

(A) Succinylcholine
(B) Vecuronium
(C) Cisatracurium
(D) Atracurium

204. What increases stroke volume?

(A) Increased ventricular end-diastolic volume
(B) Increased pulmonary vascular resistance
(C) Increased heart rate
(D) Mitral regurgitation

205. Which inhaled agent is most associated with emergence delirium in children?

(A) Sevoflurane
(B) Isoflurane
(C) Desflurane
(D) Nitrous oxide

Answers and Explanations: Advanced Principles

1. During induction of general anesthesia, the pregnant patient quickly desaturates. Which factors most likely caused the desaturation?

   (A) Increased functional residual capacity and increased oxygen consumption

   (B) Decreased residual volume and increased expiratory reserve volume

   (C) Decreased functional residual capacity and increased oxygen consumption

TABLE 4-1. Average maximum physiological changes associated with pregnancy.[1]

Parameter	Change
Neurological	
MAC	−40%
Respiratory	
Oxygen consumption	+20-50%
Airway resistance	−35%
FRC	−20%
Minute ventilation	+50%
Tidal volume	+40%
Respiratory rate	+15%
PaO_2	+10%
$PaCO_2$	−15%
HCO_3	−15%
Cardiovascular	
Blood volume	+35%
Plasma volume	+55%
Cardiac output	+40%
Stroke volume	+30%
Heart rate	+20%
Systolic blood pressure	−5%
Diastolic blood pressure	−15%
Peripheral resistance	−15%
Pulmonary resistance	−30%
Hematologic	
Hemoglobin	−20%
Platelets	−10%
Clotting factors[2]	+30-250%
Renal	
GFR	+50%

[1]MAC, minimum alveolar concentration; FRC, functional residual capacity; GFR, glomerular filtration rate.

[2]Varies with each factor.

   (D) Increased residual volume and decreased expiratory reserve volume

Rationale: Respiratory changes of pregnancy include decreased functional residual capacity (FRC), increased oxygen consumption, and decreased residual and expiratory reserve volumes. Decreased FRC and increased oxygen consumptions lead to rapid decrease in oxygen saturation.

Ref: Butterworth, J.F., Mackey, D.C., & Wasnick, J.D. (2013). Ch 41 *Morgan & Mikhail's Clinical Anesthesiology* (5th ed.). New York, NY: McGraw-Hill.

Longnecker, D.E., Brown, D.L., Newman, M.F., & Zapol, W.M. (2012). Ch 22 *Anesthesiology* (2nd ed.). San Francisco, CA: McGraw-Hill.

2. Which cardiac variable leads to heart failure resulting from obesity?

   (A) Decreased preload

   (B) Left ventricular systolic dysfunction

   (C) Decreased afterload

   (D) Hypotension

Rationale: Volume overload and vascular stiffness result from obesity. Increased preload, increased afterload, and hypertension lead to left ventricular systolic dysfunction.

Ref: Hines, R.L., & Marschall, K.E. (2012). Ch 16 *Stoelting's Anesthesia and Co-Exiting Disease* (6th ed.). Philadelphia, PA: Saunders.

3. What is the average weight of a 6-year-old?

   (A) 15 kg

   (B) 18 kg

   (C) 21 kg

   (D) 24 kg

Rationale: A simple estimation of body weight by age is: 9 + (Age × 2).

Ref: Butterworth, J.F., Mackey, D.C., & Wasnick, J.D. (2013). Ch 42 *Morgan & Mikhail's Clinical Anesthesiology* (5th ed.). New York, NY: McGraw-Hill.

4. Which of the following are considered symptomatic of fat embolism following a long bone fracture?

   Select (3) three
   (A) Dyspnea
   (B) Confusion
   (C) Petechiae
   (D) Decreased free fatty acids
   (E) One week post fracture

   Rationale: Signs of fat embolism following a long bone fracture generally occur within 72 hours of the event. Increased free fatty acids lead to capillary-alveolar membrane disturbance. Neurological symptoms result due to cerebral circulation damage and edema.
   Ref: Butterworth, J.F., Mackey, D.C., & Wasnick, J.D. (2013). Ch 38 *Morgan & Mikhail's Clinical Anesthesiology* (5th ed.). New York, NY: McGraw-Hill.

5. An 80-year-old female with moderate aortic stenosis is undergoing an emergent open reduction and internal fixation of her left hip. Preoperative vital signs include a blood pressure of 175/95 mmHg and a heart rate in sinus rhythm of 65 beats per minute. Shortly after induction with propofol and general anesthesia maintained with sevoflurane, the patient's heart rate increases to an irregular 133 beats per minute. The blood pressure decreases to 69/55 mmHg. What would be the most effective action to restore the patient to a stable hemodynamic profile?

   (A) Administer 100 μg of phenylephrine intravenously.
   (B) Request that the surgery begin immediately so that a painful stimulus may increase blood pressure.
   (C) Cardiovert the patient with a synchronized transthoracic shock of 170 joules.
   (D) Administer a 500 mL bolus of Lactated Ringer's.

   Rationale: The irregular accelerated heart rate is likely atrial fibrillation. Loss of atrial synchronized contraction can reduce ventricular filling by 20-30%. An elderly patient with atrial stenosis has a fixed outflow obstruction and can be expected to have hypertrophy, resulting in decreased ventricular compliance. The increased heart rate and decreased atrial "kick" all combine to significantly decrease this patient's left

ventricular end-diastolic volume. Hemodynamic consequences to a reduced ventricular end-diastolic volume will be most profoundly seen in a patient with concomitant reduced ventricular compliance. While all of the interventions mentioned may increase blood pressure, only synchronized cardioversion solves the underlying problem.
Ref: Butterworth, J.F., Mackey, D.C., & Wasnick, J.D. (2013). Ch 20 *Morgan & Mikhail's Clinical Anesthesiology* (5th ed.). New York, NY: McGraw-Hill.

6. What finding is most likely during preoperative examination of an awake and alert patient with a posterior cerebral artery aneurysm?

   (A) Brown–Séquard syndrome
   (B) Abnormal gaze or pupil response
   (C) Decorticate posturing
   (D) Hypertensive crisis

   Rationale: Oculomotor palsy may result from an aneurysm in this area due to close proximity of these structures.
   Ref: Butterworth, J.F., Mackey, D.C., & Wasnick, J.D. (2013). Ch 27 *Morgan & Mikhail's Clinical Anesthesiology* (5th ed.). New York, NY: McGraw-Hill.
   Moore, K.L., Dalley, A.F., & Agur, A.M.R. (Eds.) (2010). Ch 9 *Clinically Oriented Anatomy*. Philadelphia, PA: Lippincott Williams & Wilkins.

7. What is the uterine blood flow at term?

   (A) 200-300 mL/min
   (B) 300-400 mL/min
   (C) 400-500 mL/min
   (D) 600-700 mL/min

   Rationale: The normal uterine blood flow in the non-pregnant female is 50 mL/min. At term the blood flow increases to approximately 10% of the cardiac output.
   Ref: Butterworth, J.F., Mackey, D.C., & Wasnick, J.D. (2013). Ch 40 *Morgan & Mikhail's Clinical Anesthesiology* (5th ed.). New York, NY: McGraw-Hill.
   Suresh, M.S., Segal, B.S., Preston, R.L., Fernando, R., & Mason C.L. (2013). Ch 2 *Shnider and Levinson's Anesthesia for Obstetrics* (5th ed.). Philadelphia, PA: Lippincott Williams & Wilkins.

8. What is resting cerebral oxygen consumption?

   (A) 3.5 mL/100g/min
   (B) 5 mL/100g/min
   (C) 100 mL/min
   (D) 250 mL/min

Rationale: Resting cerebral oxygen demand averages 3.5 mL/100g/min.

Ref: Butterworth, J.F., Mackey, D.C., & Wasnick, J.D. (2013). Ch 26 *Morgan & Mikhail's Clinical Anesthesiology* (5th ed.). New York, NY: McGraw-Hill.

Hall, J.E. (2011). Ch 61 *Guyton and Hall Textbook of Medical Physiology* (12th ed.). Philadelphia, PA: Elsevier.

9. What dose of protamine sulfate would be appropriate to reverse 5000 units of heparin?

   (A) 500 µg
   (B) 5 mg
   (C) 50 mg
   (D) 5 µg

Rationale: Protamine is a positively charged protein that binds to and inactivates heparin. Protamine is therefore dosed according the dose of heparin given and not the degree of anticoagulation obtained. Generally 1 mg of protamine is administered for every 100 units of heparin in circulation. Therefore, this patient needs 5,000/100 = 50 mg of protamine IV.

Ref: Butterworth, J.F., Mackey, D.C., & Wasnick, J.D. (2013). Ch 22 *Morgan & Mikhail's Clinical Anesthesiology* (5th ed.). New York, NY: McGraw-Hill.

10. Which of the following may be harmful when in proximity to the Magnetic Resonance Imaging (MRI) machine?

    Select (3) three
    (A) Implanted medication pumps
    (B) Pacing wires
    (C) Cardiac pacemakers
    (D) Pulse oximeter
    (E) Precordial stethoscope

Rationale: Items containing iron (ferromagnetic) are strongly attracted to the MRI magnet. MRI-Compatible equipment lists items that are acceptable for use for patients undergoing MRI.

Ref: Nagelhout, J.J., & Plaus, K.L. Ch 52 *Nurse Anesthesia* (5th ed.). St. Louis, MO: Elsevier.

11. A patient is scheduled for bariatric surgery. What is the recommended induction dose for propofol?

    (A) Dose based on lean body weight
    (B) Dose based on total body weight
    (C) Decrease dose by 30%
    (D) Decrease dose by 10%

Rationale: The induction dose of propofol for an obese patient is based on the lean body weight (LBW). A maintenance dose of propofol is based on the total body weight.

Ref: Butterworth, J.F., Mackey, D.C., & Wasnick, J.D. (2013). Ch 34 *Morgan & Mikhail's Clinical Anesthesiology* (5th ed.). New York, NY: McGraw-Hill.

Nagelhout, J., & Plaus, K. (Eds.) (2014). Ch 43 *Nurse Anesthesia* (5th ed.). St. Louis, MO: Elsevier.

12. What is an indication of significant venous air embolism during a seated craniotomy?

    (A) Increased end-tidal carbon dioxide
    (B) Unchanged end-tidal carbon dioxide
    (C) Decreased end-tidal carbon dioxide

Rationale: Entraining large amounts of air into the venous system results in decreased end-tidal carbon dioxide.

Ref: Butterworth, J.F., Mackey, D.C., & Wasnick, J.D. (2013). Ch 27 *Morgan & Mikhail's Clinical Anesthesiology* (5th ed.). New York, NY: McGraw-Hill.

Miller, R., & Pardo, M.Jr. (Eds.) (2011). Ch 30 *Basics of Anesthesia* (6th ed.). Philadelphia, PA: Elsevier.

13. For which heart rhythm is cardioversion not indicated?

    (A) Atrial flutter
    (B) Atrial fibrillation
    (C) Stable ventricular tachycardia
    (D) Pulseless ventricular tachycardia

Rationale: Unstable ventricular tachycardia requires defibrillation.

Ref: Butterworth, J.F., Mackey, D.C., & Wasnick, J.D. (2013). Ch 22 *Morgan & Mikhail's Clinical Anesthesiology* (5th ed.). New York, NY: McGraw-Hill.

Nagelhout, J.J., & Plaus, K.L. Ch 52 *Nurse Anesthesia* (5th ed.). St. Louis, MO: Elsevier.

14. A patient with dysmenorrhea is scheduled for dilation and curettage (D & C). What preoperative testing is required?

    (A) CBC
    (B) Electrolyte panel
    (C) Chest X-ray
    (D) HCG

Rationale: A pregnancy test is needed prior to D & C.

Ref: Macksey, L.F., Sowka, W., Cipcic, E., Kaufman, P.E., & Callaway, F.D. (2012). Ch 20 *Surgical Procedures and Anesthetic Implications*. Sudbury, MA: Jones & Bartlett Learning.

15. The addition of an intravenous inotrope will tend to move the Frank–Starling curve in which direction?

(A) Up
(B) Down
(C) Left
(D) Right

Rationale: Starling's law relates preload (ventricular end-diastolic volume) with stroke volume (or cardiac output) when heart rate and contractility remain constant. If an inotrope exerts its influence on the ventricular myocardium, contractility will increase independently from preload effects. Thus the stroke volume and cardiac output will be higher for a given ventricular end-diastolic pressure.
Ref: Butterworth, J.F., Mackey, D.C., & Wasnick, J.D. (2013). Ch 20 *Morgan & Mikhail's Clinical Anesthesiology* (5th ed.). New York, NY: McGraw-Hill.

16. During an uncomplicated vaginal delivery, what is the expected blood loss?

(A) 250 mL
(B) 400 mL
(C) 750 mL
(D) 800 mL

Rationale: The normal blood loss of vaginal delivery is 400-500 mL whereas the normal blood loss during cesarean section is 700-750 mL.
Ref: Longnecker, D.E., Brown, D.L., Newman, M.F., & Zapol, W.M. (2012). Ch 62 *Anesthesiology* (2nd ed.). San Francisco, CA: McGraw-Hill.

17. What should the activated clotting time be prior to initiation of cardiopulmonary bypass (CPB)?

(A) <150 seconds
(B) >200 seconds but <350 seconds
(C) >350 seconds but <450 seconds
(D) >400 seconds

Rationale: Initiation of cardiopulmonary bypass can begin after the ACT is greater than 400-480 seconds. Failure to establish adequate anticoagulation will result in disseminated intravascular coagulation and formation of clots in the CPB pump.

Ref: Butterworth, J.F., Mackey, D.C., & Wasnick, J.D. (2013). Ch 22 *Morgan & Mikhail's Clinical Anesthesiology* (5th ed.). New York, NY: McGraw-Hill.
Nagelhout, J.J., & Plaus, K.L. (2014). Ch 24 *Nurse Anesthesia* (5th ed.). St. Louis, MO: Elsevier.

18. What level of neural blockade is needed for analgesia during the first stage of labor?

(A) T10–L1 motor level
(B) T10–S4 sensory level
(C) T10–L1 sensory level
(D) T10–S4 motor level

Rationale: A sensory level T10–L1 is needed for adequate analgesia during the first stage of labor. During the second stage of labor additional sensory levels T10–S4 require neural blockade.
Ref: Butterworth, J.F., Mackey, D.C., & Wasnick, J.D. (2013). Ch 41 *Morgan & Mikhail's Clinical Anesthesiology* (5th ed.). New York, NY: McGraw-Hill.

19. How is cardiac index calculated?

(A) $\frac{Cardiac\ Output}{Stroke\ Volume}$
(B) $\frac{Cardiac\ Output}{Systemic\ Vascular\ Resistance}$
(C) $\frac{Cardiac\ Output}{Body\ Surface\ Area}$
(D) $\frac{Cardiac\ Output}{Heart\ Rate}$

Rationale: Cardiac index is a measure of cardiac output comparable among individuals of differing body habitus. It is calculated by dividing the cardiac output by the body surface area.
Ref: Butterworth, J.F., Mackey, D.C., & Wasnick, J.D. (2013). Ch 20 *Morgan & Mikhail's Clinical Anesthesiology* (5th ed.). New York, NY: McGraw-Hill.

20. What is the goal of hemodynamic management for the patient with mitral stenosis?

(A) Avoiding bradycardia
(B) Maintenance of sinus rhythm
(C) Aggressive volume resuscitation
(D) Inotropic support with phosphodiesterase inhibitors

Rationale: The patient with mitral stenosis has impaired left ventricular filling. Sinus rhythm's atrial contractions help optimize left ventricular filling. Maintenance of sinus rhythm with a normal rate should be a perioperative goal. Tachycardia should be avoided as it will decrease diastolic left ventricular filling time and left ventricular end diastolic pressure. Mitral stenosis is associated with left atrial and pulmonary hypertension due to the stenotic transvalvular pressure gradient. Phosphodiesterase inhibitors cause vasodilation and increase left ventricular emptying which will result in severe hypotension. Noninotropic vasopressors, such as vasopressin or phenylephrine, should be used in the presence of hypotension.

Ref: Butterworth, J.F., Mackey, D.C., & Wasnick, J.D. (2013). Ch 21 *Morgan & Mikhail's Clinical Anesthesiology* (5th ed.). New York, NY: McGraw-Hill.

21. A peribulbar block was performed. There was notable resistance during the injection. The patient becomes agitated and complains of pain. What do you suspect?

    (A) Retrobulbar hemorrhage
    (B) Globe puncture
    (C) Extraocular muscle palsy
    (D) Intravascular injection

    Rationale: Globe puncture is associated with increased IOP, resistance during injection, patient agitation and pain, and hemorrhage. In a retrobulbar hemorrhage, the eye moves forward. There may be subconjunctival bleeding. Extraocular muscle palsy results in diplopia. Intravascular injection of local anesthetic during eye blocks result in seizures.

    Ref: Butterworth, J.F., Mackey, D.C., & Wasnick, J.D. (2013). Ch 36 *Morgan & Mikhail's Clinical Anesthesiology* (5th ed.). New York, NY: McGraw-Hill.

    Nagelhout, J.J., & Plaus, K.L. Ch 39 *Nurse Anesthesia* (5th ed.). St. Louis, MO: Elsevier.

22. Which sign is associated with placenta previa?

    (A) Painless vaginal bleeding
    (B) Uterine irritability
    (C) Painful vaginal bleeding
    (D) Coagulopathy

    Rationale: Placenta previa is associated with painless vaginal bleeding and in part by malpresntation of the fetus. In contrast, placenta abruption results painful vaginal bleeding, uterine irritability and is associated with coagulopathy.

    Ref: Butterworth, J.F., Mackey, D.C., & Wasnick, J.D. (2013). Ch 41 *Morgan & Mikhail's Clinical Anesthesiology* (5th ed.). New York, NY: McGraw-Hill.

23. What sign is not an effect of hyperparathyroidism?

    (A) Hypertension
    (B) Ventricular arrhythmias
    (C) Muscle weakness
    (D) Hypochloremic metabolic acidosis

    Rationale: Hyperchloremic metabolic acidosis is a renal effect of hyperparathyroidism.

TABLE 4-2. Effects of hyperparathyroidism.

Cardiovascular
  Hypertension
  Ventricular arrhythmias
  ECG[1] changes (shortened QT interval,[2] widened T wave)

Renal
  Polyuria
  Impaired renal concentrating ability
  Kidney stones
  Hyperchloremic metabolic acidosis
  Dehydration
  Polydipsia
  Kidney failure

Gastrointestinal
  Constipation
  Nausea and vomiting
  Anorexia
  Pancreatitis
  Peptic ulcer disease

Musculoskeletal
  Muscle weakness
  Osteoporosis

Neurological
  Mental status change (eg, delirium, psychosis, coma)

[1]ECG, electrocardiogram.
[2]The QT interval may be prolonged at serum calcium concentrations >16 mg/dL.

    Ref: Butterworth, J.F., Mackey, D.C., & Wasnick, J.D. (2013). Ch 34 *Morgan & Mikhail's Clinical Anesthesiology* (5th ed.). New York, NY: McGraw-Hill.

    Nagelhout, J.J., & Plaus, K.L. Ch 33 *Nurse Anesthesia* (5th ed.). St. Louis, MO: Elsevier.

24. Which factors contribute to respiratory fatigue in neonates and infants?

    (A) Respiratory musculature composed of primarily type-one muscle fibers
    (B) Increased dead space
    (C) Respiratory musculature composed of primarily type-two muscle fibers
    (D) Decreased chest wall compliance

    Rationale: Respiratory musculature in neonates is relatively lacking in type-one muscle fibers. Type-one, or slow-twitch, muscle fibers provide endurance for prolonged effort. Decreased percentage of these fibers contributes to fatigue.

Ref: Butterworth, J.F., Mackey, D.C., & Wasnick, J.D. (2013). Ch 42 *Morgan & Mikhail's Clinical Anesthesiology* (5th ed.). New York, NY: McGraw-Hill.

Hall, J.E. (2011). Ch 84 *Guyton and Hall Textbook of Medical Physiology* (12th ed.). Philadelphia, PA: Elsevier.

25. Which valvular disorder leads to the largest left ventricular volume?

(A) Mitral stenosis
(B) Aortic stenosis
(C) Mitral regurgitation
(D) Aortic regurgitation

Rationale: This question is an application of the left-ventricular pressure-volume loops for patients with valvular heart disease. Aortic regurgitation causes volume overload of the left ventricle.

Ref: Butterworth, J.F., Mackey, D.C., & Wasnick, J.D. (2013). Ch 21 *Morgan & Mikhail's Clinical Anesthesiology* (5th ed.). New York, NY: McGraw-Hill.

26. Which narcotic analgesic is not used for patient controlled analgesia (PCA)?

(A) Meperidine
(B) Morphine
(C) Fentanyl
(D) Hydromorphone

Rationale: The demerol metabolite normeperidine is neurotoxic; therefore, it is not recommended for PCA.

Ref: Butterworth, J.F., Mackey, D.C., & Wasnick, J.D. (2013). Ch 47 *Morgan & Mikhail's Clinical Anesthesiology* (5th ed.). New York, NY: McGraw-Hill.

Nagelhout, J.J., & Plaus, K.L. Ch 51 *Nurse Anesthesia* (5th ed.). St. Louis, MO: Elsevier.

27. With which patient would the anesthetist most want to maintain spontaneous ventilation while under general anesthesia?

(A) Severe aortic stenosis
(B) Severe mitral regurgitation
(C) Acute pulmonary edema
(D) Mitral valve prolapse

Rationale: Positive pressure ventilation decreases the heart's relative preload. Severe aortic stenosis leads to left ventricular diastolic dysfunction secondary to left ventricular hypertrophy. This diastolic dysfunction combined with outflow obstruction makes patients

with aortic stenosis extremely sensitive to decreases in preload (left ventricular end diastolic volume). Mitral regurgitation and pulmonary edema may benefit from positive pressure ventilation.

Ref: Butterworth, J.F., Mackey, D.C., & Wasnick, J.D. (2013). Ch 21 *Morgan & Mikhail's Clinical Anesthesiology* (5th ed.). New York, NY: McGraw-Hill.

28. The "a" wave on the central venous pressure tracing corresponds to which on the EKG tracing?

(A) P-wave
(B) QRS wave
(C) QT interval
(D) T wave

Rationale: The *a*-wave on the venous tracing corresponds to atrial contraction. The P-wave corresponds to atrial depolarization couple to atrial contraction.

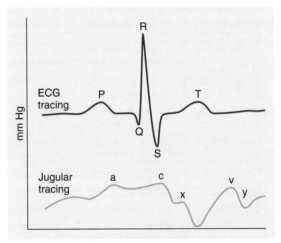

FIG. 4-1. The upward waves (*a, c, v*) and the downward descents (*x, y*) of a central venous tracing in relation to the electrocardiogram (ECG).

Ref: Butterworth, J.F., Mackey, D.C., & Wasnick, J.D. (2013). Ch 5 *Morgan & Mikhail's Clinical Anesthesiology* (5th ed.). New York, NY: McGraw-Hill.

29. What do you anticipate during laparoscopic cholecystectomy?

(A) Increased functional residual capacity
(B) Increased closing capacity
(C) Decreased functional residual capacity
(D) Decreased peak inspiratory pressure

Rationale: Due to insufflation with carbon dioxide, the functional residual capacity and closing capacity are decreased. The peak inspiratory pressure is increased.

Ref: Nagelhout, J., & Plaus, K. (Eds.) (2014). Ch 43 *Nurse Anesthesia* (5th ed.). St. Louis, MO: Elsevier.

30. Which of the following symptoms is consistent with cardiac tamponade?

   (A) Hypotension, tachycardia, tachypnea, muffled heart sounds, and pulsus paradoxus
   (B) Hypertension, tachycardia, tachypnea, and widened pulse pressure
   (C) Jugular venous distension, muffled heart sounds, and bradycardia
   (D) Hypotension, widened pulse pressure, and tachycardia

   Rationale: With cardiac tamponade, acute hypotension, tachycardia, and tachypnea develop. The heart's ability to relax is impaired by fluid compressing it; thus, diastolic pressures equalize across the heart resulting in decreased stroke volume and decreased cardiac output. Cardiac output thus becomes heart rate dependent, thus tachycardia. Decreased cardiac output and elevated left atrial and pulmonary artery pressures lead to tachypnea. Furthermore, with respiratory effort the fluctuations in venous return have a marked change on the diastolic pressures within the heart. A marked pulsus paradoxus develops for the very preload-dependent heart. Heart sounds are muffled.
   Ref: Butterworth, J.F., Mackey, D.C., & Wasnick, J.D. (2013). Ch 21 *Morgan & Mikhail's Clinical Anesthesiology* (5th ed.). New York, NY: McGraw-Hill.

31. Which of the following are absolute contraindications for electroconvulsive therapy (ECT)?

   Select (3) three
   (A) Myocardial infarction <6 weeks
   (B) Pheochromocytoma
   (C) Glaucoma
   (D) Pregnancy
   (E) Cerebrovascular accident <3 months

   Rationale: Glaucoma and pregnancy are relative contraindications to ECT. Other relative contraindications include cardiac dysfunction (angina, CHF), bone fractures, thrombophlebitis, retinal detachment, and pulmonary disease. Absolute contraindications also include intracranial mass and/or surgery, and cervical spine instability.
   Ref: Butterworth, J.F., Mackey, D.C., & Wasnick, J.D. (2013). Ch 28 *Morgan & Mikhail's Clinical Anesthesiology* (5th ed.). New York, NY: McGraw-Hill.
   Nagelhout, J.J., & Plaus, K.L. Ch 52 *Nurse Anesthesia* (5th ed.). St. Louis, MO: Elsevier.

32. What is the most common cause of acute epiglottitis?

   (A) *Streptococcus pneumoniae*
   (B) Allergic reaction
   (C) *Haemophilus influenzae B*
   (D) Viral infection

   Rationale: *Haemophilus influenzae B* bacteria are the causative agent.
   Ref: Butterworth, J.F., Mackey, D.C., & Wasnick, J.D. (2013). Ch 38 *Morgan & Mikhail's Clinical Anesthesiology* (5th ed.). New York, NY: McGraw-Hill.
   Miller, R., & Pardo, M.Jr. (Eds.) (2011). Ch 31 *Basics of Anesthesia* (6th ed.). Philadelphia, PA: Elsevier.

33. The patient is scheduled for a thyroidectomy. What are your primary anesthetic concerns?

   Select (3) three
   (A) Arrhythmias
   (B) Tachycardia
   (C) Body temperature
   (D) Hypotension
   (E) Corneal abrasion

   Rationale: Each of the options should concern the anesthetist when caring for a hyperthyroid patient. However, the primary concern focuses on decreasing sympathetic stimulation that leads to cardiac arrhythmias, hypertension, tachycardia, and increased body temperature. Corneal abrasion is possible in the patient with exophthalmos. Hypotension may result from chronic hypovolemia.
   Ref: Butterworth, J.F., Mackey, D.C., & Wasnick, J.D. (2013). Ch 34 *Morgan & Mikhail's Clinical Anesthesiology* (5th ed.). New York, NY: McGraw-Hill.
   Nagelhout, J.J., & Plaus, K.L. Ch 38 *Nurse Anesthesia* (5th ed.). St. Louis, MO: Elsevier.

34. What is the lowest recommended $PaCO_2$ if hyperventilation is used during intracranial tumor resection?

   (A) 35 mmHg
   (B) 30 mmHg
   (C) 25 mmHg
   (D) 20 mmHg

   Rationale: The recommended $PaCO_2$ range during induced hypocapnia is 30-35 mmHg.
   Ref: Butterworth, J.F., Mackey, D.C., & Wasnick, J.D. (2013). Ch 27 *Morgan & Mikhail's Clinical Anesthesiology* (5th ed.). New York, NY: McGraw-Hill.
   Nagelhout, J.J., & Plaus, K.L. (2014). Ch 28 *Nurse Anesthesia* (5th ed.). St. Louis, MO: Elsevier.

35. How is coronary perfusion pressure defined?

(A) Difference between mean arterial pressure; central venous pressure

(B) Difference between aortic diastolic pressure; left-ventricular end-diastolic pressure

(C) Difference between aortic systolic pressure; left-ventricular end-diastolic pressure

(D) Difference between systolic pressure; central venous pressure.

Rationale: Left-ventricular perfusion mostly occurs during diastole, when the force of the aortic diastolic pressure drives blood through the coronary arteries, overcoming the intramural left-ventricular end-diastolic pressure. During systole, aortic pressure is unable to overcome the higher left-ventricular systolic pressures to generate flow.

Ref: Butterworth, J.F., Mackey, D.C., & Wasnick, J.D. (2013). Ch 20 *Morgan & Mikhail's Clinical Anesthesiology* (5th ed.). New York, NY: McGraw-Hill.

36. What results when a limb tourniquet is released?

Select (3) three

(A) Temperature decrease

(B) Metabolic acidosis

(C) Metabolic alkalosis

(D) Temperature increase

(E) End-tidal CO_2 increase

Rationale: When a tourniquet is released products of cellular metabolic waste enter the circulation. Hypotension, tachycardia and increased minute ventilation occur. The end-tidal CO_2 increases along with serum potassium and lactate.

Ref: Butterworth, J.F., Mackey, D.C., & Wasnick, J.D. (2013). Ch 38 *Morgan & Mikhail's Clinical Anesthesiology* (5th ed.). New York, NY: McGraw-Hill.
Nagelhout, J.J., & Plaus, K.L. Ch 40 *Nurse Anesthesia* (5th ed.). St. Louis, MO: Elsevier.

37. Which patient faces the greatest risk of complete cardiovascular collapse?

(A) 75-year-old female with bilateral carotid artery disease with an aortic valve area of 1.1 cm² undergoing left carotid endarterectomy

(B) 82-year-old male with severe mitral regurgitation and severe tricuspid regurgitation with atrial fibrillation undergoing bowel resection for colon cancer

(C) 67-year-old male with aortic valve area of 0.7 cm² undergoing left carotid endarterectomy

(D) 59-year-old male with aortic valve area of 0.7 cm² undergoing colon resection for ischemic colon

Rationale: Aortic valve area of 0.7 cm² is indicative of severe aortic stenosis. In severe aortic stenosis, changes in intravascular volume and decreases in afterload can lead to critical coronary ischemia. Patients with advanced aortic stenosis are particularly sensitive to hypotension. Aortic stenosis leads to left ventricular hypertrophy due to elevated left ventricular pressures. This, in turn, leads to both an increase in oxygen demand (due to hypertrophy and increased left ventricular systolic pressures) and a decrease in myocardial perfusion (due to left ventricular end-diastolic pressure). Abdominal surgeries in general, and colon resections (especially with ischemia which can lead to septic shock like states) in particular, are known for fluid shifts and decreases in afterload secondary to release of vasodilatory substances. Hypotension can quickly deteriorate to ventricular dysrhythmias and complete cardiovascular collapse necessitating cardiopulmonary resuscitation, even resulting in death.

Ref: Butterworth, J.F., Mackey, D.C., & Wasnick, J.D. (2013). Ch 21 *Morgan & Mikhail's Clinical Anesthesiology* (5th ed.). New York, NY: McGraw-Hill.

38. While observing the fetal heart monitor during labor you note a decrease in the fetal heart rate. What is the probable cause?

(A) Epidural opioids

(B) Terbutaline

(C) Ritodrine

(D) Atropine

Rationale: Fetal tachycardia is linked to beta-adrenergic agonists (ritodrine, terbutaline), atropine and epinephrine. Epidural or intrathecal analgesia contributes to lowering the fetal heart rate particularly with repeated dosing.

Ref: Chestnut, D.H., Polley, L.S., Tsen, L.C., & Wong, C.A. (2009). Ch 6 & 8 *Chestnut's Obstetric Anesthesia Principles and Practice* (4th ed.). Philadelphia, PA: Elsevier.

39. Estimate the total difference in cerebral blood flow if $PaCO_2$ is decreased from 40 mmHg to 34 mmHg. Assume total brain weight is 1,400 grams.

(A) 0-50 mL/min

(B) 30-60 mL/min

(C) 60-120 mL/min

(D) 90-180 mL/min

Rationale: The change in cerebral blood flow is 1 or 2 mL/100g/min for every 1 mmHg change in $PaCO_2$.

Ref: Butterworth, J.F., Mackey, D.C., & Wasnick, J.D. (2013). Ch 26 *Morgan & Mikhail's Clinical Anesthesiology* (5th ed.). New York, NY: McGraw-Hill.

Miller, R., & Pardo, M.Jr. (Eds.) (2011). Ch 30 *Basics of Anesthesia* (6th ed.). Philadelphia, PA: Elsevier.

40. Which of the following rate control agents should be avoided in patients undergoing general anesthesia with acute onset wide-complex supraventricular tachycardia (SVT)?

(A) Digitalis

(B) Adenosine

(C) Esmolol

(D) Amiodarone

Rationale: The SVT is of an unknown type. If a reentrant pathway is present blocking the AV node with digoxin may in fact exacerbate tachycardia while limiting other treatment options (or adenosine).

Ref: Butterworth, J.F., Mackey, D.C., & Wasnick, J.D. (2013). Ch 21 *Morgan & Mikhail's Clinical Anesthesiology* (5th ed.). New York, NY: McGraw-Hill.

41. Which factors contribute to the rapid development of hypoxia during apnea in neonates?

Select (2) two

(A) Low functional residual capacity

(B) Low basal metabolic rate

(C) High oxygen reserve

(D) High oxygen demand

Rationale: Neonates and infants have relatively low functional residual capacity coupled with relatively increased oxygen demand.

Ref: Butterworth, J.F., Mackey, D.C., & Wasnick, J.D. (2013). Ch 42 *Morgan & Mikhail's Clinical Anesthesiology* (5th ed.). New York, NY: McGraw-Hill.

Nagelhout, J., & Plaus, K. (Eds.) (2014). Ch 47 *Nurse Anesthesia* (5th ed.). St. Louis, MO: Elsevier.

42. A 100-kg patient is administered 40,000 units of heparin. Five minutes later the ACT was measured to be 182 seconds. What is the next step?

(A) Proceed with cardiopulmonary bypass.

(B) Wait 5 more minutes and recheck ACT.

(C) Administer an additional 40,000 units of heparin.

(D) Administer two units of fresh frozen plasma.

Rationale: The dose administered is appropriate (300-400 units/kg) to obtain an ACT necessary for initiating cardiopulmonary bypass, 400-800 seconds. Typically, this therapeutic anticoagulation is obtained and verified within 3-5 minutes of administration. A patient may have an antithrombin III deficiency that renders them resistant to the effects of heparin. Recombinant antithrombin III can be administered, but more commonly two units of fresh frozen plasma are administered to provide the antithrombin III necessary to achieve adequate anticoagulation.

Ref: Butterworth, J.F., Mackey, D.C., & Wasnick, J.D. (2013). Ch 22 *Morgan & Mikhail's Clinical Anesthesiology* (5th ed.). New York, NY: McGraw-Hill.

43. Because you are concerned with monitoring factors contributing to cerebral ischemia during mediastinoscopy, where will you place your monitors?

(A) Blood pressure cuff on right arm; arterial line in left hand

(B) Blood pressure cuff on right arm; pulse oximeter on right hand

(C) Blood pressure cuff on left arm; arterial line in right hand

(D) Blood pressure cuff on left arm; pulse oximeter on left hand

Rationale: Because the mediastinoscope can compress the innominate artery as it passed through the upper thorax, there is concern about a decrease in blood flow to the right common carotid artery, to the right vertebral artery and a decrease in subclavian flow to the right hand; therefore, monitoring perfusion to the right hand with either a pulse oximeter waveform or radial arterial waveform can detect decreased flow to the right arm.

Ref: Butterworth, J.F., Mackey, D.C., & Wasnick, J.D. (2013). Ch 25 *Morgan & Mikhail's Clinical Anesthesiology* (5th ed.). New York, NY: McGraw-Hill.

Nagelhout, J.J., & Plaus, K.L. (2014). Ch 27 *Nurse Anesthesia* (5th ed.). St. Louis, MO: Elsevier.

44. Which symptom is not present in advanced aortic stenosis?

(A) Angina

(B) Dyspnea on exertion

(C) Orthostatic syncope

(D) Dyspnea at rest

Rationale: Angina, dyspnea on exertion, and orthostatic and/or exertional syncope are the classic triad of aortic stenosis symptoms.

Ref: Butterworth, J.F., Mackey, D.C., & Wasnick, J.D. (2013). Ch 21 *Morgan & Mikhail's Clinical Anesthesiology* (5th ed.). New York, NY: McGraw-Hill.

45. Which nerve is at greatest risk for injury during thyroid surgery?

(A) Recurrent laryngeal nerve

(B) Superior laryngeal nerve

(C) Facial nerve

(D) Glossopharyngeal nerve

Rationale: The superior laryngeal nerve injury is greatest for surgery involving the anterior neck.

Ref: Butterworth, J.F., Mackey, D.C., & Wasnick, J.D. (2013). Ch 37 *Morgan & Mikhail's Clinical Anesthesiology* (5th ed.). New York, NY: McGraw-Hill.

Nagelhout, J.J., & Plaus, K.L. Ch 38 *Nurse Anesthesia* (5th ed.). St. Louis, MO: Elsevier.

46. Which statements are true regarding gastrointestinal changes during pregnancy?

Select (3) three

(A) Pregnant patients are considered a "full stomach."

(B) Gastric acid increases.

(C) Gastric volume increases.

(D) Lower esophageal sphincter relaxation occurs due to progesterone and estrogen.

(E) Stomach elevates and rotates during pregnancy.

Rationale: Gastric acid and gastric volume are unaffected by pregnancy. Mechanical changes that affect the stomach and lower esophageal sphincter place the parturient at high risk for aspiration.

Ref: Butterworth, J.F., Mackey, D.C., & Wasnick, J.D. (2013). Ch 40 *Morgan & Mikhail's Clinical Anesthesiology* (5th ed.). New York, NY: McGraw-Hill.

Suresh, M.S., Segal, B.S., Preston, R.L., Fernando, R., & Mason C.L. (2013). Ch 1 *Shnider and Levinson's Anesthesia for Obstetrics* (5th ed.). Philadelphia, PA: Lippincott Williams & Wilkins.

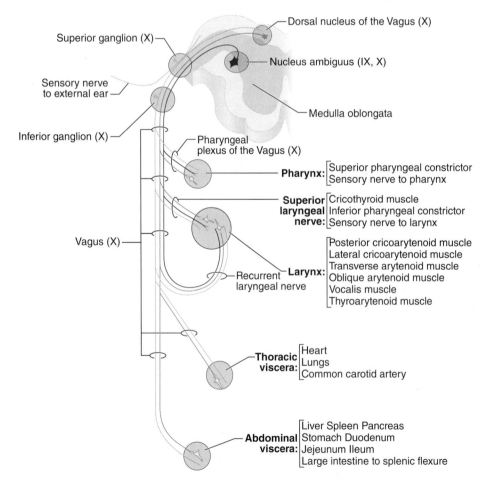

FIG. 4-2. The **vagus nerve** (cranial nerve X) originates in the medulla oblongata and then ramifies in the superior and inferior vagal ganglia in the neck. Its first major branch is the pharyngeal plexus of the vagus. The **superior laryngeal nerve** divides into the external and internal laryngeal nerves. The *internal branch* supplies sensory innervation of the laryngeal mucosa above the vocal cords, and the *external branch* innervates the inferior pharyngeal constrictor muscles and the cricothyroid muscle of the larynx. Cricothyroid muscle contraction increases the voice pitch by lengthening, tensing, and adducting the vocal folds. The superior laryngeal nerve is at risk of damage during operations of the anterior neck, especially thyroid surgery, and injury to this nerve may result in hoarseness and loss of vocal volume. The next branch of the vagus is the **recurrent laryngeal nerve**, which innervates all of the muscles of the larynx except the cricothyroid, and is responsible for phonation and glottic opening. The recurrent laryngeal nerve runs immediately behind the thyroid gland and thus is the nerve of greatest risk for injury during thyroid surgery. Unilateral recurrent laryngeal nerve damage may result in vocal changes or hoarseness, and bilateral nerve damage may result in aphonia and respiratory distress. Inferior to this nerve, the vagus nerve provides autonomic motor and sensory nerve fibers to the thoracic and abdominal viscera. (Reproduced, with permission, from Dillon FX: Electromyographic (EMG) neuromonitoring in otolaryngology-head and neck surgery. Anesthesiol Clin 2010;28:423).

47. What is the level of the larynx in a child?

    (A) C1-C3
    (B) C2-C4
    (C) C3-C5
    (D) C4-C7

    Rationale: The larynx in a small child is adjacent to cervical vertebrae 2-4 with the glottis adjacent to C4.
    Ref: Butterworth, J.F., Mackey, D.C., & Wasnick, J.D. (2013). Ch 42 *Morgan & Mikhail's Clinical Anesthesiology* (5th ed.). New York, NY: McGraw-Hill.
    Nagelhout, J., & Plaus, K. (Eds.) (2014). Ch 47 *Nurse Anesthesia* (5th ed.). St. Louis, MO: Elsevier.

48. How does obesity affect the functional residual capacity (FRC) during general anesthesia?

    (A) Increases FRC 50%
    (B) Decreases FRC 20%
    (C) Increases FRC 20%
    (D) Decreases FRC 50%

    Rationale: A 20% decrease in FRC exists for non-obese patients. For obese patients undergoing general anesthesia, FRC decreases 50%.
    Ref: Hines, R.L., & Marschall, K.E. (2012). Ch 16 *Stoelting's Anesthesia and Co-Exiting Disease* (6th ed.). Philadelphia, PA: Elsevier.

49. Which is least adaptive in an infant as compared to an adult?

    (A) Heart rate
    (B) Cardiac output
    (C) Stroke volume
    (D) Chest wall

    Rationale: Stroke volume in neonates and infants is less adaptive than in an adult. Increasing heart rate is the means of increasing cardiac output.
    Ref: Butterworth, J.F., Mackey, D.C., & Wasnick, J.D. (2013). Ch 42 *Morgan & Mikhail's Clinical Anesthesiology* (5th ed.). New York, NY: McGraw-Hill.
    Miller, R., & Pardo, M.Jr. (Eds.) (2011). Ch 34 *Basics of Anesthesia* (6th ed.). Philadelphia, PA: Elsevier Saunders.

50. A spinal anesthetic is planned for an obese patient. How will you adjust the dose of local anesthetic?

    (A) Decrease 20%.
    (B) Increase 20%.
    (C) Decrease 10%.
    (D) Increase 10%.

    Rationale: The dose of local anesthetic used for spinal or epidural anesthesia in obese patients is decreased 20-25%.
    Ref: Nagelhout, J., & Plaus, K. (Eds.) (2014). Ch 43 *Nurse Anesthesia* (5th ed.). St. Louis, MO: Elsevier.

51. What is the primary determinant of cerebral perfusion?

    (A) Position
    (B) Mean arterial pressure
    (C) Intracranial pressure
    (D) Central venous pressure

    Rationale: All of these can have some impact but the primary variable is mean arterial pressure.
    Ref: Butterworth, J.F., Mackey, D.C., & Wasnick, J.D. (2013). Ch 26 *Morgan & Mikhail's Clinical Anesthesiology* (5th ed.). New York, NY: McGraw-Hill.
    Miller, R., & Pardo, M.Jr. (Eds.) (2011). Ch 30 *Basics of Anesthesia* (6th ed.). Philadelphia, PA: Elsevier.

52. What is the efferent limb of the oculocardiac reflex?

    (A) Cranial nerve V
    (B) Cranial nerve X
    (C) Cranial nerve I
    (D) Cranial nerve III

    Rationale: Trigeminal (CN V) afferent and vagal (CN X) efferent pathways comprise the oculocardiac reflex.
    Ref: Butterworth, J.F., Mackey, D.C., & Wasnick, J.D. (2013). Ch 36 *Morgan & Mikhail's Clinical Anesthesiology* (5th ed.). New York, NY: McGraw-Hill.
    Nagelhout, J.J., & Plaus, K.L. Ch 39 *Nurse Anesthesia* (5th ed.). St. Louis, MO: Elsevier.

53. What factor is increased in a neonate as compared with an adult?

    (A) Surface area to weight ratio
    (B) Systolic blood pressure
    (C) Plasma protein concentration
    (D) Lung compliance

    Rationale: Neonates have a relatively larger body surface area to mass ratio which contributes to the risk of hypothermia. B, C, and D are all decreased in the neonate compared to the adult.
    Ref: Butterworth, J.F., Mackey, D.C., & Wasnick, J.D. (2013). Ch 42 *Morgan & Mikhail's Clinical Anesthesiology* (5th ed.). New York, NY: McGraw-Hill.
    Nagelhout, J., & Plaus, K. (Eds.) (2014). Ch 47 *Nurse Anesthesia* (5th ed.). St. Louis, MO: Elsevier.

54. When dosing medications for obese patients, what is the best weight parameter to use?

(A) Total body weight

(B) Ideal body weight

(C) Lean body weight

(D) Total body mass index

Rationale: High plasma concentrations result when administering IV medications to obese patients based on total body weight. This is due to poor blow flow to fat. Lean body weight is the parameter when dosing medications for obese patients. Lean body weight does not include fat weight. Neither ideal body weight nor body mass index is used to calculate IV medications for obese patients.

Ref: Hines, R.L., & Marschall, K.E. (2012). Ch 16 *Stoelting's Anesthesia and Co-Exiting Disease* (6th ed.). Philadelphia, PA: Elsevier.

55. Which is true regarding morbidity and mortality in pediatric anesthesia?

(A) Anesthetic risk is directly related to patient age.

(B) Anesthetic risk is greatest in patients younger than 1 year.

(C) Anesthetic risk is greater now than in the past.

(D) Anesthetic risk is similar throughout childhood.

Rationale: Pediatric anesthetic morbidity and mortality are inversely related to age with greatest risk in patients younger than 1 year.

Ref: Butterworth, J.F., Mackey, D.C., & Wasnick, J.D. (2013). Ch 42 *Morgan & Mikhail's Clinical Anesthesiology* (5th ed.). New York, NY: McGraw-Hill.

Longnecker, D., Brown, D., Newman, M., & Zapol, W. (Eds.) (2012). Ch 63 *Anesthesiology* (2nd ed.). New York, NY: McGraw-Hill.

56. With which of the following preoperative EKG findings will the anesthetist be particularly careful to avoid bradycardia?

(A) Sinus rhythm with prolonged QT interval

(B) Sinus rhythm with left bundle branch block

(C) Sinus rhythm with premature ventricular complexes

(D) Atrial fibrillation

Rationale: Long QT may precipitate torsade de pointes. QT interval is rate dependent; slow heart rate is consistent with longer QT interval. Addition-

ally, premature ventricular complexes are more common with bradycardia.

Ref: Butterworth, J.F., Mackey, D.C., & Wasnick, J.D. (2013). Ch 21 *Morgan & Mikhail's Clinical Anesthesiology* (5th ed.). New York, NY: McGraw-Hill.

57. The patient is scheduled for a total knee arthroscopy under general anesthesia. The patient's history includes retina surgery using sulfur hexafluoride 2 months ago. What will you avoid?

(A) Nitrous oxide

(B) Rocuronium

(C) Sevoflurane

(D) Fentanyl

Rationale: Nitrous oxide expands the gas bubble and may cause intraocular hypertension. There are no other medication contraindications.

Ref: Butterworth, J.F., Mackey, D.C., & Wasnick, J.D. (2013). Ch 36 *Morgan & Mikhail's Clinical Anesthesiology* (5th ed.). New York, NY: McGraw-Hill.

Nagelhout, J.J., & Plaus, K.L. Ch 39 *Nurse Anesthesia* (5th ed.). St. Louis, MO: Elsevier.

58. What is the maintenance intravenous fluid replacement rate for a toddler weighing 12 kg?

(A) 48 mL/hr

(B) 44 mL/hr

(C) 40 mL/hr

(D) 36 mL/hr

Rationale: Hourly maintenance fluid rate is calculated as 4 mL/kg/hr up to 10 kg of body weight, 2 mL/kg/hr for the second 10 kg of body weight, and 1 mL/kg/hr for every kilogram beyond 20.

Ref: Butterworth, J.F., Mackey, D.C., & Wasnick, J.D. (2013). Ch 42 *Morgan & Mikhail's Clinical Anesthesiology* (5th ed.). New York, NY: McGraw-Hill.

Nagelhout, J., & Plaus, K. (Eds.) (2014). Ch 48 *Nurse Anesthesia* (5th ed.). St. Louis, MO: Elsevier.

59. How much intravenous replacement fluid should be given in the first hour of an anesthetic for a child weighing 16 kg? The child last ate at 0400. The current time is 0700.

(A) 52 mL

(B) 104 mL

(C) 208 mL

(D) 130 mL

Rationale: The maintenance replacement rate is 52 mL/hr. The calculated fluid deficit is 52 mL/hr over 3 hours fasted (156 mL). Half of the deficit (78 mL) is given during the first hour in addition to the maintenance rate (52 mL) for a total replacement of 130 mL during the first hour.

Ref: Butterworth, J.F., Mackey, D.C., & Wasnick, J.D. (2013). Ch 42 *Morgan & Mikhail's Clinical Anesthesiology* (5th ed.). New York, NY: McGraw-Hill.

Nagelhout, J., & Plaus, K. (Eds.) (2014). Ch 48 *Nurse Anesthesia* (5th ed.). St. Louis, MO: Elsevier.

60. Which feature of a pediatric endotracheal tube will have greatest influence on work of breathing?

    (A) External diameter
    (B) Length
    (C) Internal diameter
    (D) Curvature

Rationale: The internal diameter of the tube has the greatest influence on resistance.

Ref: Butterworth, J.F., Mackey, D.C., & Wasnick, J.D. (2013). Ch 19 *Morgan & Mikhail's Clinical Anesthesiology* (5th ed.). New York, NY: McGraw-Hill.

Dorsch, J., & Dorsch, S. (Eds.) (2008). Ch 19 *Understanding anesthesia equipment* (5th ed.). Philadelphia, PA: Lippincott Williams & Wilkins.

61. During laparoscopic bariatric surgery, you apply positive end expiratory pressure (PEEP). What is the recommended upper limit?

    (A) 5 cm H_2O
    (B) 10 cm H_2O
    (C) 15 cm H_2O
    (D) 20 cm H_2O

Rationale: When using large tidal volumes, oxygenation may be impaired. Limit PEEP to 15 cm H_2O.

Ref: Butterworth, J.F., Mackey, D.C., & Wasnick, J.D. (2013). Ch 34 *Morgan & Mikhail's Clinical Anesthesiology* (5th ed.). New York, NY: McGraw-Hill.

Nagelhout, J., & Plaus, K. (Eds.) (2014). Ch 43 *Nurse Anesthesia* (5th ed.). St. Louis, MO: Elsevier.

62. Which of the following agents will cause the greatest decreased afterload?

    (A) Verapamil
    (B) Nicardipine
    (C) Metoprolol
    (D) Nitroglycerine

Rationale: All of the agents mentioned have an afterload decreasing effect. Nicardipine, however, is a calcium calcium-channel blocking agents which is very selective for vascular smooth muscle. Verapamil is a calcium-channel blocker more selective for cardiac than vascular smooth muscle. Nitroglycerine is a nitrate that causes arterial and venodilation. The dilation from nitroglycerine is much more pronounced on venous vessels. Metoprolol, a beta blocker, will have minimal to no effect on afterload. From the list, Nicardipine causes the most arterial vasodilation.

Ref: Butterworth, J.F., Mackey, D.C., & Wasnick, J.D. (2013). Ch 21 *Morgan & Mikhail's Clinical Anesthesiology* (5th ed.). New York, NY: McGraw-Hill.

TABLE 4-3. Comparison of antianginal agents.[1]

| Cardiac Parameter | Nitrates | Calcium Channel Blockers | | | β-Blockers |
		Verapamil	Nifedipine Nicardipine Nimodipine	Diltiazem	
Preload	↓↓	—	—	—	—/↑
Afterload	↓	↓	↓↓	↓	—/↓
Contractility	—	↓↓	—	↓	↓↓↓
SA node automaticity	↑/—	↓↓	↑/—	↓↓	↓↓↓
AV conduction	—	↓↓↓	—	↓↓	↓↓↓
Vasodilatation					
Coronary	↑	↑↑	↑↑↑	↑↑	—/↓
Systemic	↑↑	↑	↑↑	↑	—/↓

[1]SA, sinoatrial; AV, atrioventricular; ↑, increases; —, no change; ↓, decreases.

63. What is the correct internal diameter and depth for an endotracheal tube placed in a 4-year-old?

(A) Internal diameter 3.5 mm at a depth of 12 cm

(B) Internal diameter 5.0 cm at a depth of 10 cm

(C) Internal diameter of 4.5 mm at a depth of 13.5 cm

(D) Internal diameter of 5.0 mm at a depth of 15 cm

Rationale: The correct internal diameter for this age is 5 mm. Depth is estimated as triple the internal diameter.

Ref: Butterworth, J.F., Mackey, D.C., & Wasnick, J.D. (2013). Ch 19 *Morgan & Mikhail's Clinical Anesthesiology* (5th ed.). New York, NY: McGraw-Hill.

Miller, R., & Pardo, M.Jr. (Eds.) (2011). Ch 34 *Basics of Anesthesia* (6th ed.). Philadelphia, PA: Elsevier.

64. You are planning to add fentanyl to the epidural for labor. How much will you add to the local anesthetic solution?

(A) 5 mg

(B) 10 μg

(C) 50 μg

(D) 0.5 mg

Rationale: Fentanyl 50-150 μg is the appropriate dose as an addition to labor epidural analgesia. Morphine 5 mg is also useful as well as meperidine (50-100 μg) or Sufentanil (5-20 μg).

TABLE 4-4. Spinal opioid dosages for labor and delivery.

Agent	Intrathecal	Epidural
Morphine	0.1–0.5 mg	5 mg
Meperidine	10–15 mg	50–100 mg
Fentanyl	10–25 mcg	50–150 mcg
Sufentanil	3–10 mcg	10–20 mcg

Ref: Butterworth, J.F., Mackey, D.C., & Wasnick, J.D. (2013). Ch 41 *Morgan & Mikhail's Clinical Anesthesiology* (5th ed.). New York, NY: McGraw-Hill.

Suresh, M.S., Segal, B.S., Preston, R.L., Fernando, R., & Mason C.L. (2013). Ch 9 *Shnider and Levinson's Anesthesia for Obstetrics* (5th ed.). Philadelphia, PA: Lippincott Williams & Wilkins.

65. A patient with ischemic cardiomyopathy, with a preoperative ejection fraction of 15%, presents for a general anesthetic. After induction of general anesthesia, the vital signs include a blood pressure of 79/61 mmHg and a heart rate of 54 beats per minute. What intravenous drip is best?

(A) Epinephrine

(B) Vasopressin

(C) Phenylephrine

(D) Milrinone

Rationale: The most effective treatment would be to restore the circulating catecholamine levels through an epinephrine or norepinephrine drip, restoring an adequate blood pressure and cardiac output. Increasing afterload without simultaneously increasing contractility (with phenylephrine or vasopressin), may raise blood pressure for a time but decrease cardiac output and increase left-ventricular end-diastolic, thereby dangerously decreasing coronary perfusion in a patient already suffering from coronary ischemia. Milrinone will indeed increase cardiac output, but will only further decrease blood pressure by exacerbating vasodilation, thereby decreasing perfusion pressure to vital organs including the heart.

Ref: Butterworth, J.F., Mackey, D.C., & Wasnick, J.D. (2013). Ch 20 *Morgan & Mikhail's Clinical Anesthesiology* (5th ed.). New York, NY: McGraw-Hill.

66. Which solution is appropriate for replacement of calculated fluid deficits, blood loss, or third-space loss in the pediatric patient?

(A) Lactated Ringer's

(B) 5% dextrose in water

(C) 5% dextrose in 0.45% normal saline

(D) 25% albumin

Rationale: Lactated Ringer's is a common and appropriate choice for volume replacement.

Ref: Butterworth, J.F., Mackey, D.C., & Wasnick, J.D. (2013). Ch 42 *Morgan & Mikhail's Clinical Anesthesiology* (5th ed.). New York, NY: McGraw-Hill.

Miller, R.D., Eriksson, L.I., Fleisher, L.A., Weiner-Kronish, J.P., & Young, W.L. (Eds.) (2010). Ch 82 *Miller's Anesthesia* (7th ed.). Philadelphia, PA: Elsevier.

67. Which estimation of blood volume per kilogram is correct for a 2-week-old?

(A) 65 mL

(B) 75 mL

(C) 85 mL

(D) 95 mL

Rationale: Blood volume in the neonatal period is estimated to be between 80-90 mL/kg.

Ref: Butterworth, J.F., Mackey, D.C., & Wasnick, J.D. (2013). Ch 42 *Morgan & Mikhail's Clinical Anesthesiology* (5th ed.). New York, NY: McGraw-Hill.

Nagelhout, J., & Plaus, K. (Eds.) (2014). Ch 48 *Nurse Anesthesia* (5th ed.). St. Louis, MO: Elsevier.

68. Which patient requires the highest minimum alveolar concentration (MAC)?

    (A) Newborn of 35 weeks' gestation

    (B) A 4-month-old

    (C) An 18-month-old

    (D) A 3-year-old

    Rationale: Infants >3 but <6 months of age have the highest MAC.

TABLE 4-5. Approximate MAC[1] values for pediatric patients reported in % of an atmosphere.[2]

Agent	Neonates	Infants	Small Children	Adults
Halothane	0.90	1.1–1.2	0.9	0.75
Sevoflurane	3.2	3.2	2.5	2
Isoflurane	1.6	1.8–1.9	1.3–1.6	1.2
Desflurane	8–9	9–10	7–8	6

[1]MAC, minimum alveolar concentration.
[2]Values are derived from various sources.

Ref: Butterworth, J.F., Mackey, D.C., & Wasnick, J.D. (2013). Ch 42 *Morgan & Mikhail's Clinical Anesthesiology* (5th ed.). New York, NY: McGraw-Hill.

Miller, R.D., Eriksson, L.I., Fleisher, L.A., Weiner-Kronish, J.P., & Young, W.L. (Eds.) (2010). Ch 82 *Miller's Anesthesia* (7th ed.). Philadelphia, PA: Elsevier.

69. If intramuscular succinylcholine were indicated, what would be the correct dose for a child?

    (A) 1 mg/kg

    (B) 2 mg/kg

    (C) 3 mg/kg

    (D) 4 mg/kg

    Rationale: Intramuscular succinylcholine can be administered for emergency airway management in children. The dose is 4 mg/kg.

Ref: Butterworth, J.F., Mackey, D.C., & Wasnick, J.D. (2013). Ch 42 *Morgan & Mikhail's Clinical Anesthesiology* (5th ed.). New York, NY: McGraw-Hill.

Miller, R.D., Eriksson, L.I., Fleisher, L.A., Weiner-Kronish, J.P., & Young, W.L. (Eds.) (2010). Ch 82 *Miller's Anesthesia* (7th ed.). Philadelphia, PA: Elsevier.

70. Why does an infant require an increased induction dose (mg/kg) of propofol than an adult?

    (A) Enzyme induction

    (B) Increased central volume of distribution

    (C) Immature renal function

    (D) Decreased adipose for redistribution

    Rationale: Infants require larger per-kilogram induction doses of propofol because of a relatively larger central volume of distribution.

Ref: Butterworth, J.F., Mackey, D.C., & Wasnick, J.D. (2013). Ch 42 *Morgan & Mikhail's Clinical Anesthesiology* (5th ed.). New York, NY: McGraw-Hill.

Miller, R.D., Eriksson, L.I., Fleisher, L.A., Weiner-Kronish, J.P., & Young, W.L. (Eds.) (2010). Ch 82 *Miller's Anesthesia* (7th ed.). Philadelphia, PA: Elsevier.

71. What is the best means to avoid lung overdistension for obese ventilated patients?

    (A) Tidal volume 10-15 mL/kg

    (B) Tidal volume 12-15 mL/kg

    (C) Tidal volume 6-10 mL/kg

    (D) Tidal volume 4-8 mL/kg

    Rationale: Methods to minimize overdistension of the lung in obese patients include increasing the ventilation rate, keeping the end-inspiratory pressure <30 cm H_2O and using a tidal volume of 6-10 mL/kg.

Ref: Butterworth, J.F., Mackey, D.C., & Wasnick, J.D. (2013). Ch 34 *Morgan & Mikhail's Clinical Anesthesiology* (5th ed.). New York, NY: McGraw-Hill.

Nagelhout, J., & Plaus, K. (Eds.) (2014). Ch 43 *Nurse Anesthesia* (5th ed.). St. Louis, MO: Elsevier.

72. Which patient is at greatest risk of central apnea following anesthesia?

    (A) A 3-month-old born at 40 weeks' gestation

    (B) A 9-week-old born at 39 weeks' gestation

    (C) A 4-month-old born at 30 weeks' gestation

    (D) An 8-month-old born at 28 weeks' gestation

    Rationale: Calendar age plus gestational age yields postconceptual age. History of premature birth and postconceptual age less than 50 weeks' pose increased risk of postoperative central apnea.

Ref: Butterworth, J.F., Mackey, D.C., & Wasnick, J.D. (2013). Ch 42 *Morgan & Mikhail's Clinical Anesthesiology* (5th ed.). New York, NY: McGraw-Hill.

Miller, R., & Pardo, M.Jr. (Eds.) (2011). Ch 34 *Basics of Anesthesia* (6th ed.). Philadelphia, PA: Elsevier.

73. Following administration of intrathecal anesthesia for cesarean section the patient is unable to speak, loses consciousness and is hypotensive. What is the most likely cause?

    (A) High spinal
    (B) Use of ropivacaine
    (C) Spinal hematoma
    (D) Use of bupivacaine

    Rationale: Hypotension is a common side effect of intrathecal anesthesia. Causative factors for high spinals include lack of adjustment in dosages for pregnant patients as well as excessive spread of the local anesthetic. For cesarean section, a T4 level is desired. All local anesthetics may produce a high spinal. Spinal hematoma produces symptoms including severe back and leg pain and motor weakness.

    Ref: Butterworth, J.F., Mackey, D.C., & Wasnick, J.D. (2013). Ch 45 *Morgan & Mikhail's Clinical Anesthesiology* (5th ed.). New York, NY: McGraw-Hill.

    Longnecker, D.E., Brown, D.L., Newman, M.F., & Zapol, W.M. (2012). Ch 62 *Anesthesiology* 2nd ed.). San Francisco, CA: McGraw-Hill.

74. What is the best position for optimizing airway patency during pediatric airway management?

    (A) Small pad placed under the shoulders
    (B) Small pad placed behind the head
    (C) The "sniffing position"
    (D) "Ramp" of towels behind the back

    Rationale: A small pad under the shoulders compensates for the disproportionately large occiput.

    Ref: Butterworth, J.F., Mackey, D.C., & Wasnick, J.D. (2013). Ch 42 *Morgan & Mikhail's Clinical Anesthesiology* (5th ed.). New York, NY: McGraw-Hill.

    Longnecker, D., Brown, D., Newman, M., & Zapol, W. (Eds.). (2012). Ch 64 *Anesthesiology* (2nd ed.), New York, NY: McGraw-Hill.

75. What is the best indication for a caudal block in a pediatric patient?

    (A) Anesthesia or analgesia for procedures below the xyphoid process
    (B) Analgesia for the first stage of labor
    (C) Anesthesia or analgesia for procedures below the umbilicus
    (D) Significant deformity of the sacral region

    Rationale: Caudal anesthesia is indicated to supplement general anesthesia or provide analgesia for procedures below the level of the umbilicus.

    Ref: Butterworth, J.F., Mackey, D.C., & Wasnick, J.D. (2013). Ch 42 *Morgan & Mikhail's Clinical Anesthesiology* (5th ed.). New York, NY: Lange Medical Books McGraw-Hill.

    Miller, R.D., Eriksson, L.I., Fleisher, L.A., Weiner-Kronish, J.P., & Young, W.L. (Eds.) (2010). Ch 81 *Miller's Anesthesia* (7th ed.). Philadelphia, PA: Elsevier.

    Chestnut, D.H., Polley, L.S., Tsen, L.C., & Wong, C.A. (Eds.) (2009). Ch 12 *Chestnut's Obstetric Anesthesia Principles and Practice* (4th ed.). Philadelphia, PA: Elsevier.

76. Which valve disorder most likely predisposes a patient to coronary ischemia with hypotension?

    (A) Mitral stenosis
    (B) Mitral regurgitation
    (C) Aortic stenosis
    (D) Aortic regurgitation

    Rationale: Patients with advanced aortic stenosis are extremely sensitive to hypotension. Aortic stenosis leads to left ventricular hypertrophy due to elevated left ventricular pressures. This leads to both an increase in oxygen demand (hypertrophy and increased left ventricular systolic pressures) and a decrease in myocardial perfusion due to left ventricular end-diastolic pressure, which is elevated even early in disease progression.

    Ref: Butterworth, J.F., Mackey, D.C., & Wasnick, J.D. (2013). Ch 21 *Morgan & Mikhail's Clinical Anesthesiology* (5th ed.). New York, NY: McGraw-Hill.

77. What is the hallmark laboratory finding associated with pyloric stenosis?

    (A) Hypokalemic hypochloremic metabolic acidosis
    (B) Hypokalemic hyperchloremic metabolic alkalosis
    (C) Hyperkalemic hypochloremic metabolic acidosis
    (D) Hypokalemic hypochloremic metabolic alkalosis

    Rationale: Vomiting causes loss of stomach acid and electrolytes.

    Ref: Butterworth, J.F., Mackey, D.C., & Wasnick, J.D. (2013). Ch 42 *Morgan & Mikhail's Clinical Anesthesiology* (5th ed.). New York, NY: McGraw-Hill.

    Jaffe, R.A., Samuels, S.I., Schmiesing, C.A., & Golianu, B. (Eds.) (2009). Ch 12.5 *Anesthesiologist's Manual of Surgical Procedures* (4th ed.). Philadelphia, PA:Lippincott Williams & Wilkins.

78. Which of the following is true regarding a patient with septal defects?

(A) An increase in SVR relative to PVR will increase cyanosis.

(B) An increase in PVR relative to SVR favors right to left shunting.

(C) An increase in PVR relative to SVR will decrease risk of paradoxical air embolism.

(D) Eisenmenger syndrome is most often due to left ventricular hypertrophy.

Rationale: When right-sided pressures exceed left-sided pressures with septal defects, a mixing of unoxygenated venous blood with the oxygenated blood can lead to cyanotic states, a right to left shunting. This also can lead to right-sided air bubbles moving across the septum to the left, causing paradoxical air embolism to the cerebral or coronary arterial circulation. The reverse is true. An increase in SVR (with increased left-sided pressures) will reverse the right-to-left shunt and decrease cyanosis. Eisenmenger syndrome is the result of chronic left-to-right shunts which increase right-sided pressures, resulting in right-ventricular hypertrophy with elevated right-sided pressures. This will result in a reversal of the pressure gradient, reversing the shunt to become a right-to-left shunt.
Ref: Butterworth, J.F., Mackey, D.C., & Wasnick, J.D. (2013). Ch 21 *Morgan & Mikhail's Clinical Anesthesiology* (5th ed.). New York, NY: McGraw-Hill.

79. What is the most common site of herniation in congenital diaphragmatic hernia?

(A) Right foramen of Bochdalek

(B) Foramen of Morgagni

(C) Left foramen of Bochdalek

(D) Foramen of Luschka

Rationale: Herniation through the foramen of Bochdalek, specifically the left side, accounts for the vast majority of cases.
Ref: Butterworth, J.F., Mackey, D.C., & Wasnick, J.D. (2013). Ch 42 *Morgan & Mikhail's Clinical Anesthesiology* (5th ed.). New York, NY: Lange Medical Books McGraw-Hill.
Jaffe, R.A., Samuels, S.I., Schmiesing, C.A., & Golianu, B. (Eds.) (2009). Ch 12.5 *Anesthesiologist's Manual of Surgical Procedures* (4th ed.). Philadelphia, PA: Wolters Kluwer Lippincott Williams & Wilkins.

80. Which is the most common type of tracheoesophageal fistula?

(A) Type IIIb, esophageal atresia with a fistula between the distal esophagus and trachea

(B) Type I, proximal tracheoesophageal fistula without distal fistula between stomach and trachea

(C) Type IIIc, fistula between the trachea and both the upper and lower esophageal sections

(D) Type II, esophageal atresia without communication with the trachea

Rationale: Option A is most common. The other options are incorrectly described and/or less frequent.
Ref: Butterworth, J.F., Mackey, D.C., & Wasnick, J.D. (2013). Ch 42 *Morgan & Mikhail's Clinical Anesthesiology* (5th ed.). New York, NY: McGraw-Hill.
Nagelhout, J., & Plaus, K. (Eds.) (2014). Ch 47 *Nurse Anesthesia* (5th ed.). St. Louis, MO: Elsevier.

81. Which statement is true regarding omphalocele and gastroschisis?

(A) Gastroschisis is less common and presents with a peritoneal covering.

(B) Omphalocele is less common and presents without peritoneal covering.

(C) Gastroschisis is more common and presents without peritoneal covering.

(D) Omphalocele is more common and presents with a peritoneal covering.

Rationale: Omphalocele occurs more frequently and is contained within a peritoneal covering.
Ref: Butterworth, J.F., Mackey, D.C., & Wasnick, J.D. (2013). Ch 42 *Morgan & Mikhail's Clinical Anesthesiology* (5th ed.). New York, NY: McGraw-Hill.
Nagelhout, J., & Plaus, K. (Eds.) (2014). Ch 47 *Nurse Anesthesia* (5th ed.). St. Louis, MO: Elsevier.
Miller, R.D., Eriksson, L.I., Fleisher, L.A., Weiner-Kronish, J.P., & Young, W.L. (Eds.) (2010). Ch 82 *Miller's Anesthesia* (7th ed.). Philadelphia, PA: Elsevier.

82. Which congenital cardiac malformation is most commonly associated with Down syndrome?

(A) Transposition of the great vessels

(B) Coarctation of the aorta

(C) Endocardial cushion defect

(D) Aortic stenosis

Rationale: Endocardial cushion defects are the most common congenital cardiac malformations associated with Down syndrome.
Ref: Butterworth, J.F., Mackey, D.C., & Wasnick, J.D. (2013). Ch 42 *Morgan & Mikhail's Clinical Anesthesiology* (5th ed.). New York, NY: McGraw-Hill.
Baum, V.C., & O'Flaherty, J.E. (2007). *Anesthesia for Genetic, Metabolic, & Dysmorphic Syndromes of Childhood* (2nd ed.). Philadelphia, PA: Lippincott Williams & Wilkins.

83. Which of the following is an anatomic characteristic of the pediatric airway that distinguishes it from the adult patient?

    (A) The rime glottidis is the narrowest point of the airway until the age of 5.
    (B) The tongue is proportionately smaller.
    (C) The larynx is located at the level of C4.
    (D) The epiglottis is flat and flexible.

    Rationale: The larynx is located in a more cephalad position (C3–C4) than the adult larynx (C4–C5). Because the larynx is higher, the distance between the tongue, palate, and epiglottis are smaller and more prone to obstruction.
    Ref: Butterworth, J.F., Mackey, D.C., & Wasnick, J.D. (2013). Ch 42 *Morgan & Mikhail's Clinical Anesthesiology* (5th ed.). New York, NY: McGraw-Hill.
    Cote, C.J., Lerman, J., & Todres, D. (2013). Ch 12 *A Practice of Anesthesia for Infants and Children* (5th ed.). Philadelphia, PA: Elsevier.

84. Which type of surgical procedure will result in the greatest increase in afterload accompanied by acute hypertension during aortic cross-clamping?

    (A) Stanford Type A dissection of the ascending aorta
    (B) Suprarenal descending aortic aneurysm
    (C) Infrarenal descending aortic aneurysm
    (D) Stanford Type B dissection

    Rationale: When an aortic cross-clamp is applied, an immediate intense increase in left-ventricular afterload is experienced with a concomitant increase in blood pressure proximal to the clamp. The more proximal the clamp is applied, the more marked the effects. Since the ascending aorta is most proximal, it will experience the greatest increase in afterload if it is cross-clamped with the heart beating.
    Ref: Butterworth, J.F., Mackey, D.C., & Wasnick, J.D. (2013). Ch 22 *Morgan & Mikhail's Clinical Anesthesiology* (5th ed.). New York, NY: McGraw-Hill.

85. At what gestational age does surfactant production begin?

    (A) 30 weeks
    (B) 34 weeks
    (C) 26 weeks
    (D) 32 weeks

    Rationale: At 30 weeks, pulmonary surfactant production begins. Sufficient amounts for extrauterine life are usually present at 34 weeks.
    Ref: Butterworth, J.F., Mackey, D.C., & Wasnick, J.D. (2013). Ch 42 *Morgan & Mikhail's Clinical Anesthesiology* (5th ed.). New York, NY: McGraw-Hill.
    Cote, C.J., Lerman, J., & Todres, D. (2013). Ch 12 *A Practice of Anesthesia for Infants and Children* (5th ed.). Philadelphia, PA: Elsevier.

86. Which of the following correctly describes omphalocele?

    (A) It is due to occlusion of the omphalomesenteric artery.
    (B) 40-60% of patients have associated anomalies.
    (C) The defect is periumbilical.
    (D) Incidence is approximately 1 in 15,000 births.

    Rationale: Omphaloceles result from the failure of gut migration from the yolk sac into the abdomen. The incidence is approximately 1 in 6,000 births. The incidence of associated anomalies is approximately 40-60%. The defect lies within the umbilical cord. Problems associated with the defect are congenital heart disease, exstrophy of the bladder, and Beckwith-Wiedemann syndrome.
    Ref: Butterworth, J.F., Mackey, D.C., & Wasnick, J.D. (2013). Ch 42 *Morgan & Mikhail's Clinical Anesthesiology* (5th ed.). New York, NY: McGraw-Hill.
    Cote, C.J., Lerman, J., & Todres, D. (2013). Ch 36 *A Practice of Anesthesia for Infants and Children* (5th ed.). Philadelphia, PA: Elsevier.

87. During a repeat cesarean section a term infant is delivered. On assessment at 1 minute, the infant has a heart rate of 90, blue extremities, whimpering to stimulus, breathing regularly and active with good muscle tone. What is the 1 minute Apgar score?

    (A) 5
    (B) 6
    (C) 7
    (D) 8

Rationale: Apgar scores are calculated for this patient as such: 2 points to regular breathing and active/good muscle tone. 1 point is given each for a HR <100 bpm, acrocyanosis and whimpering. Scores 0-4 are regarded as severely depressed, 4-7 as mildly depressed, and 8-10 as vigorous.

Ref: Butterworth, J.F., Mackey, D.C., & Wasnick, J.D. (2013). Ch 41 & 42 *Morgan & Mikhail's Clinical Anesthesiology* (5th ed.). New York, NY: McGraw-Hill.

Chestnut, D.H., Polley, L.S., Tsen, L.C., & Wong, C.A. (Eds.) (2009). Ch 9 *Chestnut's Obstetric Anesthesia Principles and Practice* (4th ed.). Philadelphia, PA: Elsevier.

88. Which complications are most concerning following carotid endarterectomy?

Select (2) two

(A) Hypertension
(B) Hypoxemia
(C) Hypotension
(D) Delayed emergence

Rationale: Each of the complications poses challenges following carotid endarterectomy. Denervation of the carotid baroreceptor blunts the feedback loop in response to hypertension, thus postoperative hypertension is possible with carotid endarterectomy. The carotid baroreceptor is instrumental in respiratory stimulation in the presence of hypoxemia. For a patient dependent on the hypoxic drive for ventilation (i.e., COPD or narcotic use), unchecked hypoxemia may develop.

Ref: Butterworth, J.F., Mackey, D.C., & Wasnick, J.D. (2013). Ch 21 *Morgan & Mikhail's Clinical Anesthesiology* (5th ed.). New York, NY: McGraw-Hill.

89. Cleft palate, micrognathia, glossoptosis, and congenital heart disease are key characteristics of which syndromes?

(A) Treacher Collins
(B) VATER
(C) Pierre–Robin
(D) Prader–Willi

Rationale: The listed characteristics are those of Pierre–Robin syndrome. Glossoptosis is an important characteristic as it created a ball-valve effect in the airway that can result in asphyxiation.

Ref: Butterworth, J.F., Mackey, D.C., & Wasnick, J.D. (2013). Ch 42 *Morgan & Mikhail's Clinical Anesthesiology* (5th ed.). New York, NY: McGraw-Hill.

Cote, C.J., Lerman, J., & Todres, D. (2013). Ch 33 *A Practice of Anesthesia for Infants and Children* (5th ed.). Philadelphia, PA: Elsevier.

90. Which induction agent produces effects desirable for patients with Tetralogy of Fallot?

(A) Etomidate
(B) Ketamine
(C) Midazolam
(D) Propofol

Rationale: Tetralogy of Fallot is one of the most common cyanotic congenital heart defects. It is marked by the following four features: RV outflow tract obstruction, ventricular septal defect, a rightward aortic deviation, overriding the VSD and RVH. Due to the right ventricular outflow obstruction and coexisting VSD, patients with Tetralogy of Fallot shunt blood from right to left, ejecting deoxygenated right ventricular blood mixed with oxygenated blood into the aorta.

Ref: Butterworth, J.F., Mackey, D.C., & Wasnick, J.D. (2013). Ch 42 *Morgan & Mikhail's Clinical Anesthesiology* (5th ed.). New York, NY: McGraw-Hill.

Cote, C.J., Lerman, J., & Todres, D. (2013). Ch 16 *A Practice of Anesthesia for Infants and Children* (5th ed.). Philadelphia, PA: Elsevier.

Miller, R.D., Eriksson, L.I., Fleisher, L.A., Weiner-Kronish, J.P., & Young, W.L. (Eds.) (2010). Ch 82 *Miller's Anesthesia* (7th ed.). Philadelphia, PA: Elsevier.

91. Which of the following is true regarding a transplanted heart?

(A) No response to atropine
(B) No response to isoproterenol
(C) No response to milrinone
(D) No response to epinephrine

Rationale: A transplanted heart does not have autonomic innervation and thus is devoid of vagal influence. Therefore a vagolytic medication such as atropine or glycopyrrolate will have no effect on heart heart. Isoproterenol and epinephrine are the medications of choice to increase heart rate. Milrinone, a phosphodiesterase inhibitor, directly increase intracellular cAMP apart from any neuron-mediated or catecholamine-mediated process and thus will be an effective inotrope.

Ref: Butterworth, J.F., Mackey, D.C., & Wasnick, J.D. (2013). Ch 21 *Morgan & Mikhail's Clinical Anesthesiology* (5th ed.). New York, NY: McGraw-Hill.

92. Which inhaled agent is most suitable for a pediatric inhalation induction?

(A) Isoflurane

(B) Desflurane

(C) Sevoflurane

(D) Enflurane

Rationale: Sevoflurane is used for a pediatric inhalation induction.

Ref: Butterworth, J.F., Mackey, D.C., & Wasnick, J.D. (2013). Ch 42 *Morgan & Mikhail's Clinical Anesthesiology* (5th ed.). New York, NY: McGraw-Hill.

Barash, P.G., Cullen, B.F., Stoelting, R.K. Cahalan, M.K., & Stock, M.C. (Eds.) (2009). Ch 45 *Clinical Anesthesia* (6th ed.). Philadelphia, PA: Lippincott Williams & Wilkins.

93. Which of the following variables is not associated with aging?

(A) Increased volume of distribution for lipid soluble drugs

(B) Reduced plasma volume

(C) Decreased volume of distribution for lipid soluble drugs

(D) Reduced plasma protein binding

Rationale: Pharmacokinetics and dynamics are altered with aging. An increased volume of distribution for lipid soluble drugs, reduced plasma volume, reduced plasma protein binding, along with altered liver and renal function.

Ref: Hines, R.L., & Marschall, K.E. (2012). Ch 28 *Stoelting's Anesthesia and Co-Exiting Disease* (6th ed.). Philadelphia, PA: Elsevier.

94. An elderly patient with coronary artery disease is scheduled for an umbilical hernia repair. You note a decreased albumin level. What do you expect when administering an intravenous induction dose of propofol?

(A) Higher free drug fraction

(B) Decreased drug effect

(C) Lower free drug fraction

(D) Similar drug effect

Rationale: Plasma proteins decline with aging. Since propofol is highly protein bound, a higher free drug fraction and effect results with decreased albumin levels.

Ref: Hines, R.L., & Marschall, K.E. (2012). Ch 28 *Stoelting's Anesthesia and Co-Exiting Disease* (6th ed.). Philadelphia, PA: Elsevier.

95. What is the effect of aging on the minimum alveolar concentration (MAC)?

(A) MAC of volatile anesthetics increases 50% after age 60.

(B) MAC of volatile anesthetics decreases 10% after age 50.

(C) MAC of volatile anesthetics decreases 4% per decade after 40 years of age.

(D) MAC of volatile anesthetics increases 4% per decade after 40 years of age.

Rationale: Sensitivity to inhalational anesthetics is affected by aging. The MAC of inhalational anesthetics decreases with advancing age.

Ref: Hines, R.L., & Marschall, K.E. (2012). Ch 28 *Stoelting's Anesthesia and Co-Exiting Disease* (6th ed.). Philadelphia, PA: Elsevier.

96. What is the best induction dose for an 80-year-old weighing 100 kg?

(A) Propofol 100 mg

(B) Sodium pentathol 250 mg

(C) Etomidate 40 mg

(D) Ketamine 100 mg

Rationale: Decrease dose requirements for the elderly by 50%. Propofol 1-1.5 mg/kg is the average adult induction dose. For the aging patient, the dose was decreased. The induction dose of sodium pentothal is 2-2.5 mg/kg; ketamine 1-1.5 mg/kg; and etomidate 0.2-0.4 mg/kg. None of these doses were decreased for the 80-year-old patient.

Ref: Hines, R.L., & Marschall, K.E. (2012). Ch 28 *Stoelting's Anesthesia and Co-Exiting Disease* (6th ed.). Philadelphia, PA: Elsevier.

97. What is the definition of premature birth?

(A) Birth prior to 42 weeks' gestation

(B) Birth prior to 37 weeks' gestation

(C) Birth prior to 32 weeks' gestation

(D) Birth prior to 35 week's gestation

Rationale: A premature birth is defined as delivery prior to 37 weeks' gestation.

Ref: Butterworth, J.F., Mackey, D.C., & Wasnick, J.D. (2013). Ch 42 *Morgan & Mikhail's Clinical Anesthesiology* (5th ed.). New York, NY: McGraw-Hill.

Hines, R.L., & Marschall, K.E. (Eds.) (2012). Ch 27 *Stoelting's Anesthesia and Co-existing Disease* (6th ed.). Philadelphia, PA: Elsevier.

98. Which body mass index (BMI) is categorized as obese Class I?

(A) 18.5%

(B) 24.9%

(C) 29.9%

(D) 32.1%

Rationale: Obese class I equals a body mass index of 30-34.9; overweight equals a BMI 25-29.9; normal weight equates to 18.5-24.9, and underweight is a BMI <18.5%.

Ref: Hines, R.L., & Marschall, K.E. (2012). Ch 16 *Stoelting's Anesthesia and Co-Exiting Disease* (6th ed.) Philadelphia, PA: Elsevier.

99. Total body water will be the largest percentage of body weight in which patient?

(A) A neonate

(B) An infant

(C) A toddler

(D) A school-age child

Rationale: Total body water as a percentage of body-weight is inversely related to age.

Ref: Butterworth, J.F., Mackey, D.C., & Wasnick, J.D. (2013). Ch 42 *Morgan & Mikhail's Clinical Anesthesiology* (5th ed.). New York, NY: McGraw-Hill.

Nagelhout, J., & Plaus, K. (Eds.) (2014). Ch 48 *Nurse Anesthesia* (5th ed.). St. Louis, MO: Elsevier.

100. Which sign is associated with metabolic syndrome?

(A) High levels of high-density lipoprotein cholesterol

(B) Hypotension

(C) High triglyceride levels

(D) Small waist circumference

Rationale: Metabolic syndrome (Syndrome X) includes three of the following signs: large waist circumference, hypertension, low levels of high density lipoprotein, glucose intolerance, and high triglycerides levels.

Ref: Hines, R.L., & Marschall, K.E. (2012). Ch 16 *Stoelting's Anesthesia and Co-Existing Disease* (6th ed.). Philadelphia, PA: Elsevier.

101. The patient is undergoing a latissimus dorsi myocutaneous flap for reconstruction of the breast. What is the desired mean arterial pressure?

(A) MAP >55 mmHg

(B) MAP >60 mmHg

(C) MAP >65 mmHg

(D) MAP >70 mmHg

Rationale: A MAP >70 mmHg facilitates flap perfusion.

Ref: Macksey, L.F., Sowka, W., Cipcic, E., Kaufman, P.E., & Callaway, F.D. (2012). Ch 13 *Surgical Procedures and Anesthetic Implications*. Sudbury, MA: Jones & Bartlett Learning.

102. Which patient appropriately fasted for an anesthetic to begin at 1000?

(A) A child who had cereal at 0500

(B) A child who had clear liquids at 0900

(C) An infant who breast fed at 0500

(D) An infant who had formula at 0700

Rationale: Fasting guidelines for infants and children include 2 hours for clear liquids, 4 hours for breast milk, 6 hours for infant formula or food, and 8 hours for a heavy meal.

Ref: Butterworth, J.F., Mackey, D.C., & Wasnick, J.D. (2013). Ch 42 *Morgan & Mikhail's Clinical Anesthesiology* (5th ed.). New York, NY: McGraw-Hill.

Miller, R., & Pardo, M.Jr. (Eds.) (2011). Ch 34 *Basics of Anesthesia* (6th ed.). Philadelphia, PA: Elsevier.

103. Which dose of morphine is appropriate for intrathecal post cesarean section analgesia?

(A) 2.5 mg

(B) 50 µg

(C) 0.2 mg

(D) 100 µg

Rationale: The intrathecal dose of morphine for analgesia is 0.1-0.2 mg. The epidural dose of morphine for analgesia is 2.5-5.0 mg. Fentanyl 50-100 µg is given via the epidural route and 10-20 µg via the intrathecal route.

Ref: Longnecker, D.E., Brown, D.L., Newman, M.F., & Zapol, W.M. (2012). Ch 62 *Anesthesiology* (2nd ed.). San Francisco, CA: McGraw-Hill.

104. When is it best to avoid teratogenic drugs?

(A) 1-2 weeks' gestation

(B) 3-10 weeks' gestation

(C) 12-15 weeks' gestation

(D) 20-25 weeks' gestation

Rationale: The period of greatest fetal development occurs during the 3rd to 10th week of pregnancy.

Avoiding teratogenic drugs and chemicals is essential during this period of fetal development.
Ref: Longnecker, D.E., Brown, D.L., Newman, M.F., & Zapol, W.M. (2012). Ch 62 *Anesthesiology* (2nd ed.). San Francisco, CA: McGraw-Hill.

105. Which variable is not linked to postdural puncture headache following placement of a spinal anesthetic for cesarean section?

(A) 26-g needle
(B) Cutting needles
(C) 20-g needle
(D) Beveled needles

Rationale: Smaller gauged noncutting, nonbeveled needles are associated with a lower incidence of postdural puncture headache than larger gauged, cutting, beveled needles.
Ref: Longnecker, D.E., Brown, D.L., Newman, M.F., & Zapol, W.M. (2012). Ch 62 *Anesthesiology* (2nd ed.). San Francisco, CA: McGraw-Hill.

106. Which symptoms are associated with pregnant patients in the supine position?

(A) Hypotension, nausea
(B) Nausea, hypertension
(C) Normotension, nausea
(D) Hypertension, vomiting

Rationale: Supine hypotension syndrome results from compression of the gravid uterus on the inferior vena cava and aorta. Decreased venous return then results in decreased cardiac output. The associated symptoms include hypotension, nausea, and vomiting. The syndrome is relieved by tilting the patient thereby displacing the gravid uterus.
Ref: Longnecker, D.E., Brown, D.L., Newman, M.F., & Zapol, W.M. (2012). Ch 22 *Anesthesiology* (2nd ed.). San Francisco, CA: McGraw-Hill.

107. Which of the following physiologic changes occurs during pregnancy?

(A) Hypocoagulation
(B) Plasma volume decreases
(C) Hypercoagulation
(D) Red cell mass decreases

Rationale: Hematologic changes in pregnancy include increased plasma volume and increased red cell mass. Red cell mass increase is less than plasma volume resulting in a dilutional anemia. Coagulation factors increased

with the exception of factors XI and XIII. Pregnant patients are considered hypercoagulable.
Ref: Butterworth, J.F., Mackey, D.C., & Wasnick, J.D. (2013). Ch 41 *Morgan & Mikhail's Clinical Anesthesiology* (5th ed.). New York, NY: McGraw-Hill.
Longnecker, D.E., Brown, D.L., Newman, M.F., & Zapol, W.M. (2012). Ch 22 *Anesthesiology* (2nd ed.). San Francisco, CA: McGraw-Hill.

108. The patient requests an epidural for abdominal hysterectomy. Which sensory level is needed for epidural anesthesia?

(A) T12
(B) T10
(C) T8
(D) T6

Rationale: Intraadominal surgery requires a T4–T6 sensory block. Blocks below T6 are inadequate for pain control during intra-abdominal surgery.
Ref: Longnecker, D.E., Brown, D.L., Newman, M.F., & Zapol, W.M. (2012). Ch 62 *Anesthesiology* (2nd ed.). San Francisco, CA: McGraw-Hill.

109. The patient is scheduled for a laparoscopic cholecystectomy. Which of the following is true?

(A) Central venous pressure decreases
(B) Lung compliance increases
(C) Intra-abdominal pressure decreases
(D) Functional residual capacity decreases

Rationale: Laparoscopic procedures require insufflation of carbon dioxide increasing intraabdominal pressure. Cardiovascular effects include increased central venous pressure, stroke volume, and blood pressure. Respiratory effects include decreased functional residual capacity, increased airway pressure, and decreased lung compliance. Hypoxemia may ensue.
Ref: Longnecker, D.E., Brown, D.L., Newman, M.F., & Zapol, W.M. (2012). Ch 62 *Anesthesiology* (2nd ed.). San Francisco, CA: McGraw-Hill.

110. During a laparoscopic hernia repair, you notice a sudden drop in blood pressure and oxygen saturation and decreased end-tidal carbon dioxide. What is the most likely cause?

(A) CO_2 embolus
(B) Tension pneumothorax
(C) Hemorrhage
(D) Pneumomediastinum

Rationale: Insufflation of carbon dioxide gas during laparoscopy carries a risk for each of the complications listed above. The signs and symptoms of carbon dioxide embolus include a sudden blood pressure, oxygen saturation and notable end tidal CO_2 drop. Cardiovascular collapse and death quickly follows without prompt recognition and treatment.

Ref: Longnecker, D.E., Brown, D.L., Newman, M.F., & Zapol, W.M. (2012). Ch 62 *Anesthesiology* (2nd ed.). San Francisco, CA: McGraw-Hill.

111. Which of the following is true about the infant airway?

(A) The tongue is small in relation to the mandible.

(B) The larynx is located at the C2–C3 vertebrae.

(C) The epiglottis is stiff and flat.

(D) The larynx is located at C5–C6.

Rationale: Infants airways differ significantly from older children and adults. The tongue is large in relation to the mandible. The epiglottis is floppy and omega shaped. Location of the larynx is at the C2–C3 vertebrae as compared to adults whose larynx is located at C5–C6.

Ref: Butterworth, J.F., Mackey, D.C., & Wasnick, J.D. (2013). Ch 42 *Morgan & Mikhail's Clinical Anesthesiology* (5th ed.). New York, NY: McGraw-Hill.

Longnecker, D.E., Brown, D.L., Newman, M.F., & Zapol, W.M. (2012). Ch 63 *Anesthesiology* (2nd ed.). San Francisco, CA: McGraw-Hill.

112. While reversing heparin, the anesthetist notes that the blood pressure has dropped precipitously to 42/23 mmHg. What will you do first?

(A) Administer 100 μg of epinephrine IV.

(B) Administer 10 μg of epinephrine IV

(C) Administer 50 mg of Benadryl and 125 mg of methylprednisolone IV.

(D) Begin chest compressions.

Rationale: Heparin is reversed with protamine. Protamine reactions are immunologic (anaphylactic or anaphylactoid) in nature. It is accompanied by severe pulmonary artery vasoconstriction, myocardial depression, and severe systemic hypotension. First line treatment for an anaphylactic/anaphylactoid reaction is epinephrine. After administration of epinephrine and hemodynamic improvement (chest compressions may be necessary in order for epinephrine to travel to heart), then the other treatments may be initiated.

Ref: Butterworth, J.F., Mackey, D.C., & Wasnick, J.D. (2013). Ch 22 *Morgan & Mikhail's Clinical Anesthesiology* (5th ed.). New York, NY: McGraw-Hill.

113. By how much are neuraxial requirements for cesarean section decreased?

(A) 10%

(B) 20%

(C) 30%

(D) 50%

Rationale: Because of increased sensitivity to local anesthetics by pregnant patients, local anesthetic dosages should be decreased by 30-40%.

Ref: Butterworth, J.F., Mackey, D.C., & Wasnick, J.D. (2013). Ch 40 *Morgan & Mikhail's Clinical Anesthesiology* (5th ed.). New York, NY: McGraw-Hill.

Suresh, M.S., Segal, B.S., Preston, R.L., Fernando, R., & Mason C.L. (2013). Ch 1 *Shnider and Levinson's Anesthesia for Obstetrics* (5th ed.). Philadelphia, PA: Lippincott Williams & Wilkins.

114. What are the normal physiological changes associated with pregnancy?

Select (3) three

(A) MAC decreases by 50%.

(B) Functional Residual Capacity decreases by 20%.

(C) Respiratory rate decreases by 15%.

(D) Plasma volume increases by 55%.

(E) Heart rate increases by 20%.

(F) Hemoglobin increases by 10%.

Rationale: Minimum alveolar concentration (MAC) decreases by 30-40%. The respiratory rate increases by 15% and hemoglobin decreases by 20%.

Ref: Butterworth, J.F., Mackey, D.C., & Wasnick, J.D. (2013). Ch 40 *Morgan & Mikhail's Clinical Anesthesiology* (5th ed.). New York, NY: McGraw-Hill.

Suresh, M.S., Segal, B.S., Preston, R.L., Fernando, R., & Mason C.L. (2013). Ch 1 *Shnider and Levinson's Anesthesia for Obstetrics* (5th ed.). Philadelphia, PA: Lippincott Williams & Wilkins.

115. What is the best size endotracheal tube used for a patient undergoing general anesthesia for cesarean section?

(A) 5.5 mm

(B) 6.5 mm

(C) 7.5 mm

(D) 8.5 mm

Rationale: Due to the changes during pregnancy, the airway becomes swollen and friable, and visualization of airway structure is difficult. A 6-6.5 mm endotracheal tube facilitates intubation.

Ref: Butterworth, J.F., Mackey, D.C., & Wasnick, J.D. (2013). Ch 40 *Morgan & Mikhail's Clinical Anesthesiology* (5th ed.). New York, NY: McGraw-Hill.

Suresh, M.S., Segal, B.S., Preston, R.L., Fernando, R., & Mason C.L. (2013). Ch 1 *Shnider and Levinson's Anesthesia for Obstetrics* (5th ed.). Philadelphia, PA: Lippincott Williams & Wilkins.

116. How does propofol affect uterine blood flow (UBF)?

   (A) Decreases UBF

   (B) No change on UBF

   (C) Dose-related increase in UBF

   (D) Dose-related decrease in UBF

Rationale: Propofol has little or no effect on UBF. Medications with alpha adrenergic activity as well as endogenous catecholamines cause vasoconstriction decreasing UBF.

Ref: Butterworth, J.F., Mackey, D.C., & Wasnick, J.D. (2013). Ch 40 *Morgan & Mikhail's Clinical Anesthesiology* (5th ed.). New York, NY: McGraw-Hill.

Suresh, M.S., Segal, B.S., Preston, R.L., Fernando, R., & Mason C.L. (2013). Ch 2 *Shnider and Levinson's Anesthesia for Obstetrics* (5th ed.). Philadelphia, PA: Lippincott Williams & Wilkins.

117. What statement is false regarding the use of metoclopramide in pregnant patients?

   (A) Speeds gastric emptying

   (B) Increases pH

   (C) Decreases gastric volume

   (D) Increases lower esophageal sphincter tone

Rationale: Metoclopramide has no effect on gastric pH.

Ref: Butterworth, J.F., Mackey, D.C., & Wasnick, J.D. (2013). Ch 17 & 41 *Morgan & Mikhail's Clinical Anesthesiology* (5th ed.). New York, NY: McGraw-Hill.

118. A patient is scheduled for a radical neck dissection. History includes neck radiation. How will you manage this patient's airway?

   (A) Standard IV induction

   (B) Rapid sequence induction

   (C) Laryngeal mask airway

   (D) Awake fiberoptic intubation

Rationale: Radiation to the neck may cause anatomical changes that pose challenges for intubation. The best approach is to use an awake fibertopic intubation or fibertoptic approach following inhaled anesthetic whereby the patient maintains spontaneous ventilation.

Ref: Butterworth, J.F., Mackey, D.C., & Wasnick, J.D. (2013). Ch 37 *Morgan & Mikhail's Clinical Anesthesiology* (5th ed.). New York, NY: McGraw-Hill.

Nagelhout, J.J., & Plaus, K.L. Ch 38 *Nurse Anesthesia* (5th ed.). St. Louis, MO: Elsevier.

119. Within 1 minute following the epidural test dose, the patient complains of heavy legs. What is the most likely cause?

   (A) Intravascular injection

   (B) Incomplete epidural analgesia

   (C) Unintentional intrathecal block

   (D) Local anesthetic toxicity

Rationale: Motor blocks following an epidural test dose typically herald inadvertant intrathecal injection. The onset of the motor block occurs 3-5 minutes following the test dose. Preceding the motor block, signs, and symptoms of a sensory block will occur.

Ref: Butterworth, J.F., Mackey, D.C., & Wasnick, J.D. (2013). Ch 41 *Morgan & Mikhail's Clinical Anesthesiology* (5th ed.). New York, NY: McGraw-Hill.

120. The patient is receiving echothiophate eye drops for glaucoma. You plan to use succinylcholine. What should you expect?

   (A) Shortened onset of action

   (B) Shortened duration of action

   (C) Prolonged duration of action

   (D) Prolonged onset of action

Rationale: Use of echothiophate decreases plasma cholinesterase activity. For this reason there may be prolonged action of succinylcholine.

Ref: Butterworth, J.F., Mackey, D.C., & Wasnick, J.D. (2013). Ch 36 *Morgan & Mikhail's Clinical Anesthesiology* (5th ed.). New York, NY: McGraw-Hill.

Nagelhout, J.J., & Plaus, K.L. Ch 39 *Nurse Anesthesia* (5th ed.). St. Louis, MO: Elsevier.

121. The patient has severe preeclampsia. When will you avoid regional anesthesia?

   (A) Platelet count 100,000/µL

   (B) Platelet count 150,000/µL

   (C) Platelet count 125,000/µL

   (D) Platelet count 75,000/µL

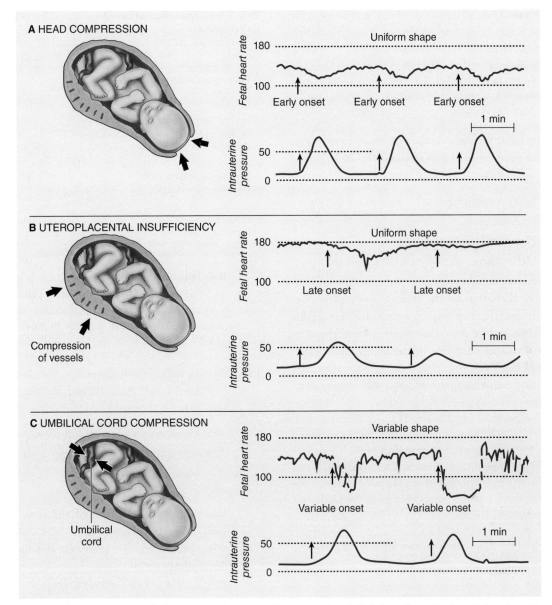

A HEAD COMPRESSION

Uniform shape

Fetal heart rate

180

100

Early onset   Early onset   Early onset

1 min

Intrauterine pressure

50

0

B UTEROPLACENTAL INSUFFICIENCY

Uniform shape

Fetal heart rate

180

100

Late onset   Late onset

Compression of vessels

1 min

Intrauterine pressure

50

0

C UMBILICAL CORD COMPRESSION

Variable shape

Fetal heart rate

180

100

Variable onset   Variable onset

Umbilical cord

1 min

Intrauterine pressure

50

0

FIG. 4-3. Periodic changes in fetal heart rate related to uterine contraction. **A**: Early (type I) decelerations. **B**: Late (type II) decelerations. **C**: Variable (type III) decelerations. (Reproduced, with permission, from Danforth DN, Scott JR: *Obstetrics and Gynecology*, 5th ed. Lippincott, 1986.)

Rationale: Before starting regional anesthesia for a parturient with severe preeclampsia, obtain a platelet count. Platelet counts greater than 100,000/μL are considered acceptable. Although there are exceptions, platelet counts less than 100,000/μL require additional testing and patient assessment.

Ref: Butterworth, J.F., Mackey, D.C., & Wasnick, J.D. (2013). Ch 41 *Morgan & Mikhail's Clinical Anesthesiology* (5th ed.). New York, NY: Lange Medical Books McGraw-Hill.

Suresh, M.S., Segal, B.S., Preston, R.L., Fernando, R., & Mason C.L. (2013). Ch 28 *Shnider and Levinson's Anesthesia for Obstetrics* (5th ed.). Philadelphia, PA: Lippincott Williams & Wilkins.

122. What fetal monitoring pattern is associated with umbilical cord compression?

(A) Variable decelerations

(B) Late decelerations

(C) Early decelerations

(D) Increased variability

Rationale: Umbilical cord compression evidenced by variable decelerations. Early decelerations are associated with head compression. Late decelerations evidence fetal compromise including uteroplacental insufficiency.

Ref: Butterworth, J.F., Mackey, D.C., & Wasnick, J.D. (2013). Ch 41 *Morgan & Mikhail's Clinical Anesthesiology* (5th ed.). New York, NY: McGraw-Hill.

Suresh, M.S., Segal, B.S., Preston, R.L., Fernando, R., & Mason C.L. (2013). Ch 9 *Shnider and Levinson's Anesthesia for Obstetrics* (5th ed.). Philadelphia, PA: Lippincott Williams & Wilkins.

123. During labor the patient experiences an abrupt onset of constant abdominal pain accompanied by hypotension. What is the most likely cause?

    (A) Uterine rupture
    (B) Placenta previa
    (C) Placenta abruption
    (D) Hemorrhage

    Rationale: Uterine rupture, placenta previa, and placenta abruption are the main causes of maternal hemorrhage. The new onset constant abdominal pain and hypotension are indicative of uterine rupture leading to significant antepartum hemorrhage. Painless vaginal bleeding points to placenta previa, whereas painful vaginal bleeding with uterine contractions point to placental abruption.
    Ref: Butterworth, J.F., Mackey, D.C., & Wasnick, J.D. (2013). Ch 41 *Morgan & Mikhail's Clinical Anesthesiology* (5th ed.). New York, NY: McGraw-Hill.

    Suresh, M.S., Segal, B.S., Preston, R.L., Fernando, R., & Mason C.L. (2013). Ch 10 *Shnider and Levinson's Anesthesia for Obstetrics* (5th ed.). Philadelphia, PA: Lippincott Williams & Wilkins.

124. Which of the following increases intraocular pressure?

    Select (2) two
    (A) Hypotension
    (B) Hypoventilation
    (C) Hypertension
    (D) Hyperventilation

    Rationale: Hypoventilation increases $PaCO_2$ thereby increasing intraocular pressure. Hypertension and increased CVP increase intraocular pressure.

TABLE 4-6. The effect of cardiac and respiratory variables on intraocular pressure (IOP).[1]

Variable	Effect on IOP
Central venous pressure	
Increase	↑↑↑
Decrease	↓↓↓
Arterial blood pressure	
Increase	↑
Decrease	↓
$PaCO_2$	
Increase (hypoventilation)	↑↑
Decrease (hyperventilation)	↓↓
PaO_2	
Increase	0
Decrease	↑

[1] ↓, decrease (mild, moderate, marked); ↑, increase (mild, moderate, marked); 0, no effect.

Ref: Butterworth, J.F., Mackey, D.C., & Wasnick, J.D. (2013). Ch 36 *Morgan & Mikhail's Clinical Anesthesiology* (5th ed.). New York, NY: McGraw-Hill.

Nagelhout, J.J., & Plaus, K.L. Ch 39 *Nurse Anesthesia* (5th ed.). St. Louis, MO: Elsevier.

125. During radical neck dissection, you note new onset bradycardia, arrhythmias, and prolonged QT intervals. What is the probable cause of these symptoms?

    (A) Denervation of carotid sinus
    (B) Manipulation of the carotid sinus
    (C) Venous air embolism
    (D) Denervation of carotid bodies

    Rationale: Manipulation of the carotid sinus and stellate ganglion may lead to bradycardia, arrhythmias, prolonged QT intervals, and blood pressure fluctuation.
    Ref: Butterworth, J.F., Mackey, D.C., & Wasnick, J.D. (2013). Ch 37 *Morgan & Mikhail's Clinical Anesthesiology* (5th ed.). New York, NY: McGraw-Hill.

    Nagelhout, J.J., & Plaus, K.L. Ch 38 *Nurse Anesthesia* (5th ed.). St. Louis, MO: Elsevier.

126. The patient is scheduled for laser removal of vocal cord papilloma. What will you avoid?

    (A) Eye protection with colored glasses
    (B) Nitrous oxide
    (C) Eye protection with wet gauze
    (D) Oxygen and air mixture

    Rationale: Nitrous oxide supports combustion so should be avoided. A low concentration of oxygen mixed with air helps avoid airway fire. Using wet gauze or colored glasses protects the eyes during laser surgery.

Ref: Butterworth, J.F., Mackey, D.C., & Wasnick, J.D. (2013). Ch 37 *Morgan & Mikhail's Clinical Anesthesiology* (5th ed.). New York, NY: McGraw-Hill.

Nagelhout, J.J., & Plaus, K.L. Ch 38 *Nurse Anesthesia* (5th ed.). St. Louis, MO: Elsevier.

127. Fifteen minutes ago you transported a patient to the post anesthesia care unit following tonsillectomy. The patient is bleeding. How will you induce this patient?

    (A) Rapid sequence induction

    (B) Standard induction

    (C) Awake intubation

    (D) Standard induction with a glidescope

    Rationale: Patients who experience post-tonsillectomy bleeding are considered a full stomach. A rapid sequence induction is indicated. Depending on the extent of the bleeding, an awake intubation may be needed.

    Ref: Butterworth, J.F., Mackey, D.C., & Wasnick, J.D. (2013). Ch 37 *Morgan & Mikhail's Clinical Anesthesiology* (5th ed.). New York, NY: McGraw-Hill.

    Nagelhout, J.J., & Plaus, K.L. Ch 38 *Nurse Anesthesia* (5th ed.). St. Louis, MO: Elsevier.

128. Which of the following is associated with a peribulbar block?

    Select (3) three

    (A) Intraconal procedure

    (B) Patient gaze is supranasal.

    (C) Extraconal procedure

    (D) Patient gaze is straight ahead.

    (E) 5-8 mL local anesthetic is used.

    Rationale: Because the peribulbar block is extraconal, it is considered a safer block than retrobulbar. The patient is supine and looks straight ahead. In a retrobulbar block 2-4 mL of local anesthetic is used.

    Ref: Butterworth, J.F., Mackey, D.C., & Wasnick, J.D. (2013). Ch 36 *Morgan & Mikhail's Clinical Anesthesiology* (5th ed.). New York, NY: McGraw-Hill.

    Nagelhout, J.J., & Plaus, K.L. Ch 39 *Nurse Anesthesia* (5th ed.). St. Louis, MO: Elsevier.

129. Which statement is true regarding the use of inhalational agents during pregnancy?

    (A) Uterine blood flow is increased.

    (B) Uteroplacental blood flow is increased.

    (C) Uteroplacental blood flow is decreased.

    (D) Uterine blood flow is unchanged.

    Rationale: Inhalational agents cause a dose-related decreased in blood pressure thereby decreasing uterine blood flow and blood flow to through the placenta. The recommendation is to use less than 1 MAC to minimize the neonatal effects.

    Ref: Butterworth, J.F., Mackey, D.C., & Wasnick, J.D. (2013). Ch 40 *Morgan & Mikhail's Clinical Anesthesiology* (5th ed.). New York, NY: McGraw-Hill.

    Suresh, M.S., Segal, B.S., Preston, R.L., Fernando, R., & Mason C.L. (2013). Ch 2 *Shnider and Levinson's Anesthesia for Obstetrics* (5th ed.). Philadelphia, PA: Lippincott Williams & Wilkins.

130. The patient is scheduled for an endoscopic sinus surgery. Which of the following will not minimize blood loss?

    (A) Head-up position

    (B) Cocaine 4%

    (C) Supine position

    (D) Hypotensive technique

    Rationale: The head-up position rather than the supine position assists with minimizing blood loss. Cocaine 4% or 10% or epinephrine soaked pledgets minimize blood loss. In some cases, hypotensive techniques are used to lessen blood loss.

    Ref: Butterworth, J.F., Mackey, D.C., & Wasnick, J.D. (2013). Ch 37 *Morgan & Mikhail's Clinical Anesthesiology* (5th ed.). New York, NY: McGraw-Hill.

    Nagelhout, J.J., & Plaus, K.L. Ch 38 *Nurse Anesthesia* (5th ed.). St. Louis, MO: Elsevier.

131. A patient is scheduled for surgery involving a Le Fort II fracture. During the preoperative interview, periorbital edema, and raccoon eyes hematoma are noted. What is your main anesthetic concern?

    (A) Securing the airway

    (B) Bleeding

    (C) Emergence with a wired jaw

    (D) Postoperative respiratory compromise

    Rationale: Each of the options poses challenges for surgery involving a Le Fort II fracture. Securing the airway may be problematic due to the nature of the fracture. Nasal endotracheal tubes are commonly used in dental reconstruction; however, care should be taken with a Le Fort II or III fracture due to the possibility of additional skull fractures, brain damage or meningitis.

Ref: Butterworth, J.F., Mackey, D.C., & Wasnick, J.D. (2013). Ch 37 *Morgan & Mikhail's Clinical Anesthesiology* (5th ed.). New York, NY: McGraw-Hill.
Nagelhout, J.J., & Plaus, K.L. Ch 38 *Nurse Anesthesia* (5th ed.). St. Louis, MO: Elsevier.

132. What are the clinical signs of hyperthyroidism?

Select (3) three

(A) Polyuria

(B) Weight gain

(C) Nervousness

(D) Paresthesias

(E) Hypertension

Rationale: Weight gain and paresthesias are signs of hypothyroidism. Other signs of hyperthyroidism include bone pain and muscle weakness, gastrointestinal and cognitive disturbances, and altered renal function.

Ref: Butterworth, J.F., Mackey, D.C., & Wasnick, J.D. (2013). Ch 34 *Morgan & Mikhail's Clinical Anesthesiology* (5th ed.). New York, NY: McGraw-Hill.
Nagelhout, J.J., & Plaus, K.L. Ch 38 *Nurse Anesthesia* (5th ed.). St. Louis, MO: Elsevier.

133. What is the hemodynamic priority for anesthetic management of an unrepaired aortic dissection?

(A) Decrease blood pressure with arterial vasodilators to decrease risk of rupture or further dissection.

(B) Increase blood pressure to ensure adequate perfusion distal to the aneurysm.

(C) Decrease shear force on the aneurysm using beta-blockers to decrease risk of rupture of further dissection.

(D) Decrease heart rate with medications in order to decrease myocardial oxygen demand.

Rationale: Aortic dissections grow due to hemodynamic shear forces related to the rate of rise of blood pressure (dP/dt). Management of an unrepaired aortic aneurysm is focused on avoiding propagation of dissection and avoiding rupture. Hemodynamic management focuses on decreasing shear forces related to quick changes in blood pressure on systole. This is accomplished by reducing systolic pressure (arterial vasodilators) and decreasing the strength of contraction (beta-blockers). Arterial vasodilators alone may actually increase the shear force by decreasing the resistance against systolic ejection.

Ref: Butterworth, J.F., Mackey, D.C., & Wasnick, J.D. (2013). Ch 21 *Morgan & Mikhail's Clinical Anesthesiology* (5th ed.). New York, NY: McGraw-Hill.

134. The patient is scheduled for a laryngeal endoscopy. Jet ventilation is planned. What statement is false regarding jet ventilation?

(A) High-pressure (30-60 psi) is used.

(B) FiO_2 of 30% or less is used.

(C) End-tidal CO_2 is accurate.

(D) Expiration is passive.

Rationale: A dilution of alveolar gas results in variable CO_2 readings.

Ref: Butterworth, J.F., Mackey, D.C., & Wasnick, J.D. (2013). Ch 37 *Morgan & Mikhail's Clinical Anesthesiology* (5th ed.). New York, NY: McGraw-Hill.
Nagelhout, J.J., & Plaus, K.L. Ch 38 *Nurse Anesthesia* (5th ed.). St. Louis, MO: Elsevier.

135. A patient undergoing repair of a descending thoracic aortic aneurysm is found postoperatively to exhibit loss of lower extremity motor function bilaterally. What is the most likely cause?

(A) Blood flow to the motor cortex of the brain was decreased during cross-clamp.

(B) Blood flow to the anterior spinal cord was damaged during the surgery.

(C) Blood flow to the posterior spinal cord was damaged during the surgery.

(D) This is a normal occurrence when blood flow to the lower extremities has been restricted as in aortic cross clamping.

Rationale: The patient has experienced anterior spinal cord ischemia and is experiencing anterior spinal artery syndrome. The anterior spinal cord is responsible for motor control and that the anterior spinal cord is perfused by the vertebral arteries and from arterial flow from the thoracic and abdominal aorta. The artery of Adamkiewicz along with many other smaller vessels may be covered or ligated during aortic repair. If the degree of flow impairment is large, the patient may develop anterior spinal artery syndrome secondary to spinal cord ischemia. Classic symptoms of this syndrome include loss of motor function, loss of pinprick sensation, but retained vibration sensation and proprioception.

Ref: Butterworth, J.F., Mackey, D.C., & Wasnick, J.D. (2013). Ch 21 *Morgan & Mikhail's Clinical Anesthesiology* (5th ed.). New York, NY: McGraw-Hill.

136. The patient is undergoing a mediastinoscopy. What will you consider for this patient?

    Select (3) three

    (A) Blood pressure in the left arm

    (B) Large bore IV

    (C) Blood pressure in the right arm

    (D) Air embolism

    (E) Superior laryngeal nerve damage

    Rationale: Hemorrhage, air embolism, injury to the recurrent laryngeal and phrenic nerves, pneumothorax, and reflex bradycardia may result during mediastinoscopy. The blood pressure is taken in the left arm because of possible compression of the innominate artery.

    Ref: Butterworth, J.F., Mackey, D.C., & Wasnick, J.D. (2013). Ch 25 *Morgan & Mikhail's Clinical Anesthesiology* (5th ed.). New York, NY: McGraw-Hill.
    Nagelhout, J.J., & Plaus, K.L. Ch 27 *Nurse Anesthesia* (5th ed.). St. Louis, MO: Elsevier.

137. What statements are true regarding cardioversion?

    Select (2) two

    (A) 50-100 joules are used initially for atrial flutter.

    (B) Electrical shock is synchronized with the "R" wave.

    (C) 200-300 joules are used initially to convert atrial flutter.

    (D) Electrical shock is asynchronous.

    (E) Electrical shock is synchronized with the "Q" wave.

    Rationale: Conversion of atrial rhythms begins at 50-100 joules but may increase incrementally when needed. Shocks are given synchronously with the "R" wave of the QRS complex.

    Ref: Butterworth, J.F., Mackey, D.C., & Wasnick, J.D. (2013). Ch 22 *Morgan & Mikhail's Clinical Anesthesiology* (5th ed.). New York, NY: McGraw-Hill.
    Nagelhout, J.J., & Plaus, K.L. Ch 52 *Nurse Anesthesia* (5th ed.). St. Louis, MO: Elsevier.

138. What do you anticipate with distention of the bowel during colonoscopy?

    (A) Tachycardia

    (B) Hypertension

    (C) Bradycardia

    (D) EKG changes

    Rationale: Vagal stimulation is likely with insufflations of the bowel during colonoscopy. Bradycardia, hypotension and arrhythmias may occur.

    Ref: Nagelhout, J.J., & Plaus, K.L. Ch 52 *Nurse Anesthesia* (5th ed.). St. Louis, MO: Elsevier.

139. The patient is scheduled for computed tomography (CT) scan with intravenous contrast media (ICM). What is your main concern?

    (A) Patient must not move during the CT.

    (B) Patient anxiety

    (C) Hypothermia

    (D) Allergic reaction

    Rationale: ICM causes anaphylactic and anaphylactoid reactions. Renal dysfunction is possible. Patients at risk for reaction to ICM include asthmatics, numerous comorbidities, and allergic reaction.

    Ref: Nagelhout, J.J., & Plaus, K.L. Ch 52 *Nurse Anesthesia* (5th ed.). St. Louis, MO: Elsevier.

140. A patient is scheduled for electroconvulsive therapy. What is your main anesthetic concern when calculating dosages for induction agents?

    (A) Anterograde amnesia

    (B) Seizure quality

    (C) Parasympathetic stimulation

    (D) Sympathetic stimulation

    Rationale: Patients undergoing ECT experience initial bradycardia and secretions (parasympathetic) followed by tachycardia and hypertension (sympathetic surge) as well as anterograde amnesia. The quality of the seizure is considered key to the treatment. Induction agents increase the seizure threshold and decrease the duration of the seizure; therefore, lower dosages improve the likelihood that the seizure will result in the quality necessary for the treatment.

    Ref: Butterworth, J.F., Mackey, D.C., & Wasnick, J.D. (2013). Ch 28 *Morgan & Mikhail's Clinical Anesthesiology* (5th ed.). New York, NY: McGraw-Hill.
    Nagelhout, J.J., & Plaus, K.L. Ch 52 *Nurse Anesthesia* (5th ed.). St. Louis, MO: Elsevier.

141. A patient with an intestinal obstruction is scheduled for surgery. The patient's history includes pancreatitis and GERD. What is the best approach to airway management?

   (A) Awake fiberoptic intubation

   (B) Endotracheal intubation

   (C) LMA

   (D) Intubating LMA

Rationale: Protecting the airway is required for patients with intestinal obstruction and GERD. There is no indication for an awake fiberoptic intubation.
Ref: Nagelhout, J., & Plaus, K. (Eds.) (2014). Ch 43 *Nurse Anesthesia* (5th ed.). St. Louis, MO: Elsevier.

142. When is cardiac output greatest?

   (A) Immediately following delivery

   (B) Third trimester

   (C) Second trimester

   (D) First trimester

Rationale: Cardiac output increases progressively during pregnancy. During the third trimester there is a 45% increase in cardiac output. The greatest increase is immediately following delivery.
Ref: Butterworth, J.F., Mackey, D.C., & Wasnick, J.D. (2013). Ch 40 *Morgan & Mikhail's Clinical Anesthesiology* (5th ed.). New York, NY: McGraw-Hill.

143. Which of the following would be the most appropriate induction technique for a patient undergoing drainage of a severe cardiac tamponade via subxiphoid approach or pericardiocentesis?

   (A) Propofol, high dose fentanyl, succinylcholine, and intubate. Maintain with light sevoflurane and positive pressure ventilation.

   (B) Ketamine, high dose fentanyl, succinylcholine, and intubate. Maintain with light sevoflurane.

   (C) Inhalational induction and LMA insertion. Maintain with light sevoflurane and ketamine supplementation.

   (D) High dose fentanyl, midazolam, and mask ventilate patient.

Rationale: The cardiac output is heart rate dependent and blood pressure is dependent on arterial vasoconstriction. The anesthetic technique should ensure that sympathetic tone is maintained. High-dose fentanyl would be contraindicated. Positive pressure ventilation should be avoided if possible as it will decrease venous return, severely reducing cardiac output. Ketamine is a choice agent for induction and maintenance. Consider epinephrine use as well, as it will both increase heart rate and arterial vasoconstriction.
Ref: Butterworth, J.F., Mackey, D.C., & Wasnick, J.D. (2013). Ch 21 *Morgan & Mikhail's Clinical Anesthesiology* (5th ed.). New York, NY: McGraw-Hill.

144. A sedated patient experiences headache, nausea and vomiting during stereotactic Gamma knife surgery. What is the most likely cause?

   (A) Hemorrhage

   (B) Perforated aneurysm

   (C) Radiocontrast reaction

   (D) Embolization

Rationale: Each of the causes is possible with Gamma Knife surgery. Hemorrhage is the most likely cause.
Ref: Nagelhout, J.J., & Plaus, K.L. Ch 52 *Nurse Anesthesia* (5th ed.). St. Louis, MO: Elsevier.

145. Which of the following medications shortens the duration of a seizure during electroconvulsive therapy (ECT)?

   (A) Caffeine

   (B) Etomidate

   (C) Ketamine

   (D) Propofol

Rationale: Propofol when given in low doses does not affect the seizure activity with ECT.
Ref: Butterworth, J.F., Mackey, D.C., & Wasnick, J.D. (2013). Ch 28 *Morgan & Mikhail's Clinical Anesthesiology* (5th ed.). New York, NY: McGraw-Hill.
Nagelhout, J.J., & Plaus, K.L. Ch 52 *Nurse Anesthesia* (5th ed.). St. Louis, MO: Elsevier.

146. The patient is undergoing a mastectomy. During surgery, isosulfan blue dye is injected. What do you expect?

   (A) Tachycardia

   (B) Increased oxygen saturation

   (C) Bradycardia

   (D) Decreased oxygen saturation

Rationale: Isosulfan blue dye causes a 3% decrease in oxygen saturation.

Ref: Hines, R.L., & Marschall, K.E. (2012). Ch 23 *Stoelting's Anesthesia and Co-Existing Disease* (6th ed.). Philadelphia, PA: Elsevier.

147. Following cystoscopy the patient's blood pressure falls. What is the most likely cause?

   (A) Sympathectomy
   (B) Blood loss
   (C) Vasoconstriction due to spinal anesthesia
   (D) Lowering legs from lithotomy position

   Rationale: Lithotomy position is frequently used
   Ref: Butterworth, J.F., Mackey, D.C., & Wasnick, J.D. (2013). Ch 28 *Morgan & Mikhail's Clinical Anesthesiology* (5th ed.). New York, NY: McGraw-Hill.
   Nagelhout, J.J., & Plaus, K.L. Ch 29 *Nurse Anesthesia* (5th ed.). St. Louis, MO: Elsevier.

148. Pain relief during the second stage of labor requires neural blockade at what sensory level?

   (A) T10 to T12
   (B) T12 to S1
   (C) T10 to S1
   (D) T10 to S4

   Rationale: During the first stage of labor neural blockade of sensory fibers T10 to L1 are targeted. However, the second stage of labor requires neural blockade of sensory fibers that extend to S4.
   Ref: Butterworth, J.F., Mackey, D.C., & Wasnick, J.D. (2013). Ch 41 *Morgan & Mikhail's Clinical Anesthesiology* (5th ed.). New York, NY: McGraw-Hill.
   Suresh, M.S., Segal, B.S., Preston, R.L., Fernando, R., & Mason C.L. (2013). Ch 9 *Shnider and Levinson's Anesthesia for Obstetrics* (5th ed.). Philadelphia, PA: Lippincott Williams & Wilkins.

149. Which condition benefits most from epidural steroid Injections?

   (A) Radiculopathy
   (B) Intractable cancer pain
   (C) Intra-abdominal neoplasms
   (D) Phantom limb pain

   Rationale: Patients with nerve root compression benefit from epidural steroid injections. Conditions that benefit from epidural steroids include chronic low back and neck pain, rheumatoid arthritis, and herpetic neuralgia. Neurolytic blocks are used for patients with intractable cancer pain including intraabdominal and pelvic neoplasms, and rib metas-

tasis. Patients with phantom limb pain benefit from spinal cord stimulation.
   Ref: Butterworth, J.F., Mackey, D.C., & Wasnick, J.D. (2013). Ch 47 *Morgan & Mikhail's Clinical Anesthesiology* (5th ed.). New York, NY: McGraw-Hill.
   Nagelhout, J.J., & Plaus, K.L. Ch 51 *Nurse Anesthesia* (5th ed.). St. Louis, MO: Elsevier.

150. Which of the following has mainly analgesic and anytipyretic properties?

   (A) Acetaminophen
   (B) Ketorolac
   (C) Fentanyl
   (D) Codeine

   Rationale: The nonselective COX inhibitor Ketorolac possesses anti-inflammatory, antipyretic, and analgesic properties. Opioids including fentanyl and morphine are analgesics.
   Ref: Butterworth, J.F., Mackey, D.C., & Wasnick, J.D. (2013). Ch 47 *Morgan & Mikhail's Clinical Anesthesiology* (5th ed.). New York, NY: McGraw-Hill.
   Nagelhout, J.J., & Plaus, K.L. Ch 51 *Nurse Anesthesia* (5th ed.). St. Louis, MO: Elsevier.

151. Which statement regarding the use of epidural analgesia and anesthesia for preeclamptic patients is true?

   (A) Circulating catecholamines are decreased.
   (B) Decreases intervillous blood flow.
   (C) Epidural block should be avoided.
   (D) Epidural blocks are difficult to place.

   Rationale: Epidural blocks are suitable for patients with preeclampsia. The block decreases circulating catecholamines and improves intervillous blood flow. The epidural block also allows for control of systemic blood pressure.
   Ref: Longnecker, D.E., Brown, D.L., Newman, M.F., & Zapol, W.M. (2012). Ch 22 *Anesthesiology* (2nd ed.). San Francisco, CA: McGraw-Hill.

152. The patient is taking duloxetine and fluoxetine for chronic neuropathic pain. The patient complains of fever, agitation, sweating, and anxiety. What is the most likely cause?

   (A) Duloxetine overdose
   (B) Fluoxetine sensitivity
   (C) Combined use of Fluoxetine and Duloxetine
   (D) Allergic reaction to Duloxetine

Rationale: Using selective serotonin reuptake inhibitors and selective serotonin–norepinephrine reuptake inhibitors in combination may lead to serotonin syndrome. Toxic levels of serotonin cause symptoms listed above but also delirium, seizures, hyperdynamic states, hyperreflexia, muscle rigidity, and myoclonus.

Ref: Butterworth, J.F., Mackey, D.C., & Wasnick, J.D. (2013). Ch 47 *Morgan & Mikhail's Clinical Anesthesiology* (5th ed.). New York, NY: Lange Medical Books McGraw-Hill.

Nagelhout, J.J., & Plaus, K.L. Ch 51 *Nurse Anesthesia* (5th ed.). St. Louis, MO: Elsevier Saunders.

153. A patient is receiving tocolytic therapy for preterm labor. Which of the following is most concerning for this patient?

    (A) Hyperkalemia
    (B) Hypoglycemia
    (C) Pulmonary edema
    (D) Increased systemic vascular resistance

    Rationale: Tocolytic therapy that includes terbutaline and ritodrine is associated with hypokalemia, hyperglycemia, and decreased systemic vascular resistance. Pulmonary edema leads to maternal death.

    Ref: Longnecker, D.E., Brown, D.L., Newman, M.F., & Zapol, W.M. (2012). Ch 22 *Anesthesiology* (2nd ed.) San Francisco, CA: McGraw-Hill.

154. Which of the following are systemic effects of hydrocortisone?

    Select (3) three
    (A) Adrenal-pituitary insufficiency
    (B) Cushing syndrome
    (C) Hypertension
    (D) Sodium depletion
    (E) Hypotension

    Rationale: Corticosteroids affect multiple body systems. Sodium and water are retained. Hypertension develops as well as the potential for congestive heart failure and cardiomyopathy. Musculoskeletal effects include truncal obesity, muscle and bone weakness as well as fractures. Hyperglycemia, dermatologic, gastrointestinal, and neurologic or psychological effects are also prevalent. Long-term use of steroids rather than a single injection such as epidural administration foster the systemic effects.

    Ref: Nagelhout, J.J., & Plaus, K.L. Ch 33 *Nurse Anesthesia* (5th ed.). St. Louis, MO: Elsevier.

155. How is the renal system affected by pregnancy?

    Select (2) two
    (A) Renal plasma flow increases.
    (B) Glomerular filtration rate increases.
    (C) Tubular absorption of glucose increases.
    (D) Renal blood flow decreases.

    Rationale: The absorption of glucose via the proximal tubules decrease. This results in normal glucosuria. Renal blood flow increases early in pregnancy by 50-80%.

    Ref: Butterworth, J.F., Mackey, D.C., & Wasnick, J.D. (2013). Ch 40 *Morgan & Mikhail's Clinical Anesthesiology* (5th ed.). New York, NY: McGraw-Hill.

    Suresh, M.S., Segal, B.S., Preston, R.L., Fernando, R., & Mason C.L. (2013). Ch 1 *Shnider and Levinson's Anesthesia for Obstetrics* (5th ed.). Philadelphia, PA: Lippincott Williams & Wilkins.

156. When giving epidural steroid injections what dose will you use to avoid systemic effects?

    (A) Methylprednisolone acetate 40 mg
    (B) Triamcinolone diacetate 100 mg
    (C) Methylprednisolone acetate 20 mg
    (D) Triamcinolone diacetate 120 mg

    Rationale: The effective dose for epidural steroid injection is 40-80 mg for each drug. Exceeding the doses increases the likelihood of systemic effects. Decreasing the dose lessens the likelihood of effective treatment.

    Ref: Butterworth, J.F., Mackey, D.C., & Wasnick, J.D. (2013). Ch 47 *Morgan & Mikhail's Clinical Anesthesiology* (5th ed.). New York, NY: McGraw-Hill.

    Nagelhout, J.J., & Plaus, K.L. Ch 51 *Nurse Anesthesia* (5th ed.). St. Louis, MO: Elsevier.

157. The patient is scheduled for in vitro fertilization (IVF). Which medications are considered safe for this patient?

    Select (3) three
    (A) Morphine
    (B) Fentanyl
    (C) Demerol
    (D) NSAIDs
    (E) Nitrous oxide

    Rationale: Morphine may affect fertilization. NSAIDs may affect implantation of the embryo.

    Ref: Nagelhout, J.J., & Plaus, K.L. Ch 52 *Nurse Anesthesia* (5th ed.). St. Louis, MO: Elsevier.

158. Which statement is false regarding open breast biopsy?

(A) Postoperative nausea and vomiting is increased.

(B) Smooth emergence minimizes hematoma formation.

(C) Monitor the EKG for ST-segment changes when local anesthetic with epinephrine is used.

(D) The blood pressure cuff is placed on the nonoperative arm and IV placed on the operative side.

Rationale: The blood pressure cuff and IV are placed on the nonoperative side.

Ref: Macksey, L.F., Sowka, W., Cipcic, E., Kaufman, P.E., & Callaway, F.D. (2012). Ch 13 *Surgical Procedures and Anesthetic Implications.* Sudbury, MA: Jones & Bartlett Learning.

159. The patient is undergoing a modified radical mastectomy. When planning the general anesthetic, why would you check with the surgeon?

(A) Determine the patient's risk for postoperative nausea and vomiting.

(B) Type and cross-match preoperatively.

(C) Determine what if any neuromuscular blockers will be used.

(D) Determine when to give antiemetics.

Rationale: Nerve injury is possible with this surgery. The surgeon may prefer that no neuromuscular blockers are used.

Ref: Macksey, L.F., Sowka, W., Cipcic, E., Kaufman, P.E., & Callaway, F.D. (2012). Ch 13 *Surgical Procedures and Anesthetic Implications.* Sudbury, MA: Jones & Bartlett Learning.

160. What is your primary concern when caring for a patient undergoing hysteroscopy?

(A) Vasovagal response to uterine traction

(B) Postoperative pain

(C) Lithotomy positioning

(D) Absorption of glycine or saline solution

Rationale: Each of the items poses anesthetic concerns for this patient. Absorption of glycine or saline solutions predisposes the patient to fluid overload as well as electrolyte imbalance. Electrolyte testing should be done preoperatively.

Ref: Macksey, L.F., Sowka, W., Cipcic, E., Kaufman, P.E., & Callaway, F.D. (2012). Ch 20 *Surgical Procedures and Anesthetic Implications.* Sudbury, MA: Jones & Bartlett Learning.

161. The patient is scheduled for a total abdominal hysterectomy. Why is the patient likely to become hypotensive following induction?

(A) Bowel prep

(B) Chronic bleeding

(C) Anemia

(D) Position changes

Rationale: Dehydration following a bowel prep is common for these patients. These patients may also be anemic due to chronic bleeding.

Ref: Macksey, L.F., Sowka, W., Cipcic, E., Kaufman, P.E., & Callaway, F.D. (2012). Ch 20 *Surgical Procedures and Anesthetic Implications.* Sudbury, MA: Jones & Bartlett Learning.

162. During a cystoscopy, the patient complains of upper abdominal pain and nausea. The patient is diaphoretic. What is the most likely cause?

(A) Bladder perforation

(B) Stent placement

(C) Biopsy

(D) Stone removal

Rationale: Stent placement, biopsy, and stone removal may be performed with cystoscopy. The symptomology in an awake patient is consistent with bladder or ureteral perforation. Other symptoms include referred pain (diaphragmatic or shoulder) or hemodynamic changes.

Ref: Macksey, L.F., Sowka, W., Cipcic, E., Kaufman, P.E., & Callaway, F.D. (2012). Ch 19 *Surgical Procedures and Anesthetic Implications.* Sudbury, MA: Jones & Bartlett Learning.

163. What emergency medication is essential for penile surgery?

(A) Midazolam

(B) Propofol

(C) Fentanyl

(D) Glycopyrrolate

Rationale: For procedures involving the penis and testes, manipulation may result in profound bradycardia due to vagal stimulation. Atropine or glycopyrrolate should be immediately available.

Ref: Macksey, L.F., Sowka, W., Cipcic, E., Kaufman, P.E., & Callaway, F.D. (2012). Ch 19 *Surgical Procedures and Anesthetic Implications.* Sudbury, MA: Jones & Bartlett Learning.

164. What is the primary anesthetic concern for patients undergoing rectal surgery?

(A) Postoperative pain

(B) Relaxation of the anal sphincter

(C) Fluid and electrolyte balance

(D) Postoperative nausea and vomiting

Rationale: Each of the items poses concerns for the patient. The patients are often dehydrated due to the bowel prep.

Ref: Macksey, L.F., Sowka, W., Cipcic, E., Kaufman, P.E., & Callaway, F.D. (2012). Ch 16 *Surgical Procedures and Anesthetic Implications*. Sudbury, MA: Jones & Bartlett Learning.

165. During a total knee arthroplasty with spinal anesthesia the patient develops hypotension, arrhythmias, and loses consciousness. What is the most likely cause?

(A) Hemorrhage

(B) Fluid imbalance

(C) Tourniquet pain

(D) Methyl methacrylate

Rationale: Bone cement (methyl methacrylate) is used during total joint procedures to cement the prosthetic components. In addition to the symptoms for this patient, hypoxia, pulmonary hypertension and decreased cardiac output occur. A decreased end-tidal CO_2 is the first sign of bone cement implantation syndrome for patients undergoing joint replacement with general anesthesia.

Ref: Butterworth, J.F., Mackey, D.C., & Wasnick, J.D. (2013). Ch 38 *Morgan & Mikhail's Clinical Anesthesiology* (5th ed.). New York, NY: McGraw-Hill.

Nagelhout, J.J., & Plaus, K.L. Ch 40 *Nurse Anesthesia* (5th ed.). St. Louis, MO: Elsevier.

166. Which is the preferred method of airway management in a child with acute epiglottitis?

(A) Rapid sequence induction followed by laryngoscopy

(B) Awake laryngoscopy

(C) Inhalation induction maintaining spontaneous respiration

(D) Urgent tracheostomy

Rationale: Spontaneously breathing inhalation induction is the preferred method.

Ref: Butterworth, J.F., Mackey, D.C., & Wasnick, J.D. (2013). Ch 38 *Morgan & Mikhail's Clinical Anesthesiology* (5th ed.). New York, NY: McGraw-Hill.

Miller, R., & Pardo, M. Jr. (Eds.) (2011). Ch 34 *Basics of Anesthesia* (6th ed.). Philadelphia, PA: Elsevier.

167. Which factor does not contribute to decreased uterine blood flow?

(A) Systemic hypotension

(B) Uterine vasoconstriction

(C) Uterine contractions

(D) Uterine vasodilation

Rationale: Decreased uterine blood flow is caused by factors including hypotension, uterine vasoconstriction and uterine contractions, sympathetic block, hypovolemia, supine hypotensive syndrome, and vasoconstrictors. Maternal conditions including pre-eclampsia, hypertension, use of cocaine, and abruptio placenta also decrease uterine blood flow.

Ref: Butterworth, J.F., Mackey, D.C., & Wasnick, J.D. (2013). Ch 40 *Morgan & Mikhail's Clinical Anesthesiology* (5th ed.). New York, NY: Lange Medical Books McGraw-Hill.

Suresh, M.S., Segal, B.S., Preston, R.L., Fernando, R., & Mason C.L. (2013). Ch 2 *Shnider and Levinson's Anesthesia for Obstetrics* (5th ed.). Philadelphia, PA: Lippincott Williams & Wilkins.

168. Which of the following physiologic changes occur with limb tourniquets?

(A) Cellular acidosis

(B) Metabolic alkalosis

(C) Cellular alkalosis

(D) Metabolic acidosis

Rationale: Limb tourniquets produce cellular acidosis due to ischemia. Hypoxia develops within 2 minutes of inflation. Endothelial capillary leak occurs with inflation of 2 hours or more.

Ref: Butterworth, J.F., Mackey, D.C., & Wasnick, J.D. (2013). Ch 38 *Morgan & Mikhail's Clinical Anesthesiology* (5th ed.). New York, NY: McGraw-Hill.

Nagelhout, J.J., & Plaus, K.L. Ch 40 *Nurse Anesthesia* (5th ed.). St. Louis, MO: Elsevier.

169. While undergoing a shoulder arthroscopy with regional anesthesia the patient exhibits tachycardia, agitation, diaphoresis, hypotension, and jugular vein distention. What is the most likely cause?

(A) Tension pneumothorax

(B) Subcutaneous emphysema

(C) Pneumomediastinum

(D) Failed regional block

Rationale: Each of the items may occur during shoulder arthroscopy. The symptoms are consistent with tension pneumothorax. Other signs include absence of breath sounds on the affected side, hypoxemia, increased central venous pressure, cyanosis, and increased airway pressure (general anesthesia).

Ref: Butterworth, J.F., Mackey, D.C., & Wasnick, J.D. (2013). Ch 38 *Morgan & Mikhail's Clinical Anesthesiology* (5th ed.). New York, NY: McGraw-Hill.
Nagelhout, J.J., & Plaus, K.L. Ch 40 *Nurse Anesthesia* (5th ed.). St. Louis, MO: Elsevier Saunders.

170. Which of the following risk factors are linked to postoperative vision loss (POVL)?

Select (3) three

(A) Female

(B) Thin

(C) Obese

(D) Male

(E) <18 years

(F) >18 years

Rationale: Postoperative vision loss may occur in all patients. Risk factors include male, obesity, <18 and >65 years, spinal surgery (prone position), prolonged surgery, large blood loss, and hypotension.

Ref: Nagelhout, J.J., & Plaus, K.L. Ch 21 & 40 *Nurse Anesthesia* (5th ed.). St. Louis, MO: Elsevier.

171. The patient is scheduled for a total hip arthroplasty (THR). What are your anesthetic concerns?

Select (3) three

(A) Hemorrhage

(B) Thromboembolism

(C) Tourniquet pain

(D) Bone cement implantation syndrome

(E) Postoperative pain

Rationale: Tourniquets are not used for THR. Reaming the femur results in significant blood loss. Bone cement (methyl methacrylate) induces an exothermic reaction that results in vasodilation and decreased systemic vascular resistance. Pulmonary or thromboembolism due to venous stasis may result in patients undergoing lower extremity surgery. Postoperative pain is concerning, but it is not a life-threatening event as are the other options.

Ref: Butterworth, J.F., Mackey, D.C., & Wasnick, J.D. (2013). Ch 38 *Morgan & Mikhail's Clinical Anesthesiology* (5th ed.). New York, NY: McGraw-Hill.
Nagelhout, J.J., & Plaus, K.L. Ch 40 *Nurse Anesthesia* (5th ed.). St. Louis, MO: Elsevier.

172. How are hypotensive bradycardic episodes (HBEs) that occur during shoulder surgery defined?

Select (2) two

(A) Any heart rate <50 bpm

(B) Any systolic blood pressure <90 mmHg

(C) Heart rate decrease of 30 bpm in 3 minutes

(D) Heart rate decrease of 20 bpm in 5 minutes

Rationale: In addition to A and B, a heart rate decrease of 50 bpm in 5 minutes defines HBEs.

Ref: Nagelhout, J.J., & Plaus, K.L. Ch 40 *Nurse Anesthesia* (5th ed.). St. Louis, MO: Elsevier.

173. Your patient is undergoing an elective coronary artery bypass graft (CABG). The patient was managed on heparin therapy for 5 days preoperatively. The patient is now on cardiopulmonary bypass and the perfusionist is having difficulty maintaining total heparinization. What is the most likely cause?

(A) Antithrombin deficiency

(B) Factor V deficiency

(C) Factor VIII deficiency

(D) Factor IV deficiency

Rationale: Patients who have recently been managed on heparin therapy may become "heparin-resistant," thus, requiring higher than usual doses to obtain therapeutic anticoagulation on bypass.

Ref: Butterworth, J.F., Mackey, D.C., & Wasnick, J.D. (2013). Ch 22 *Morgan & Mikhail's Clinical Anesthesiology* (5th ed.). New York, NY: McGraw-Hill.
Nagelhout, J.J., & Plaus, K.L. (2014). Ch 24 *Nurse Anesthesia* (5th ed.). St. Louis, MO: Elsevier.

174. Which condition is associated with carbamazepine taken during pregnancy?

(A) Spina bifida

(B) Pyloric stenosis

(C) Biliary atresia

(D) Hypospadias

Rationale: Antiepileptic drugs taken during pregnancy are associated with ventricular septal defects, mid face and mouth abnormalities, and digital or nail-bed hypoplasia. Carbamazepine is specifically associated with spina bifida.

Ref: Stoelting, R.K., & Hillier, S.C. (2006). Ch 30 *Pharmacology and Physiology in Anesthetic Practice* (4th ed.). Philadelphia, PA: Elsevier.

175. A patient is undergoing an elective abdominal aortic aneurysm (AAA) repair. What drug are you most likely to administer after aortic clamping?

    (A) Nitroglycerin
    (B) Phenylephrine
    (C) Milrinone
    (D) Dopamine

    Rationale: Because of the acute hypertension that develops above the clamp, a vasodilator infusion is often necessary to prevent excessive increases in blood pressure.

    Ref: Butterworth, J.F., Mackey, D.C., & Wasnick, J.D. (2013). Ch 22 *Morgan & Mikhail's Clinical Anesthesiology* (5th ed.). New York, NY: McGraw-Hill.

    Nagelhout, J.J., & Plaus, K.L. (2014). Ch 25 *Nurse Anesthesia* (5th ed.). St. Louis, MO: Elsevier.

176. A 5-year-old requires endotracheal intubation for an exploratory laparotomy. What size ETT will you select?

    (A) 6
    (B) 5
    (C) 4
    (D) 3

    Rationale: To determine the oral tracheal tube size, use the equation: 4 plus the child's age/4.

TABLE 4-7. Oral tracheal tube size guidelines.

Age	Internal Diameter (mm)	Cut Length (cm)
Full-term infant	3.5	12
Child	$4 + \dfrac{Age}{4}$	$14 + \dfrac{Age}{4}$
Adult		
Female	7.0–7.5	24
Male	7.5–9.0	24

Ref: Butterworth, J.F., Mackey, D.C., & Wasnick, J.D. (2013). Ch 19 *Morgan & Mikhail's Clinical Anesthesiology* (5th ed.). New York, NY: McGraw-Hill.

Nagelhout, J.J., & Plaus, K.L. (2014). Ch 48 *Nurse Anesthesia* (5th ed.). St. Louis, MO: Elsevier.

177. Which of the following is linked to late decelerations?

    (A) Fetal head compression
    (B) Begins 10-30 seconds following the peak of a contraction
    (C) Begin with the contraction
    (D) Umbilical cord compression

    Rationale: Variable decelerations are associated with umbilical cord compression and occur abruptly. Early decelerations occur at the beginning of a contraction and are associated with head compression. Late decelerations occur just after the peak of the contraction and are associated with uteroplacental insufficiency.

    Ref: Butterworth, J.F., Mackey, D.C., & Wasnick, J.D. (2013). Ch 41 *Morgan & Mikhail's Clinical Anesthesiology* (5th ed.). New York, NY: McGraw-Hill.

    Chestnut, D.H., Polley, L.S., Tsen, L.C., & Wong, C.A. (2009). Ch 6 & 8 *Chestnut's Obstetric Anesthesia Principles and Practice* (4th ed.). Philadelphia, PA: Elsevier.

178. Which neurosurgical procedure places the patient at highest risk for postoperative diabetes insipidus?

    (A) Resection of intracranial aneurysm in the anterior Circle of Willis
    (B) Stereotactic biopsy of a lesion in the parietal lobe
    (C) Tumor resection within the posterior fossa
    (D) Transsphenoidal hypophysectomy

    Rationale: Diabetes insipidus is a known postoperative complication of pituitary resection.

    Ref: Butterworth, J.F., Mackey, D.C., & Wasnick, J.D. (2013). Ch 28 *Morgan & Mikhail's Clinical Anesthesiology* (5th ed.). New York, NY: McGraw-Hill.

    Jaffe, R.A., Samuels, S.I., Schmiesing, C.A., & Golianu, B. (Eds.). Ch 1.1 *Anesthesiologist's Manual of Surgical Procedures* (4th ed.). Philadelphia, PA: Lippincott Williams & Wilkins.

179. What is the correct placement of a precordial Doppler to monitor for venous air embolism?

    (A) Midclavicular line at the first intercostal space
    (B) Right sternal border at the third intercostal space
    (C) Right midaxillary line at the fifth intercostal space
    (D) Left sternal border at the fifth intercostal space

Rationale: Correct placement is third intercostal space and right of the sternum.

Ref: Butterworth, J.F., Mackey, D.C., & Wasnick, J.D. (2013). Ch 27 *Morgan & Mikhail's Clinical Anesthesiology* (5th ed.). New York, NY: McGraw-Hill.

Miller, R., & Pardo, M.Jr. (Eds.) (2011). Ch 30 *Basics of Anesthesia* (6th ed.). Philadelphia, PA: Elsevier.

180. What is average total cerebral blood flow?

(A) 550 mL/min

(B) 650 mL/min

(C) 750 mL/min

(D) 850 mL/min

Rationale: Cerebral blood flow can be estimated as 15% of cardiac output or 50 mL/min/100 g; either totals roughly 750 mL/min.

Ref: Butterworth, J.F., Mackey, D.C., & Wasnick, J.D. (2013). Ch 26 *Morgan & Mikhail's Clinical Anesthesiology* (5th ed.). New York, NY: McGraw-Hill.

Hall, J.E. (2011). Ch 61 *Guyton and Hall Textbook of Medical Physiology* (12th ed.). Philadelphia, PA: Saunders.

181. How is Minimum Alveolar Concentration (MAC) affected for inhaled anesthetics during pregnancy?

(A) MAC is increased 30%.

(B) MAC is decreased 15%.

(C) MAC is increased 25%.

(D) MAC is decreased 40%.

Rationale: MAC is decreased to 40% for all inhalational agents during pregnancy.

Ref: Longnecker, D.E., Brown, D.L., Newman, M.F., & Zapol, W.M. (2012). Ch 22 *Anesthesiology* (2nd ed.). San Francisco, CA: McGraw-Hill.

182. Calculate cerebral perfusion pressure (CPP) using the information provided and correctly interpret the result. Blood pressure is 130/90 mmHg, intracranial pressure is 12 mmHg, central venous pressure is 6 mmHg.

(A) CPP = 110 mmHg, high

(B) CPP = 97 mmHg, normal

(C) CPP = 105 mmHg, high

(D) CPP = 91 mmHg, normal

Rationale: Cerebral perfusion pressure is estimated by subtracting either intracranial pressure or central venous pressure, the greater value of the two, from mean the arterial pressure. The normal range is 80-100 mmHg.

Ref: Butterworth, J.F., Mackey, D.C., & Wasnick, J.D. (2013). Ch 26 *Morgan & Mikhail's Clinical Anesthesiology* (5th ed.). New York, NY: McGraw-Hill.

Miller, R., & Pardo, M.Jr. (Eds.) (2011). Ch 30 *Basics of Anesthesia* (6th ed.). Philadelphia, PA: Elsevier.

183. Inhalational anesthetic agents have what effects on the hearts conduction?

(A) Decrease AV node refractoriness

(B) Suppress SA node automaticity

(C) Increase pacing thresholds

(D) All of the above

Rationale: Inhalational agents depress AV node automaticity. This can be observed in everyday practice both by a reduction of heart rate during anesthesia and the frequency of junctional rhythm during anesthesia. Inhalational agents mildly increase AV node refractoriness. They have no effect reported on pacing thresholds.

Ref: Butterworth, J.F., Mackey, D.C., & Wasnick, J.D. (2013). Ch 20 *Morgan & Mikhail's Clinical Anesthesiology* (5th ed.). New York, NY: McGraw-Hill.

184. For Frank–Starling's law what does the *x*-axis and *y*-axis represent?

(A) Heart rate; cardiac output

(B) Ventricular end-diastolic volume; cardiac output

(C) Cardiac output; ventricular end-diastolic volume

(D) Afterload; systemic vascular resistance

Rationale: Frank–Starling's law relates preload (ventricular end-diastolic volume) with stroke volume (or cardiac output) when heart rate and contractility remain constant. With increasing preload, cardiac output will rise until a maximum ability for the heart chamber to respond is reached. After this excessive point is reached, increasing end-diastolic volume will not increase cardiac output, and may even decrease it.

Ref: Butterworth, J.F., Mackey, D.C., & Wasnick, J.D. (2013). Ch 20 *Morgan & Mikhail's Clinical Anesthesiology* (5th ed.). New York, NY: McGraw-Hill.

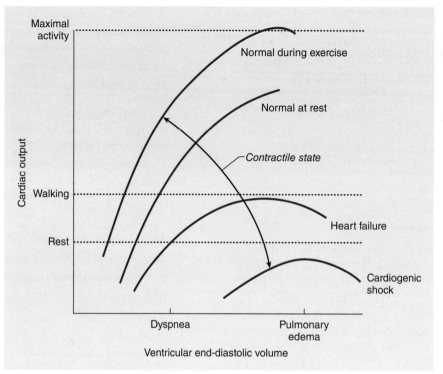

FIG. 4-4. Starling's law of the heart.

185. The fetal scalp pH is 7.25. How would you interpret this value?

(A) Normal infant pH

(B) Abnormal infant pH

(C) Needs to be repeated to ensure accuracy

(D) Requires neonatal resuscitation

Rationale: A fetal scalp pH >7.25 is considered normal. A pH of 7.20 is marginal so should be repeated to ensure accuracy. A pH <7.20 indicates neonatal depression.

Ref: Butterworth, J.F., Mackey, D.C., & Wasnick, J.D. (2013). Ch 41 *Morgan & Mikhail's Clinical Anesthesiology* (5th ed.). New York, NY: McGraw-Hill.

Chestnut, D.H., Polley, L.S., Tsen, L.C., & Wong, C.A. (2009). Ch 6 & 8 *Chestnut's Obstetric Anesthesia Principles and Practice* (4th ed.). Philadelphia, PA: Elsevier.

186. What does the formula,
$$\frac{\text{(end-diastolic volume)} - \text{(end-systolic volume)}}{\text{end-diastolic volume}}, \text{represent?}$$

(A) Stroke volume

(B) Cardiac index

(C) Cardiac output

(D) Ejection fraction

Rationale: Ejection fraction is defined by the proportion of ventricular blood ejected during systole. Therefore, ejection fraction is calculated as the volume of blood ejected during systole (end-diastolic volume minus end-systolic volume) is divided by volume of blood present prior to systole (end-diastolic volume). Clinically, ejection fraction can be obtained using echocardiography and is a valuable indication of systolic function.

Ref: Butterworth, J.F., Mackey, D.C., & Wasnick, J.D. (2013). Ch 20 *Morgan & Mikhail's Clinical Anesthesiology* (5th ed.). New York, NY: McGraw-Hill.

187. A pacemaker is placed in a patient with symptomatic sinus bradycardia with a normally functioning atrioventricular node. What settings would be most appropriate?

(A) AAI

(B) AOO

(C) DDD

(D) DDI

Rationale: Since the AV node is functioning normally, the atrial signal will be conducted to the ventricles normally. The pacemaker only needs to ensure an adequate ventricular rate. Therefore, dual pacing

TABLE 4-8. Classification of pacemakers.

Chamber-Paced	Chamber-Sensed	Response to Sensing	Programmability	Antitacharrhythmia Function
O = none	O = none	O = none	O = none	O = none
A = atrium	A = atrium	T = triggered	P = simple	P = pacing
V = ventricle	V = ventricle	I = inhibited	M = multiprogrammable	S = shock
D = dual (atrium and ventricle)	D = dual (atrium and ventricle)	D = dual (triggered and inhibited)	C = communicating R = rate modulation	D = dual (pacing and shock)

is unnecessary. AOO is inappropriate as that would be asynchronous pacing of the atrium, pacing which occurs regardless of the intrinsic atrial rate. AAI is appropriate because in this demand mode the atrium is sensed, the atrium will be paced if needed, and the pacemaker will be inhibited (i.e., not pace) if the patient's own atrial signal is detected.

Ref: Butterworth, J.F., Mackey, D.C., & Wasnick, J.D. (2013). Ch 21 *Morgan & Mikhail's Clinical Anesthesiology* (5th ed.). New York, NY: McGraw-Hill.

188. Which of the following agents possesses combined alpha- and beta-adrenergic blocking affects?

(A) Metoprolol
(B) Esmolol
(C) Propranolol
(D) Labetalol

Rationale: Labetalol has both alpha and beta blocking properties. The other agents are beta-blocking agents without direct effects on alpha receptors.

Ref: Butterworth, J.F., Mackey, D.C., & Wasnick, J.D. (2013). Ch 21 *Morgan & Mikhail's Clinical Anesthesiology* (5th ed.). New York, NY: McGraw-Hill.

189. Which of the following would be appropriate anesthesia induction techniques for a severely hypertensive patient with coronary artery disease and moderate ventricular dysfunction?

(A) Inhalational induction with sevoflurane
(B) Inhalational induction with desflurane
(C) Intravenous induction with ketamine
(D) Intravenous induction with propofol

Rationale: An inhalational induction with desflurane will likely cause catecholamine release, further increasing blood pressure and heart rate. Ketamine alone may cause severe hypertension. It can be combined with other agents such as propofol to make an appro-priate induction agent. Propofol alone in a severely hypertensive patient will likely cause severe hypotension in a dose large enough to attenuate a hypertensive response to laryngoscopy. An inhalational induction with sevoflurane will allow a general anesthetic depth of anesthesia, minimizing hypertension with laryngoscopy, without the quick and profound hypotension associated with propofol induction.

Ref: Butterworth, J.F., Mackey, D.C., & Wasnick, J.D. (2013). Ch 21 *Morgan & Mikhail's Clinical Anesthesiology* (5th ed.). New York, NY: McGraw-Hill.

190. Which arrhythmia is best treated with magnesium sulfate?

(A) Ventricular fibrillation
(B) Polymorphic ventricular tachycardia in the presence of prolonged QT syndrome
(C) Atrioventricular nodal reentrant tachycardia
(D) Polymorphic ventricular tachycardia in the absence of prolonged QT syndrome

Rationale: Polymorphic ventricular tachycardia in the presence of prolonged QT syndrome is also known as torsade de pointes. Torsade de pointes typically responds best to magnesium or pacing. Polymorphic ventricular tachycardias in the absence of long QT interval typically respond to conventional antiarrhythmics.

Ref: Butterworth, J.F., Mackey, D.C., & Wasnick, J.D. (2013). Ch 21 *Morgan & Mikhail's Clinical Anesthesiology* (5th ed.). New York, NY: McGraw-Hill.

191. What is the goal of hemodynamic management for the patient with severe mitral valve regurgitation?

(A) Aggressive volume resuscitation
(B) Inotropic support
(C) Afterload reduction
(D) Maintenance of moderate bradycardia

Rationale: Mitral regurgitation results in retrograde flow into the left atrium on systole. This results in decreased forward stroke volume. Hemodynamic management should focus on maintaining forward blood flow, accomplished by reducing after load. Increases in afterload will increase retrograde flow and should be avoided. Bradycardia and volume overload will both increase left-ventricular end-diastolic volume which can exacerbate regurgitation through mitral annular dilation.

Ref: Butterworth, J.F., Mackey, D.C., & Wasnick, J.D. (2013). Ch 21 *Morgan & Mikhail's Clinical Anesthesiology* (5th ed.). New York, NY: McGraw-Hill.

192. Which patient is most at risk for catastrophic bleeding upon midline sternotomy?

  (A) Patient with ischemic cardiomyopathy on multiple vasopressor therapies undergoing aortic valve replacement
  (B) Patient with heparin induced thrombocytopenia to be treated with argatroban for cardiopulmonary bypass undergoing coronary artery bypass grafts
  (C) Patient with previous coronary artery bypass grafting undergoing mitral valve repair
  (D) Obese patient with severe aortic stenosis undergoing aortic valve replacement

Rationale: In patients with previous sternotomy, right ventricle surface or grafts (if present) may be attached to the sternum. The pericardium has been removed and scar tissue may develop adhering cardiac structures to the posterior sternum. This is often referred to as a "redo." The anesthetist should have blood immediately available and be aware that the "redo" sternotomy may enter the heart or coronary structures, leading to massive bleeding necessitating emergent transfusion and repair.

Ref: Butterworth, J.F., Mackey, D.C., & Wasnick, J.D. (2013). Ch 22 *Morgan & Mikhail's Clinical Anesthesiology* (5th ed.). New York, NY: McGraw-Hill.

193. What is the approximate mean arterial blood pressure for the patient whose pressure is 115/70 mmHg?

  (A) 100 mmHg
  (B) 85 mmHg
  (C) 92.5 mmHg
  (D) 80 mmHg

Rationale: Mean arterial pressure is the average pressure. The most accurate way to measure this is to determine that area under a pressure wave divided by the time over which that wave occurred. This can generally be estimated by the formula,

$$MAP = Diastolic\ Pressure + \frac{Pulse\ Pressure}{3} =$$
$$70 + \frac{115-70}{3} = 70 + \frac{45}{3} = 85\ mmHg.$$

Another commonly memorized form of this formula is

$$MAP = \frac{Systolic\ Pressure + 2 \times Diastolic\ Pressure}{3} =$$
$$\frac{115 + 2 \times 70}{3} = \frac{115 + 140}{3} = \frac{255}{3} = 85\ mmHg.$$

Ref: Butterworth, J.F., Mackey, D.C., & Wasnick, J.D. (2013). Ch 5 & 20 *Morgan & Mikhail's Clinical Anesthesiology* (5th ed.). New York, NY: Lange Medical Books McGraw-Hill.

194. In which valvular disorder is the left ventricular volume approximately normal, but left ventricular pressure higher than normal?

  (A) Mitral stenosis
  (B) Aortic stenosis
  (C) Mitral regurgitation
  (D) Aortic regurgitation

Rationale: This question is an application of the pressure-volume loops for patients with valvular heart disease. With aortic stenosis, left ventricular pressures are elevated as a result of the added resistance. Left ventricular volumes are approximately normal despite hypertrophy.

Ref: Butterworth, J.F., Mackey, D.C., & Wasnick, J.D. (2013). Ch 21 *Morgan & Mikhail's Clinical Anesthesiology* (5th ed.). New York, NY: McGraw-Hill.

195. Measured systolic and pulse pressure will appear greatest when transduced and measured at which point?

  (A) Aortic root
  (B) Brachial artery
  (C) Radial artery
  (D) Dorsalis pedis

Rationale: Arterial blood pressure waveform is distorted as it moves distally. As the waveform moves distally the waveform becomes narrowed and heightened. Therefore, the measured systolic pressure and pulse pressure are highest at the most distal point measured. The dorsalis pedis is the most distal artery among the selections.

Ref: Butterworth, J.F., Mackey, D.C., & Wasnick, J.D. (2013). Ch 21 *Morgan & Mikhail's Clinical Anesthesiology* (5th ed.). New York, NY: McGraw-Hill.

196. Which of the following is a relative contraindication to pulmonary artery catheter placement?

    (A) Atrial fibrillation
    (B) Left bundle branch block
    (C) Complete heart block
    (D) 1st-degree block

    Rationale: The pulmonary artery catheter passes through the right ventricle and can lead to arrhythmias or right bundle branch block. In the presence of left bundle branch block, an additional right bundle branch block will lead to complete heart block. A patient in complete heart block or atrial fibrillation may make placement technically difficult, but placement is not contraindicated.
    Ref: Butterworth, J.F., Mackey, D.C., & Wasnick, J.D. (2013). Ch 21 *Morgan & Mikhail's Clinical Anesthesiology* (5th ed.). New York, NY: McGraw-Hill.

197. Which law explains the effect of postintubation airway edema in children?

    (A) Poiseuille's equation
    (B) Dalton's law
    (C) The Ideal Gas Law
    (D) Avogadro's number

    Rationale: Poiseuille's equation describes the direct relationship between flow and the radius of the tube raised to the fourth power. This principle can be applied to illustrate the effect of edema on small neonatal and pediatric airways.
    Ref: Butterworth, J.F., Mackey, D.C., & Wasnick, J.D. (2013). Ch 42 *Morgan & Mikhail's Clinical Anesthesiology* (5th ed.). New York, NY: McGraw-Hill.
    Shubert, D., & Leyba, J. (Eds.) (2013). Ch 5 *Chemistry and Physics for Nurse Anesthesia* (2nd ed.). New York, NY: Springer Publishing.

198. Which medication used for preeclampsia may extend the duration of rocuronium?

    (A) Nitroglycerin
    (B) Hydralazine
    (C) Labetolol
    (D) Magnesium

    Rationale: Nitroglycerin, hydralazine and labetolol are commonly used to control high blood pressure associated with preeclampsia. Magnesium also used to control high blood pressure and seizures in preeclampsia, may extend the duration of muscle relaxants. For this reason, the dose of muscle relaxants should be decreased.
    Ref: Longnecker, D.E., Brown, D.L., Newman, M.F., & Zapol, W.M. (2012). Ch 62 *Anesthesiology* (2nd ed.). San Francisco, CA: McGraw-Hill.

199. What is the normal fetal heart rate?

    (A) 80-100 bpm
    (B) 100-110 bpm
    (C) 110-160 bpm
    (D) >160

    Rationale: The normal fetal heart rate is 110-160.
    Ref: Butterworth, J.F., Mackey, D.C., & Wasnick, J.D. (2013). Ch 41 *Morgan & Mikhail's Clinical Anesthesiology* (5th ed.). New York, NY: McGraw-Hill.
    Chestnut, D.H., Polley, L.S., Tsen, L.C., & Wong, C.A. (2009). Ch 6 & 8 *Chestnut's Obstetric Anesthesia Principles and Practice* (4th ed.). Philadelphia, PA: Elsevier.

200. What is the best choice to improve hypotension resulting from aortocaval compression?

    (A) Give oxygen via facemask.
    (B) Turn the patient on his/her side.
    (C) Give ephedrine.
    (D) Give phenylephrine.

    Rationale: Each of the choices will improve hypotension; however, the first measure is to reposition the patient. Turning the patient on his/her side will relieve the compression of the gravid uterus on the inferior vena cava. Venous return improves.
    Ref: Butterworth, J.F., Mackey, D.C., & Wasnick, J.D. (2013). Ch 40 *Morgan & Mikhail's Clinical Anesthesiology* (5th ed.). New York, NY: Lange Medical Books McGraw-Hill.
    Suresh, M.S., Segal, B.S., Preston, R.L., Fernando, R., & Mason C.L. (2013). Ch 1 *Shnider and Levinson's Anesthesia for Obstetrics* (5th ed.). Philadelphia, PA: Lippincott Williams & Wilkins.

201. Which opioid causes the greatest respiration depression in newborns?

    (A) Meperidine
    (B) Morphine
    (C) Fentanyl
    (D) Remifentanil

    Rationale: Most opioids cross the placenta and may produce respiratory depression. Neonates are most sensitive to morphine followed by meperidine. Fentanyl has minimal effect on neonatal respiration when using low doses.

Ref: Butterworth, J.F., Mackey, D.C., & Wasnick, J.D. (2013). Ch 41 *Morgan & Mikhail's Clinical Anesthesiology* (5th ed.). New York, NY: McGraw-Hill.

Suresh, M.S., Segal, B.S., Preston, R.L., Fernando, R., & Mason C.L. (2013). Ch 2 *Shnider and Levinson's Anesthesia for Obstetrics* (5th ed.). Philadelphia, PA: Lippincott Williams & Wilkins.

202. The patient is scheduled for a parathyroidectomy. What is the anesthetic implication for hyperparathyroidism and neuromuscular blockade (NMB)?

(A) Decrease NMB dose.

(B) Titrate NMB carefully.

(C) No relationship exists.

(D) No change in the response to NMB.

Rationale: Patient's with hyperparathyroid disease experience muscle weakness and atrophy. Response to neuromuscular blockade is variable. For this reason, titrate nondepolarizers carefully using a peripheral nerve stimulator.

Ref: Butterworth, J.F., Mackey, D.C., & Wasnick, J.D. (2013). Ch 34 *Morgan & Mikhail's Clinical Anesthesiology* (5th ed.). New York, NY: McGraw-Hill.

Nagelhout, J.J., & Plaus, K.L. Ch 33 *Nurse Anesthesia* (5th ed.). St. Louis, MO: Elsevier.

203. A patient undergoes bronchoscopy for removal of a foreign body. What neuromuscular blocker (NMB) is the best choice for this procedure?

(A) Succinylcholine

(B) Vecuronium

(C) Cisatracurium

(D) Atracurium

Rationale: A short-acting NMB is the best choice.

Ref: Butterworth, J.F., Mackey, D.C., & Wasnick, J.D. (2013). Ch 25 *Morgan & Mikhail's Clinical Anesthesiology* (5th ed.). New York, NY: McGraw-Hill.

Nagelhout, J.J., & Plaus, K.L. Ch 38 *Nurse Anesthesia* (5th ed.). St. Louis, MO: Elsevier Saunders.

204. What increases stroke volume?

(A) Increased ventricular end-diastolic volume

(B) Increased pulmonary vascular resistance

(C) Increased heart rate

(D) Mitral regurgitation

Rationale: Stroke volume is defined by $SV = \dfrac{CO}{HR}$ (this is just an algebraic manipulation of the formula $CO = SV \times HR$ the blood that moves retrograde in the atria is not included in the commonly understood definition of stroke volume. Thus "ventricular end-diastolic volume" is the most appropriate answer.

Ref: Butterworth, J.F., Mackey, D.C., & Wasnick, J.D. (2013). Ch 20 *Morgan & Mikhail's Clinical Anesthesiology* (5th ed.). New York, NY: McGraw-Hill.

205. Which inhaled agent is most associated with emergence delirium in children?

(A) Sevoflurane

(B) Isoflurane

(C) Desflurane

(D) Nitrous oxide

Rationale: As compared to adults emergence delirium is documented for children during emergence with sevoflurane.

Ref: Barash, P.G., Cullen, B.F., Stoelting, R.K. Cahalan, M.K., & Stock, M.C. (Eds.) (2009). Ch 45 *Clinical Anesthesia* (6th ed.). Philadelphia, PA: Lippincott Williams & Wilkins.

Miller, R.D., Eriksson, L.I., Fleisher, L.A., Weiner-Kronish, J.P., & Young, W.L. (Eds.) (2010). Ch 82 *Miller's Anesthesia* (7th ed.). Philadelphia, PA: Elsevier.

Index

post-intubation airway edema in, 232
spinal cord, 164, 211
chloroprocaine, cardiac contractility and, 13, 62
Cholecystectomy, cisatracurium for, 8
Cholinesterase inhibitors, muscarinic side effects of, 15, 66
Chronic bronchitis
clinical diagnosis of, 30, 103
PaCO$_2$, elevated level, 15, 65
smoking and, 4
Chronic neuropathic pain, 145, 168
Chronic obstructive pulmonary disease (COPD), 2
air trapping in, 13, 63
cor pulmonale and, 13, 63
FEV$_1$/FVC ratio, 14, 63–64
mechanical ventilation modalities for, 14, 64
Cigarette smoking, 27, 96
bronchitis and, 12, 61
Cirrhosis
cisatracurium in, 33, 109
laboratory findings, 29, 101, 102
manifestations of, 101
thromboelastography, 144, 164
Cisatracurium
for cholecystectomy, 8
in severe cirrhosis, 33, 109
Cisplatin, and magnesium wasting, 60
Clindamycin, for penicillin-allergic patients, 12, 60–61
Closed Claims Project database, 117, 137
Closed waste gas scavenging system, 116, 135
Coagulopathies, asparaginase, 60
Codeine *vs.* morphine, 10, 56
Colonoscopy, bowel distention during, 226, 261
Color, of air cylinders, 111, 121
Combitube, 113, 128
Complete cardiovascular collapse, 216, 240
Compound A, 118, 140
Computed tomography (CT) scan
with intravenous contrast media (ICM), 226, 261
Congenital cardiac malformation, 221, 249–250
Congenital diaphragmatic hernia, 220, 249
Coronary artery bypass graft (CABG), 229, 267
Coronary blood flow, 7
at rest, 7
Coronary ischemia with hypotension, 220, 248
Coronary perfusion pressure, 5, 216, 240
Cor pulmonale
adenotonsillar hypertrophy, 30, 103
cause of, 13, 63
COPD and, 13, 30, 63, 103
obesity, 30, 103
pathology of, 1, 35

Corticosteroids
glucocorticoid activity, 211
intravenous, 62
systemic effects of, 264
COX-1
aspirin and, 57
vs. COX-2 enzymes, 10, 57
COX inhibitors, 57
CPB. *See* Cardiopulmonary bypass (CPB)
Cranial nerve (CN)
tongue, 144, 165
Craniotomy, seated, air embolism and, 214, 232, 235
Cryoprecipitate, 146, 170
Current leak, in operating room, 111, 120
Cushing's syndrome
clinical sign, 13, 62
glucocorticoids excess and, 25, 91
Cyclophosphamide, side effects of, 55
Cylinder pressure delivered to anesthesia machine, 116, 136

D
Dantrolene, 7
reconstituting vial of, 12, 60
Dead space increases, heat and moisture exchangers, 111, 120
Decelerations
early, 257
late, 230, 257, 268
variable, 268
Delirium in children, 232, 275
Demerol
MAO inhibitor and, 24, 90
renal dysfunction and, 28, 100
Deoxyhemoglobin, 71
Desaturation, 213, 233
Desflurane, 118, 140
and vaporizer, 112, 124
Dexamethasone, 69
glucocorticoid potency of, 211
Diabetes insipidus, 230, 268
Diameter-index safety system (DISS), 119, 140–141
Diastolic heart failure, 6
Difficult Airway Algorithm, 127, 128
Digital flow meter displays, 124
Digitalis, supraventricular tachycardia (SVT), 217, 241
Digoxin, for atrial arrhythmias, 24, 88
Dilation and curettage (D&C)
pregnancy test and, 235–236
Diltiazem
for atrial fibrillation, 57
electrophysiologic effects of, 13, 62
for flutter, 57
Dobutamine, for systolic heart failure, 57
Donor blood test, 146, 170
Dorsalis pedis, 231, 272
Doxepin, 25, 90
Doxorubicin, 55
Droperidol, 69

Duchenne muscular dystrophy, 31, 105
malignant hyperthermia and, 32, 107
Duloxetine, 145, 168
Dysmenorrhea, preoperative testing, 214, 235–236
Dyspnea, postoperative pulmonary complications, 13, 63
Dyspnea at rest, in aortic stenosis, 217, 241–242

E
Eaton-Lambert syndrome, 33, 109–110
Echinacea, 12, 59
Echothiophate
with glycopyrrolate, 33, 109
with succinylcholine, 33, 109
Echothiophate eye drops, glaucoma, 224, 256
E-cylinder, 116, 118, 135, 139
nitrous oxide capacity in, 111, 117, 121, 138
oxygen in, 117, 137
Edema, goldenseal and, 60
Edrophonium, and atropine, 66
Efferent limb, of oculocardiac reflex, 218, 243
Efferent vagal response, cardiovascular reflex and, 11, 58
Ejection fraction, 230, 270
EKG tracing, P-wave, 215, 238
Elderly patients
complete cardiovascular collapse, 216, 240
with coronary artery disease, 222, 252
obesity, 222
Electrical wall outlet power, 112, 124
Electroconvulsive therapy (ECT), 226, 261
contraindications, 216, 239
propofol and, 227, 262
seizure duration, 227, 262
Emphysema, 12, 60
alpha-1 antitrypsin and, 14, 64
cigarette smoking and, 12, 61
hyperinflation of the lungs and, 14, 64
protease inhibitor and, 14, 64
Endocardial cushion defect, 221, 249–250
Endotracheal intubation, for exploratory laparotomy, 230, 268
Endotracheal tube, 218, 219, 224, 246, 255–256, 259
End-tidal carbon dioxide, 115, 133
Ephedrine, 12, 59
Epidural hematomas, 28, 97
Epidural opioids
fetal heart rate during labor, 216, 240
Epidural steroid injections
avoiding systemic effects, 228, 264
benefits, 227, 264
Epinephrine, to local anesthetics, 9
Epinephrine and ischemic cardiomyopathy, 219, 246
Eschmann Stylet, 113, 128